# Edge AI for Industry 5.0 and Healthcare 5.0 Applications

Edge AI is the seamless and spontaneous combination of edge or fog computing and AI. It enables acquiring real-time insights, which, in turn, leads to the realization of real-time, people-centric, event-driven, business-critical, process-aware, and knowledge-filled software services and applications.

***Edge AI for Industry 5.0 and Healthcare 5.0 Applications*** looks at the unique contributions of edge AI for developing solutions for Industry 5.0 and Healthcare 5.0. It explains how Industry 5.0 fine-tunes the human-machine connection and leverages tiny, high-performance AI-centric processors in IoT edge devices for real-time decision-making and application processing.

Focusing on explainable AI (XAI), the book discusses:

- The role of XAI in Healthcare 5.0
- Best practices, challenges, and opportunities of applying XAI in healthcare setting
- How to enhance transparency and trust of XAI in Healthcare 5.0
- XAI and its methods in predicting healthcare outcomes

Other highlights of the book include:

- 5G communication networks requirements
- The fusion of IoT, AI, edge computing, cloud, and blockchain
- Trustworthiness of blockchain technology in Healthcare 5.0 and Industry 5.0
- The future of trust and the potential of blockchain technology

By explaining how edge AI can transform healthcare and industry, this book empowers researchers and professionals to envisage and implement sophisticated and smart digital solutions.

# Edge AI for Industry 5.0 and Healthcare 5.0 Applications

Edited by
Pethuru Raj, B. Sundaravadivazhagan,
A. Saleem Raja and Mohammed M. Alani

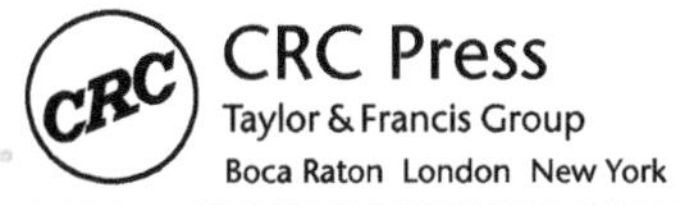

CRC Press
Taylor & Francis Group
Boca Raton  London  New York

CRC Press is an imprint of the
Taylor & Francis Group, an **informa** business

AN AUERBACH BOOK

First edition published 2025
by CRC Press
2385 NW Executive Center Drive, Suite 320, Boca Raton FL 33431

and by CRC Press
4 Park Square, Milton Park, Abingdon, Oxon, OX14 4RN

*CRC Press is an imprint of Taylor & Francis Group, LLC*



ISBN: 978-1-032-57794-4 (hbk)
ISBN: 978-1-032-58013-5 (pbk)
ISBN: 978-1-003-44206-6 (ebk)

DOI: 10.1201/9781003442066

Typeset in Times
by Apex CoVantage, LLC

# Contents


Preface............................................................................................................................xvii
Editor Biographies .........................................................................................................xix
List of Contributors.........................................................................................................xxi

**Chapter 1** Digital Twins for Smart Grids....................................................................1

Pooja Jain, Tapan Kumar, Yaman Birla, and Anshul Mishra

1.1 Introduction ...............................................................................................1
1.2 Concept of Digital Twin, Digital Model, Digital Shadow ........................................................................2
1.3 Digital Twin as an Emerging Technology ................................................3
1.4 A Glance of IIoT.......................................................................................4
1.5 Digital Twin in Smart Cities.....................................................................4
1.6 Digital Twin in Healthcare .......................................................................6
1.7 Digital Twin in Supply Chain Management..............................................7
1.8 Digital Twins in Manufacturing Industries..............................................8
    1.8.1 Smart Manufacturing by Digital Twins .....................................8
    1.8.2 Production Management in Industries........................................10
    1.8.3 Future of Manufacturing Industry.............................................11
1.9 Versatile Production Systems..................................................................12
1.10 Conclusions.............................................................................................14

**Chapter 2** Delineating the Healthcare 5.0................................................................17

Nancy Deborah R, Gobinath A, Soundarya M, and Manjula Devi C

2.1 Introduction to Healthcare 5.0...............................................................17
2.2 Key Characteristics of Healthcare 5.0...................................................17
2.3 Technological Advancements in Healthcare 5.0 ....................................19
2.4 Patient-Centered Care in Healthcare 5.0...............................................20
2.5 Data-Driven Healthcare in Healthcare 5.0 ............................................22
2.6 Ethical and Regulatory Considerations in Healthcare 5.0...............................................................................23
2.7 Conclusions.............................................................................................26

**Chapter 3** Virus Dispersion in Environment: Fuzzy Approach for Infectious Diseases............27

Dilip Kumar Jaiswal and Sudhakar Kumar Chaubey

3.1 Introduction .............................................................................................27
3.2 Spatially Dependent Dispersion along the Non-Uniform Flow ......................................................................28
    3.2.1 Deterministic (Analytical) Solution ..........................................29
    3.2.2 Indeterministic (Fuzzy) Solution...............................................29
3.3 Numerical Example and Discussions......................................................30
3.4 Conclusions.............................................................................................34

**Chapter 4** Revolutionizing COVID-19 Diagnosis: A Hybrid Quantum Neural Network-Based Framework for Accurate Detection of Lung Abnormalities from CT Scans Using Custom Computer Vision Model and AI Edge Device ........................36

*Senthilkumar Vijayakumar*

4.1 Motivation and Solution Overview........................................................37
    4.1.1 Model Training Pipeline................................................37
    4.1.2 Lesser Training Time ....................................................37
    4.1.3 Real-Time Inferencing for Real-World Deployments....................38
4.2 System Design and Framework...........................................................38
    4.2.1 Medical Mild to Severe Lung CT Scan Data Collection and Orchestration ..............................................................38
    4.2.2 Design and Development of Transfer Learning Framework...........39
    4.2.3 Deployment and Real-Time Inferencing on AI Edge Device...........42
4.3 Conclusion .......................................................................................43

**Chapter 5** The Role of Explainable AI for Healthcare 5.0: Best Practices, Challenges, and Opportunities........................................................45

*Srija Chattopadhyay, Subhadeep Barman, and Lakshmi D*

5.1 Introduction .....................................................................................45
    5.1.1 Review of Literature......................................................46
5.2 Rationale of the Study ......................................................................46
5.3 Types of XAI....................................................................................46
    5.3.1 Methods .....................................................................49
    5.3.2 Model-Agnostic Methods ..............................................50
    5.3.3 Global Interpretability Method ......................................50
    5.3.4 Attention Mechanism ...................................................51
    5.3.5 Visual Explanations......................................................52
    5.3.6 Human-in-the-Loop Explanations....................................52
5.4 Use Cases.........................................................................................53
    5.4.1 Rule-Based Systems .....................................................53
    5.4.2 Model Introspection Techniques .....................................54
    5.4.3 Local Interpretable Model-Agnostic Explanations (LIME)...........55
    5.4.4 Counterfactual Explanations .........................................57
    5.4.5 Interactive Visualizations ..............................................58
5.5 Successful Case Study.......................................................................60
    5.5.1 DeepPatient....................................................................60
    5.5.2 Predicting Diabetic Retinopathy and Its Progression Using XAI and Deep Learning....................................................64
5.6 How XAI Redefines Healthcare AI Landscape .....................................66
    5.6.1 Bias and Fairness.........................................................66
    5.6.2 Lack of Transparency ...................................................66
    5.6.3 Safety and Reliability ...................................................67
    5.6.4 Data Privacy and Security.............................................67
    5.6.5 Human-AI Collaboration...............................................69
    5.6.6 Regulatory and Ethical Challenges .................................71
5.7 How XAI Helps in Cancer Prediction and Treatment............................73
5.8 Comparison of AI vs. XAI ................................................................73
5.9 Legal Perspective..............................................................................74
5.10 Challenges .......................................................................................75

5.11  Opportunities or Future Direction ..................................................77
5.12  Conclusion and Future Scope ......................................................77

**Chapter 6**  Explainable AI for Healthcare 5.0—Enhancing Transparency and Trust ................81

*Deepa S, Vinay M, Jayapriya J, and Sundaravadivazhagan B*

6.1  Introduction ................................................................................81
    6.1.1  Background of AI in Healthcare ......................................81
    6.1.2  Evolution of Healthcare toward Version 5.0 ...................82
    6.1.3  Importance of Explainable AI in Healthcare ..................84
    6.1.4  Research Objective and Scope of This Chapter ..............84
6.2  Fundamentals of Explainable AI .................................................85
    6.2.1  Definition and Concepts of Explainable AI ....................85
    6.2.2  Techniques and Approaches for Explainability ...............86
    6.2.3  Challenges and Trade-offs in Achieving Explainability ....86
6.3  Explainable AI in Healthcare 5.0 ...............................................87
    6.3.1  Applications of AI in Healthcare 5.0 ...............................87
    6.3.2  Limitations of Black Box AI Systems in Healthcare ......88
    6.3.3  Benefits of Explainability for Healthcare 5.0 ..................89
    6.3.4  Ethical Considerations in Explainable AI for Healthcare ....89
6.4  Explainability Techniques for Healthcare 5.0 .............................90
    6.4.1  Rule-Based and Logic-Based Systems .............................90
    6.4.2  Symbolic Reasoning and Expert Systems ........................90
    6.4.3  Interpretable Machine Learning Models ..........................90
    6.4.4  Model-Agnostic Explanation Techniques .........................91
6.5  Case Studies and Use Cases .......................................................91
    6.5.1  Explainable AI for Clinical Decision Support Systems ....91
    6.5.2  Interpretable Deep Learning Models for
           Medical Imaging ..............................................................93
    6.5.3  Use Case: Interpretable Deep Learning Models for Breast
           Cancer Detection .............................................................94
    6.5.4  Case Study: Predictive Modeling with Explainable AI in
           Healthcare ........................................................................95
    6.5.5  Use Case: Predictive Modeling with Explainable AI for
           Hospital Readmission ......................................................96
    6.5.6  Case Study: Explainable AI for Personalized Medicine .....98
6.6  Evaluating and Assessing Explainable AI Systems .....................99
    6.6.1  Evaluation Metrics for Explainability .............................99
    6.6.2  Assessing Performance and Interpretability Trade-offs ....99
    6.6.3  User-Centric Evaluation and Human Factors in Explainability ....100
6.7  Challenges and Future Directions ..............................................100
    6.7.1  Technical Challenges in Developing Explainable AI Models .....100
    6.7.2  Adoption Challenges and Integration in
           Healthcare Systems .........................................................100
    6.7.3  Future Research Directions for Explainable
           AI in Healthcare 5.0 .......................................................101
6.8  Conclusion .................................................................................101
    6.8.1  Significance and Implications for the Healthcare Industry ....101
    6.8.2  Recommendations for Implementing Explainable AI in
           Healthcare 5.0 .................................................................101

**Chapter 7**    A Complete Analysis of Explainable AI and Its Methods for Healthcare
Prediction ............................................................................................... 104

*Vinora A, Lloyds E, and Soundarya M*

7.1    AI in Healthcare .................................................................... 105
7.2    Explainable AI (XAI).............................................................. 106
       7.2.1    Principles behind XAI............................................ 107
       7.2.2    XAI Methods ......................................................... 107
7.3    Key Benefits of XAI in Healthcare 5.0 .................................. 109
7.4    Drawbacks/Limitations .......................................................... 114
7.5    Applications of XAI in Healthcare......................................... 116
7.6    Conclusion ............................................................................. 117

**Chapter 8**    Artificial Intelligence (AI) Algorithms and Approaches for Edge AI.................... 119

*Samar Mouti and Samer Rihawi*

8.1    Introduction ........................................................................... 119
8.2    AI Algorithms and Approaches for Edge Computing in the Industry and
       Healthcare Sectors.................................................................. 120
8.3    Use Cases of Edge AI in the Industry and Healthcare Sectors .................... 121
8.4    Key Challenges and Limitations of Edge AI in the Industry and
       Healthcare Sectors.................................................................. 121
       8.4.1    Heterogeneous Data.............................................. 123
       8.4.2    Resource Management .......................................... 123
       8.4.3    Environmental Sustainability ............................... 123
       8.4.4    Security................................................................. 123

**Chapter 9**    Integrating Fuzzy Clustering into CNN for Improved Brain Tumor Detection ..........127

*Kannaki Devi B, Ramyachitra D, and Akalya T*

9.1    Overview of Brain Tumor, CNN, RNN, and FCM ................................. 127
       9.1.1    Significance of Brain Tumor Detection................. 127
       9.1.2    Challenges in Brain Tumor Detection ................... 129
9.2    Conventional Imaging Techniques ......................................... 130
       9.2.1    Role of Machine Learning in Medical Imaging...... 131
       9.2.2    Convolutional Neural Networks (CNNs)............... 134
       9.2.3    Fuzzy Clustering in Medical Image Analysis ........ 134
9.3    Fuzzy C-Means Clustering Algorithm .................................... 135
       9.3.1    Incorporating Fuzzy Clustering into CNN Architecture ............. 136
       9.3.2    Benefits of Combining Fuzzy Clustering and CNN...................... 137
9.4    Integrating Fuzzy Clustering with CNN ................................. 138
       9.4.1    Training the Integrated Model ............................... 139
       9.4.2    Results of Using FCM and with CNN.................... 141
9.5    Conclusion ............................................................................. 141

**Chapter 10**    Leveraging Edge AI for Real-Time Detection and Prevention of Online
Harassment and Cyberbullying: Enhancing Women's Safety and Mental Health........ 144

*Kathiravan Pannerselvam, Saranya Rajiakodi, and Shanmugavadivu Pichai*

10.1    Introduction ......................................................................... 144
        10.1.1    Edge AI................................................................ 145

10.1.2    Applications of Edge AI................................................................145
10.1.3    Edge AI in Real-Time Data Processing........................................145
10.2    Related Works on Cyberbullying .............................................................146
10.3    Natural Language Processing for Cyberbullying....................................147
10.4    Reinforcing Detection Mechanisms .........................................................148
10.4.1    A Swift and Proactive Approach.................................................148
10.4.2    Enhanced Privacy Protection ......................................................148
10.4.3    Customizable Models and Reduced False Positives....................148
10.4.4    Adaptability and Scalability ........................................................148
10.4.5    Empowering Users and Reducing Moderator Workload..............149
10.4.6    Creating Safer and More Inclusive Online Environments ...........149
10.5    Privacy Considerations and Regulatory Compliance..............................149
10.6    Conclusion ................................................................................................149

**Chapter 11**    Leveraging Artificial Intelligence and IoT for Healthcare 5.0: Use Cases, Applications, and Challenges..................................................................................153

*Gnanasankaran Natarajan, Elakkiya Elango, Sandhya Soman, and Shirley Chellathurai Pon Anna Bai*

11.1    Introduction ..............................................................................................153
11.1.1    Overview of Artificial Intelligence .............................................153
11.1.2    Explainable Artificial Intelligence—a Next-Level
AI Platform..................................................................................154
11.2    Introduction to Modern Healthcare Systems...........................................155
11.2.1    Accessible and Equitable Care ....................................................155
11.2.2    Interdisciplinary Collaboration ...................................................155
11.2.3    Technological Advancements.......................................................155
11.2.4    Preventive and Population Health ................................................155
11.2.5    Evidence-Based Medicine ...........................................................156
11.2.6    Patient-Centered Care..................................................................156
11.2.7    Quality Improvement and Safety .................................................156
11.2.8    Health Information Exchange and Privacy ..................................156
11.2.9    Health Policy and Governance .....................................................156
11.2.10    Research and Innovation ..............................................................156
11.3    Artificial Intelligence Advances in Modern Healthcare Systems.................156
11.3.1    Medical Imaging and Diagnostics................................................157
11.3.2    Predictive Analytics and Early Detection ...................................157
11.3.3    Personalized Medicine .................................................................157
11.3.4    Virtual Assistants and Chatbots ..................................................157
11.3.5    Robotics and Surgical Assistance................................................157
11.3.6    Drug Discovery and Development ...............................................157
11.3.7    Health Monitoring and Wearable Devices ..................................157
11.3.8    Health Data Analytics and Decision Support..............................157
11.3.9    Workflow Optimization and Operational Efficiency...................158
11.3.10    Clinical Research and Insights.....................................................158
11.4    Internet of Things—a Preview .................................................................158
11.5    Collaboration Between IoT and Modern Healthcare Systems .....................159
11.5.1    Remote Patient Monitoring .........................................................159
11.5.2    Telemedicine and Virtual Care ....................................................159
11.5.3    Real-Time Health Data Collection ..............................................159
11.5.4    Health and Wellness Tracking.....................................................160
11.5.5    Improved Medication Management..............................................160

|        | 11.5.6  | Operational Efficiency and Asset Management | 160 |
|        | 11.5.7  | Enhanced Patient Safety and Security | 160 |
|        | 11.5.8  | Predictive Analytics and Preventive Care | 160 |
|        | 11.5.9  | Smart Hospitals and Infrastructure | 160 |
|        | 11.5.10 | Data Analytics and Decision Support | 160 |
| 11.6   | Role of IoT in Modern Medical Equipment Manufacturing | | 161 |
|        | 11.6.1  | Remote Monitoring and Real-Time Data | 161 |
|        | 11.6.2  | Predictive Maintenance | 161 |
|        | 11.6.3  | Enhanced Connectivity and Interoperability | 161 |
|        | 11.6.4  | Automated Inventory Management | 161 |
|        | 11.6.5  | Quality Control and Compliance | 161 |
|        | 11.6.6  | Data-Driven Product Improvement | 162 |
|        | 11.6.7  | Remote Software Updates and Upgrades | 162 |
|        | 11.6.8  | Enhanced Patient Safety | 162 |
|        | 11.6.9  | Research and Development | 162 |
|        | 11.6.10 | Regulatory Compliance and Reporting | 162 |
| 11.7   | Modern Sensors Used in Healthcare Systems | | 162 |
|        | 11.7.1  | Temperature Sensors | 163 |
|        | 11.7.2  | Heart Rate Sensors | 163 |
|        | 11.7.3  | Blood Pressure Sensors | 163 |
|        | 11.7.4  | Oxygen Sensors | 163 |
|        | 11.7.5  | Glucose Sensors | 163 |
|        | 11.7.6  | Motion Sensors | 165 |
|        | 11.7.7  | Imaging Sensors | 165 |
|        | 11.7.8  | Gas and Chemical Sensors | 165 |
|        | 11.7.9  | Pressure Sensors | 166 |
|        | 11.7.10 | Proximity and Contact Sensors | 166 |
|        | 11.7.11 | pH Sensors | 166 |
|        | 11.7.12 | Infrared and Thermal Sensors | 168 |
| 11.8   | Industry 5.0—a Modern Era in Technology Invasion | | 168 |
| 11.9   | Medical Advancements Combined with Industry 5.0 | | 169 |
|        | 11.9.1  | Customized Medicine | 169 |
|        | 11.9.2  | Cooperative Robotics in Surgery | 169 |
|        | 11.9.3  | Telemedicine and Isolated Care | 169 |
|        | 11.9.4  | Human-Machine Interfaces | 169 |
|        | 11.9.5  | Smart Medical Devices and IoT Integration | 170 |
|        | 11.9.6  | Data Analytics and Predictive Models | 170 |
|        | 11.9.7  | Patient-Centric Practice | 170 |
|        | 11.9.8  | Ethical Attentions and Data Privacy | 170 |
| 11.10  | Applications of Industry 5.0 in Modern Healthcare | | 170 |
|        | 11.10.1 | Robot Supported Surgery | 171 |
|        | 11.10.2 | AI in Diagnostics | 172 |
|        | 11.10.3 | Remote Patient Monitoring | 173 |
|        | 11.10.4 | Predictive Analytics and Precautionary Care | 173 |
|        | 11.10.5 | Smart Hospital Setup | 173 |
|        | 11.10.6 | Telemedicine and Virtual Care | 174 |
|        | 11.10.7 | 3D Printing in Medical Engineering | 174 |
| 11.11  | Challenges Faced by Industry 5.0 to Integrate with Healthcare Systems | | 174 |
|        | 11.11.1 | Data Interoperability | 174 |
|        | 11.11.2 | Concerns about Privacy and Security | 175 |
|        | 11.11.3 | Cost and Infrastructure Requirements | 175 |

      11.11.4   Workforce Readiness and Training .................................. 175
      11.11.5   Ethical and Regulatory Considerations ......................... 175
      11.11.6   User Acceptance and Adoption ..................................... 175
  11.12  Conclusion ............................................................................. 175

**Chapter 12**  Unleashing Patient Insights: Leveraging Edge AI in Sentiment Analysis for Enhanced Healthcare Experiences ................................................................. 178

*Kathiravan Pannerselvam, Saranya Rajiakodi, and Shanmugavadivu Pichai*

  12.1  Introduction ............................................................................. 178
  12.2  Healthcare Data ...................................................................... 178
      12.2.1   The Social Media Revolution ...................................... 179
      12.2.2   Edge AI: Revolutionizing Sentiment Analysis in Healthcare ............................................................... 179
      12.2.3   Enhanced Privacy and Security .................................... 179
      12.2.4   Personalized Care Delivery .......................................... 179
  12.3  Ethical Considerations and Responsible Use of Data ............. 180
      12.3.1   Data Protection and Consent ........................................ 180
      12.3.2   Privacy Compliance ...................................................... 180
      12.3.3   Bias Mitigation ............................................................ 180
      12.3.4   Algorithm Explainability ............................................. 181
  12.4  Potential Implications and Future Directions ......................... 181
      12.4.1   Improved Patient Satisfaction and Loyalty .................. 181
      12.4.2   More Efficient and Responsive Healthcare Systems ..... 181
  12.5  Enhanced Decision-Making and Resource Allocation ............ 181
      12.5.1   A Shift toward Proactive Healthcare ............................ 182
      12.5.2   Greater Transparency and Trust ................................... 182
  12.6  Challenges and Considerations for the Future ....................... 182
  12.7  Conclusion ............................................................................. 182

**Chapter 13**  Edge AI in LoRa-Based Health Monitoring ............................. 185

*Manjula Devi C, Sivakarthi G, Srinivasan A, Gobinath A, and Rajeswari P*

  13.1  Introduction ............................................................................. 185
      13.1.1   Defining Edge AI ......................................................... 185
      13.1.2   The Role of LoRa Technology in IoT Devices ............. 186
  13.2  Fundamentals of Edge AI and LoRa Technology ................... 187
      13.2.1   Advantages of Edge AI ................................................ 188
      13.2.2   The Synergy between Edge AI and IoT Is Evident due to Several Factors .................................................. 188
  13.3  Key Features of LoRa Technology, Including Its Range, Data Rate, and Energy Efficiency ......................................... 189
  13.4  Health Monitoring in the IoT Era ........................................... 190
      13.4.1   The Challenges of Traditional Health Monitoring Methods and the Potential Benefits of IoT-Enabled Solutions ..... 191
  13.5  Convergence of Edge AI and LoRa for Health Monitoring ...... 191
      13.5.1   Real-Time Data Analysis with Edge AI ....................... 192
      13.5.2   Long-Range Communication and Energy Efficiency with LoRa ................................................... 192
      13.5.3   Enhancing Health Monitoring ..................................... 192

13.6     Examples of Practical Applications ............................................................. 192
13.7     The Integration of AI Processing with LoRa
         Communication Protocols ........................................................................ 193
13.8     Proposed Solutions for Overcoming These Challenges ............................ 194
13.9     Case Studies.............................................................................................. 195
13.10    Conclusions............................................................................................... 196

**Chapter 14**   IoT-Based Smart Health Monitoring with Convolutional Neural Network
(CNN) Using Edge Computing ........................................................................... 198

*Rajeswari P, Gobinath A, Suresh Kumar N, and Anandan M*

14.1     Introduction .............................................................................................. 198
14.2     Introduction to CNNs: Applications in Image Analysis
         and Recognition........................................................................................ 199
14.3     Architecture of an IoT-Based Health Monitoring System........................ 201
14.4     Convolutional Neural Networks (CNNs).................................................. 203
14.5     Edge Computing in Health Monitoring..................................................... 204
14.6     Case Studies.............................................................................................. 206
14.7     Conclusions............................................................................................... 207

**Chapter 15**   Enhancing Healthcare Monitoring Through IoT, CNN, and
Edge Computing Technologies............................................................................ 209

*Feroz Khan AB*

15.1     Introduction .............................................................................................. 209
         15.1.1     Background and Motivation ..................................................... 209
         15.1.2     Objectives of the Chapter ........................................................ 209
15.2     Challenges in Elderly Care........................................................................ 210
         15.2.1     Aging Population and Healthcare Demands ............................. 210
         15.2.2     Specific Healthcare Needs of Elderly Individuals.................... 211
15.3     Overview of Edge AI and Deep Convolutional Neural Networks .............. 211
         15.3.1     Edge AI and Its Advantages in Healthcare .............................. 211
         15.3.2     Deep Convolutional Neural Networks for Health Monitoring...... 211
15.4     System Implementation ............................................................................ 212
         15.4.1     Data Preprocessing for Elderly Health Monitoring..................... 212
         15.4.2     Model Training and Optimization Techniques for
                    Deep CNN Models .................................................................. 212
         15.4.3     Edge AI Deployment for Real-Time Data Processing................. 213
15.5     Applications in Elderly Care ..................................................................... 213
         15.5.1     Fall Detection and Prevention ................................................. 213
         15.5.2     Activity Monitoring and Personalized Care............................. 214
         15.5.3     Vital Sign Tracking and Health Anomaly Detection ................ 214
15.6     Results and Performance Evaluation.......................................................... 214
         15.6.1     Evaluation Metrics for Elderly Health Monitoring ..................... 214
         15.6.2     Evaluation Metrics for Vital Sign Tracking and
                    Anomaly Detection................................................................. 215
         15.6.3     Impact on Quality of Life for Elderly Individuals..................... 215
15.7     Privacy and Security Considerations.......................................................... 216
         15.7.1     Data Protection Measures for Healthcare Applications.............. 217
         15.7.2     Ensuring Confidentiality and Compliance ............................... 217
15.8     Conclusion ................................................................................................ 217

**Chapter 16** Delineating the Need of 5G Communication Networks ...................220

*Wasim Haidar SK, Sudhakar Kumar Chaubey, and Mohammed Bakhit Al-Mahri*

16.1 Introduction ...................220
16.2 Applications of 5G ...................222
16.3 5G E2E Network Design ...................223
16.4 Slicing Network Architecture ...................223
16.5 Crucial Functions of the vEPC Network ...................225
16.6 Management and Orchestration for NFV ...................225
16.7 Planning for the 5G Mobile System ...................225
16.8 Communications and Networks on the Bandwidth of the
5G Standard ...................226
16.9 Heterogeneous Network ...................228
16.10 Conclusion and Future Scope ...................228

**Chapter 17** The Fusion of IoT, AI, Edge Cloud, and Blockchain ...................231

*Alwyn Rajiv S, Nancy Deborah R, Vinora A, Gobinath A, Sivakarthi G, and
Soundarya M*

17.1 Introduction ...................231
   17.1.1 Internet of Things (IoT) ...................231
   17.1.2 Artificial Intelligence (AI) ...................231
   17.1.3 Edge Cloud ...................232
   17.1.4 Blockchain ...................232
17.2 The Fusion ...................233
17.3 AI as the Brain for Industry Automation ...................234
17.4 IoT Devices as Data Generators in Industry Automation ...................235
17.5 5G as the Data Carrier in Industry Automation ...................236
17.6 Blockchain as the Memory in Industry Automation ...................237
17.7 Fusion of AI and Blockchain ...................238
17.8 Fusion of AI and Edge Cloud ...................240
17.9 Convergence of IoT and Edge Cloud ...................240
17.10 Convergence of IoT and AI ...................241
17.11 Conclusion ...................242

**Chapter 18** Trustworthiness of Blockchain Technology in Healthcare
5.0 and Industry 5.0 ...................244

*Kalaiselvi Thiruvenkadam and Veerakumar Pandi*

18.1 Introduction ...................244
18.2 Related Works ...................245
18.3 Methodology ...................247
18.4 Evolution of Healthcare 5.0 ...................247
18.5 Evolution of Industry 5.0 ...................249
18.6 Distributed Ledger Technology ...................249
18.7 Blockchain Basics ...................251
18.8 Impact of Blockchain in Healthcare 5.0 ...................252
18.9 Impact of Blockchain in Industry 5.0 ...................256
18.10 Security Challenges ...................257
18.11 The Quantum Impact in Strengthening of Blockchain Technology ...................259
18.12 Conclusion ...................261

**Chapter 19** The Future of Trust: Exploring the Potential of Blockchain Technology ...............269

*Divyajyothi MG, Rachappa Jopate, and Lenin J*

19.1 Introduction ................................................................................................269
19.2 Blockchain Technology Applications .........................................................269
    19.2.1 Finance Sector ..............................................................................269
    19.2.2 Healthcare......................................................................................270
    19.2.3 Supply Chain Management ...........................................................271
    19.2.4 Intellectual Property Protection ...................................................272
    19.2.5 Voting and Governance .................................................................272
19.3 Implementation of Blockchain ...................................................................272
    19.3.1 Role of EdgeAI in Blockchain Technology .................................273
    19.3.2 Role of Machine Learning Algorithms in Blockchain
            Technology .....................................................................................273
    19.3.3 Role of IoT in Blockchain Technology ........................................274
    19.3.4 Role of Cloud Services in Blockchain Technology ......................274
19.4 Challenges to Blockchain Adoption ...........................................................275
    19.4.1 Regulatory Hurdles.......................................................................275
    19.4.2 Scalability Issues ..........................................................................275
    19.4.3 Interoperability Challenges ..........................................................275
    19.4.4 Security Concerns .........................................................................275
    19.4.5 Lack of Standardization ...............................................................276
    19.4.6 User Experience.............................................................................276
    19.4.7 Energy Consumption .....................................................................276
    19.4.8 Privacy and Anonymity.................................................................276
    19.4.9 Costs and Resource Constraints ...................................................276
    19.4.10 Resistance to Change.....................................................................277
    19.4.11 Tokenization Challenges...............................................................277
    19.4.12 Blockchain Education....................................................................277
    19.4.13 Network Security...........................................................................277
    19.4.14 Cross-Border Challenges..............................................................277
    19.4.15 Ethical Concerns ..........................................................................277
19.5 Conclusion ..................................................................................................278

**Chapter 20** Demystifying the Industry 5.0 Version ...............................................................282

*Venkatesan Ramachandran, Feroze Ahamed Zahir Ahamed,
Thanga Helina Stalin, and Shirley Chellathurai Pon Anna Bai*

20.1 Introduction ................................................................................................282
    20.1.1 Background and Context ...............................................................282
    20.1.2 Significance of Industry 5.0..........................................................283
20.2 Foundations of Industry 5.0........................................................................283
    20.2.1 Historical Evolution of Industrial Revolutions ...........................283
    20.2.2 Industry 4.0 vs. Industry 5.0.........................................................284
    20.2.3 Key Principles and Concepts........................................................284
20.3 Human-Machine Collaboration...................................................................286
    20.3.1 The Role of Humans in Industry 5.0 ............................................286
    20.3.2 Synergies between Humans and Machines ...................................287
20.4 Technological Underpinnings......................................................................288
    20.4.1 Cyber-Physical Systems................................................................288

20.4.2    Artificial Intelligence in Industry 5.0 ...........288

20.4.3    Internet of Things Integration ...........289

20.5    Real-World Applications ...........289

20.5.1    Case Studies in Manufacturing ...........289

20.5.2    Impact on Productivity and Efficiency ...........290

20.5.3    Socioeconomic Impacts and Challenges ...........291

20.5.4    Opportunities for Inclusive Growth ...........292

20.6    Future Trends and Predictions ...........294

20.6.1    Emerging Technologies in Industry 5.0 ...........294

20.6.2    Anticipated Transformations in Industrial Practices ...........295

20.7    Conclusion ...........296

**Chapter 21**   Edge AI for Connected Healthcare in Internet of Medical Things for Smart Cities ...........299

*Mohamed Sirajudeen Mohamed Hanifa, Karima Salim Hashil Alnaamani, Gnanasankaran Natarajan, and Elakkiya Elango*

21.1    Introduction ...........299

21.1.1    Background ...........299

21.1.2    Significance of Edge AI and IoMT Integration in Healthcare ...........300

21.1.3    Contextualizing within Smart Cities ...........301

21.1.4    Foundations of Edge AI and IoMT ...........301

21.2    Synergy in Connected Healthcare ...........303

21.2.1    Proximity Computing in Healthcare ...........303

21.2.2    Advanced Diagnostics through Edge AI ...........304

21.2.3    Personalized Treatment and Proactive Healthcare ...........304

21.2.4    Challenges and Considerations ...........306

21.3    Impact on Resource Utilization and Patient Outcomes ...........308

21.3.1    Optimizing Resource Allocation in Healthcare ...........308

21.3.2    Improving Patient Outcomes with Data-Driven Insights ...........309

21.3.3    Future Directions and Innovations ...........310

21.4    Conclusion ...........311

**Index** ...........315

# Preface

All physical, mechanical, and electrical systems in our everyday environments are digitized through various digitization and edge technologies such as sensors, actuators, tags, codes, microcontrollers, stickers, etc. To accomplish more, electronic devices are increasingly empowered with computational, memory, storage, communication, and security resources. In short, ordinary and dumb elements extensively found in our living, walking, working, and socializing environments are technologically enabled to be digitized. That is, digitized entities gain the power to find one another in the vicinity and are integrated with remote digital assets through one or other networking methods. Such local and remote networking empowers edge devices to correspond and share their unique capabilities. Thus, the flourishing concept of the Internet of Things (IoT) talks about all kinds of ordinary, casual, and cheap things in our everyday environments (homes, offices, hospitals, retail stores, airports, educational campuses, eating joints, entertainment plazas, etc.) are methodically digitized (instrumented) and connected to exhibit intelligent capabilities.

AI models are meticulously engineered, evaluated, optimized, deployed, and observed. They are honed to be highly efficient, primarily through optimization and compression techniques such as pruning, quantization, and knowledge distillation. These lightweight models can be swiftly deployed in edge devices to infer valuable insights quickly.

Deploying and running artificial intelligence (AI) models has become more manageable. The development processes for AI models are constantly refined and simplified, accelerating the creation of competent and cognitive AI models. These models and systems have the unique and reassuring ability to continuously learn from various data sources, including environmental, performance, and operational data. This adaptability and resilience through continuous learning empower IoT edge devices to automate various needs.

The unique capacities and capabilities of IoT, edge computing, and AI are being realized through a series of advancements. These include multifaceted AI-centric processors, integrated platforms, facilitating frameworks, automated toolsets, and enabling libraries. These technologies and tools are paving the way for the development of pioneering AI models and systems. This chapter will explore how these advancements in AI, IoT, edge computing, and 5G communication, a high-speed, low-latency network crucial for connecting and transferring data between IoT devices, are shaping the future of technology. These advancements can potentially revolutionize various industries, bringing unprecedented capabilities and opportunities.

This book discusses how on-device data is processed quickly and how this state-of-the-art technique contributes immensely to envisaging real-world and real-time services and applications. Especially how the path-breaking edge AI concept (the strategically sound combination of edge data processing and AI's analytical, generative, transformative, and creative power) helps in visualizing and implementing Industry 4.0 and 5.0 systems is detailed in this book. Without an iota of doubt, multiple industry verticals are empowered through real-time data capture, processing, decision-making, and action. Edge AI has the innate power to open up fresh possibilities and opportunities. This book describes the recent trends and transitions in the edge AI space. Scores of evolutionary and revolutionary concepts combine well to prepare the field of edge AI to assimilate and accomplish better and bigger things for society's empowerment and betterment.

# Editor Biographies

**Pethuru Raj** is a chief architect at Reliance Jio Platforms Ltd. (JPL) Bangalore. Previously. worked in IBM global cloud center of excellence (CoE), Wipro consulting services (WCS), and Robert Bosch corporate research (CR). He has more than 22 years of IT industry experience and 8 years of research experience.

**B. Sundaravadivazhagan** obtained a PhD in computer science from Anna University, Chennai, India. Currently, he is a faculty member of the Department of Information Technology at the University of Technology and Applied Science-AL Mussanah in Oman. He has professional memberships in ISACA and ISTE and is a senior member of IEEE. His academic and research background spans more than 21 years at many institutions.

**A. Saleem Raja** is an associate professor in the Department of Information Technology at the Shinas University of Technology and Applied Sciences in the Sultanate of Oman. He obtained a PhD in 2017 in the general field of data mining as well as an MTech in information technology from Bharathidasan University in Tamil Nadu, India. He has published more than 25 research papers in national and international journals, conferences, and book chapters.

**Mohammed M. Alani** holds a PhD in computer engineering with specialization in network security. He has worked as a professor and a cybersecurity expert in many countries around the world. His experience includes serving as VP of academic affairs in the United Arab Emirates, working in network and security consultancies in the Middle East, and being a cybersecurity program manager in Toronto, Canada. He currently works as a cybersecurity professor at Seneca College and a research fellow at Toronto Metropolitan University, Toronto, Canada.

# Contributors

**Gobinath A**
Velammal College of Engineering and
    Technology
Department of Information Technology,
    Madurai
Tamil Nadu, India

**Srinivasan A**
Velammal College of Engineering and
    Technology
Department of Information Technology
Madurai, Tamil Nadu, India

**Vinora A**
Velammal College of Engineering and
    Technology
Department of Information Technology
Madurai, Tamil Nadu, India

**Feroz Khan AB**
Syed Hameedha Arts and Science College
Department of Computer Science
Kilakarai, India

**Feroze Ahamed Zahir Ahamed**
College of Computing and Information Sciences
University of Technology and Applied
    Sciences-Al-Musannah, Information
    Technology Department
Al-Musannah, Sultanate of Oman

**Mohammed Bakhit Al-Mahri**
College of Computing and Information Sciences
University of Technology and Applied
    Sciences-Salalah, IT Department
Salalah, Sultanate of Oman

**Karima Salim Hashil Alnaamani**
College of Computing and Information Sciences
University of Technology and Applied
    Sciences-Al-Musannah Information
    Technology Department
Al-Musannah, Sultanate of Oman

**Shirley Chellathurai Pon Anna Bai**
Karunya Institute of Technology and Sciences,
    Computer Science and Engineering
Coimbatore, Tamil Nadu, India

**Kannaki Devi B**
Bharathiar University
Department of Computer Science, Coimbatore
Tamil Nadu, India

**Sundaravadivazhagan B**
College of Computing and Information Sciences
University of Technology and Applied
    Sciences-Al-Musannah, Information
    Technology Department
Al-Musannah, Sultanate of Oman

**Subhadeep Barman**
IIIT NR University, School of Computing
    Science and Engineering
Chhattisgarh, India

**Yaman Birla**
Shri Govindram Seksaria Institute of
    Technology and Science
Department of Computer Science and Engineering
Indore, India

**Srija Chattopadhyay**
VIT Bhopal University
School of Computing Science and Engineering
    (SCSE)
Madhya Pradesh, India

**Sudhakar Kumar Chaubey**
University of Technology and Applied
    Sciences-Shinas Mathematics Section
Information Technology Department
Shinas, Sultanate of Oman

**Lakshmi D**
VIT Bhopal University
School of Computing Science and Engineering
    (SCSE)
Madhya Pradesh, India

**Ramyachitra D**
Bharathiar University
Department of Computer Science
Coimbatore, Tamil Nadu, India

**Manjula Devi C**
Velammal College of Engineering and Technology

Department of Information Technology
Madurai, Tamil Nadu, India

**Lloyds E**
Government Sivagangai Medical College,
    Inpatient Ward
Madurai, Tamil Nadu, India

**Elakkiya Elango**
Government Arts College for Women
Department of Computer Science
Sivaganga, Tamil Nadu, India

**Sivakarthi G**
Velammal College of Engineering and
    Technology
Department of Information Technology
Madurai, Tamil Nadu, India

**Jayapriya J**
Christ University
Department of Computer Science
Bangalore, Karnataka, India

**Lenin J**
College of Computing and Information Sciences
University of Technology and Applied
    Sciences-Al-Musannah
Al-Musannah, Sultanate of Oman

**Pooja Jain**
Indian Institute of Information Technology
Department of Computer Science and Engineering
Nagpur, India

**Dilip Kumar Jaiswal**
Institute of Natural Sciences and Humanities
Shri Ramswaroop Memorial University,
    Mathematical and Statistical Sciences
    Lucknow-Deva Road
Barabanki, India

**Rachappa Jopate**
College of Computing and Information Sciences
University of Technology and Applied
    Sciences-Al-Musannah
Information Technology Department
Al-Musannah, Sultanate of Oman

**Tapan Kumar**
Indian Institute of Information Technology
Department of Electronics and
    Communication Engineering
Nagpur, India

**Suresh Kumar N**
Velammal College of Engineering and
    Technology
Department of Information Technology
Madurai, Tamil Nadu, India

**Anandan M**
Vel Tech Rangarajan Dr. Sagunthala R&D
    Institute of Science and Technology
Department of Information Technology
Chennai, Tamil Nadu, India

**Soundarya M**
Velammal College of Engineering and
    Technology
Department of Information Technology
Madurai, Tamil Nadu, India

**Vinay M**
Christ University
Department of Computer Science
Bangalore, Karnataka, India

**Divyajyothi MG**
College of Computing and Information Sciences
University of Technology and Applied
    Sciences-Al-Musannah Information
    Technology Department
Al-Musannah, Sultanate of Oman

**Anshul Mishra**
Shri Govindram Seksaria Institute of
    Technology and Science
Department of Computer Science and
    Engineering
Indore, India

**Mohamed Sirajudeen Mohamed Hanifa**
Nilgiri College of Arts and Science Dean-PG
    and Research Thaloor
The Nilgiris
Tamil Nadu, India

**Samar Mouti**
Liwa College, Information Technology
  Department
Abu Dhabi, United Arab Emirates

**Gnanasankaran Natarajan**
Thiagarajar College
Department of Computer Science
Madurai, Tamil Nadu, India

**Rajeswari P**
Velammal College of Engineering and
  Technology
Department of Information Technology
Madurai, Tamil Nadu, India

**Veerakumar Pandi**
The Gandhigram Rural Institute (Deemed to be
  University)
Department of Computer Science and
  Applications
Gandhigram, Dindigul, Tamil Nadu, India

**Kathiravan Pannerselvam**
Central University of Tamil Nadu
Department of Computer Science
Thiruvarur, Tamil Nadu, India

**Shanmugavadivu Pichai**
Gandhigram Rural Institute
Department of Computer Science and
  Applications
Gandhigram, Dindigul, Tamil Nadu, India

**Nancy Deborah R**
Velammal College of Engineering and Technology
Department of Information Technology
Madurai, Tamil Nadu, India

**Saranya Rajiakodi**
Central University of Tamil Nadu
Department of Computer Science
Thiruvarur, Tamil Nadu, India

**Venkatesan Ramachandran**
Karunya Institute of Technology and Sciences,
  Computer Science and Engineering
Coimbatore, Tamil Nadu, India

**Samer Rihawi**
Liwa College, Information Technology
  Department
Abu Dhabi, United Arab Emirates

**Alwyn Rajiv S**
Kamaraj College of Engineering and
  Technology
Department of Electronics and Communication
  Engineering
Virudhunagar, Tamil Nadu, India

**Deepa S**
Christ University, Department of Computer
  Science
Bangalore, Karnataka, India

**Wasim Haidar SK**
College of Computing and Information Sciences
University of Technology and Applied
  Sciences-Salalah, IT Department
Salalah, Sultanate of Oman

**Sandhya Soman**
GITAM University
Department of Computer Science
Bangalore, Karnataka, India

**Thanga Helina Stalin**
KPR College of Arts Science and Research
Department of Commerce with Computer
  Applications
Coimbatore, Tamil Nadu, India

**Akalya T**
Bharathiar University
Department of Computer Science
Coimbatore, Tamil Nadu, India

**Kalaiselvi Thiruvenkadam**
The Gandhigram Rural Institute (Deemed to be
  University)
Department of Computer Science and
  Applications
Gandhigram, Dindigul, Tamil Nadu, India

**Senthilkumar Vijayakumar**
IEEE Senior Member, USA

# 1 Digital Twins for Smart Grids

*Pooja Jain, Tapan Kumar, Yaman Birla, and Anshul Mishra*

## Ethical Statement

The submitted work is original and has not been published elsewhere in any form or language (partially or in full).

## Author Contribution

All authors whose names appear on the submission

1. made substantial contributions to the conception or design of the work; or the acquisition, analysis, or interpretation of data; or the creation of new software used in the work;
2. drafted the work or revised it critically for important intellectual content;
3. approved the version to be published; and
4. agree to be accountable for all aspects of the work in ensuring that questions related to the accuracy or integrity of any part of the work are appropriately investigated and resolved.

## Data Availability

The datasets generated during and/or analyzed during the current study are available from the corresponding author on reasonable request.

## 1.1  INTRODUCTION

The fourth industrial revolution (Industry 4.0) has been accelerated by the rapid advancement of digital technology and intelligence. Industrial IoT (IIoT) and digital twins are two of Industry 4.0's most cutting-edge concepts. The IIoT enables real-time data collection, processing, and analytics of massive amounts of sensor data feed created by smart factory sensors [1]. The authors [2] state that the digital twin (DT) is created as a virtual and computerized element of a physical system that may be applied by means of a real-time synchronizing between sensed data from a field to simulate sensed data in various ways. In addition, in [3], the authors define DT as "a detailed digital representation of a single product." Through models and data, it involves the features, status, and behavior of the real-life object. The digital twin is a collection of realistic models that can be used to imitate the product's actual behavior in the context." It is possible for such synchronization with the enabling technologies of Industry 4.0. The cyber-physical integration of production is facilitated with the use of a digital twin. With the use of a digital twin, Industry 4.0's technical base is rooted in the IoT that advocated the incorporation of electronics, software, sensors, and connections to objects (i.e., "things") so that the data may be collected and sent via the Internet.

Industry 4.0 was extensively researched and essential technologies, including smart embedded and networked systems in production systems, were identified despite the latest trend. Cyber-physical systems (CPS) were also proposed. They are working at virtual and physical levels to communicate with, monitor, feel, and act in the real world. In order to fully exploit the potential of CPS and IoT, appropriate data modeling is available in scientific literature.[4]

DOI: 10.1201/9781003442066-1

The digital twin technique aims to generate a digital representation of a real-world object that concentrates on the object itself. When every physical source has a digital twin equivalent (such as an automobile, an industry, or a human), the spatial-temporal relationships between the digital twins take priority over the individual digital twins. Object interactions will be improved at a system-of-systems level, rather than locally and individually, as is currently done. This will result in huge efficiency gains. The usage of digital twins in the industrial Internet of Things is examined in-depth in this paper. The review attempted to capture important papers from 2012 onwards across three areas—manufacturing, supply chain, and production—because the literature's center of gravity is manufacturing application.

## 1.2  CONCEPT OF DIGITAL TWIN, DIGITAL MODEL, DIGITAL SHADOW

Digital Twins are important instruments for dealing with today's industrial difficulties. In many cases, they provide a one-of-a-kind opportunity for increased efficiency and cost savings. For power trains predictive, digital twins allow for the creation of a novel solution or service—typically tasks that were previously thought to be unattainable [5]. The terms digital twin, digital model, and digital shadow are frequently used interchangeably in smart manufacturing. However, the extent of data flow between physical and digital counterparts varies between these systems.

A digital model represents a digital representation that does not comprise an automated exchange of information between the digital and physical subject matter of an existing or future physical object. Data from physical objects are used to create a digital model, which is manually shared. As a result, a change in an object's physical condition has no effect on its digital representation and vice versa.[6]

As per the definition of the digital model, when there is an automated one-way data flow between a physical object and a digital object, a digital shadow is formed. As a result, a change in the physical object produces a change in the state of a digital object, but the other way around is not the case.[6]

Moreover, if the data flow between an existing physical object and a digital object in both directions, this is referred to as the digital twin. In this model, the digital object and physical object both act as a controlling instance of each other. A change in the state of a physical object leads to a change in the state of the digital object and vice versa.[6]

In the next paragraph [7], we are going to discuss some computation properties of the digital twin.

- Physical things (**P**): In every physical thing $p \in \mathbf{P}$ we consider it composed of seven elements (S, A, F, E, N, P, D), where $S \rightarrow$ sensors, $A \rightarrow$ actuators, $F \rightarrow$ processes sensory values, $E \rightarrow$ events, $D \rightarrow$ data storage, $P \rightarrow$ power supply, $N \rightarrow$ network interface.

$$P \equiv \{P_j, j = 1. \ldots . |\mathbf{P}|\} \tag{1.1}$$

As inputs, several sensor data are used, $I \subseteq S$ to a state initiates a transfer function $\lambda$ to other states. Every state has a corresponding output O following the output function $\delta$, So event $O \subseteq E$ can be determined.

$$\lambda: Q \times I \rightarrow Q \tag{1.2}$$

$$: Q \rightarrow O \tag{1.3}$$

Here, Q is Various states of function.

- Virtual things (**V**): Just like in physical twin, here the seven elements in virtual twin are $(S_V, A_V, F_V, E_V, N_V, P_V, D_V)$, where $S \rightarrow$ virtual sensors, $A \rightarrow$ virtual actuators, $F_v \rightarrow$ functional units, $E_v \rightarrow$ observed events, $D_v \rightarrow$ data storage, $N_v \rightarrow$ virtual interface, $P_v \rightarrow$ virtual power supply. In this context, the virtual interface refers to the communication channel of the digital twin that is linked to the real entity.

$$V \equiv \{V_m, m = 1. . . . . . |V|\} \tag{1.4}$$

$$\mathbf{P} \rightarrow \mathbf{V} \tag{1.5}$$

As a sequential state machine consists of six parameters, the authors represent any functional unit fv [8]. (same parameters for physical systems) (equation—6). The Figure 1.1 shows the digital twin framework.

$$f_V = (Q_V, I_V, O_V, q0_V, \lambda_V, \delta_V) \tag{1.6}$$

$$\lambda_v: Q_v \times I_v \rightarrow Q_v \tag{1.7}$$

$$\delta_v: Q_v \rightarrow O_v \tag{1.8}$$

## 1.3 DIGITAL TWIN AS AN EMERGING TECHNOLOGY

The concept of digital twins was derived from the hardware of twins composed from two identical space cars developed in the NASA Apollo program "where at least two identical space vehicles were designed to enable mirroring of the spacecraft's circumstances during the operation"[9]. The aim of NASA in this technology is to replicate the mirror life of flying twins completely for a successful mission.

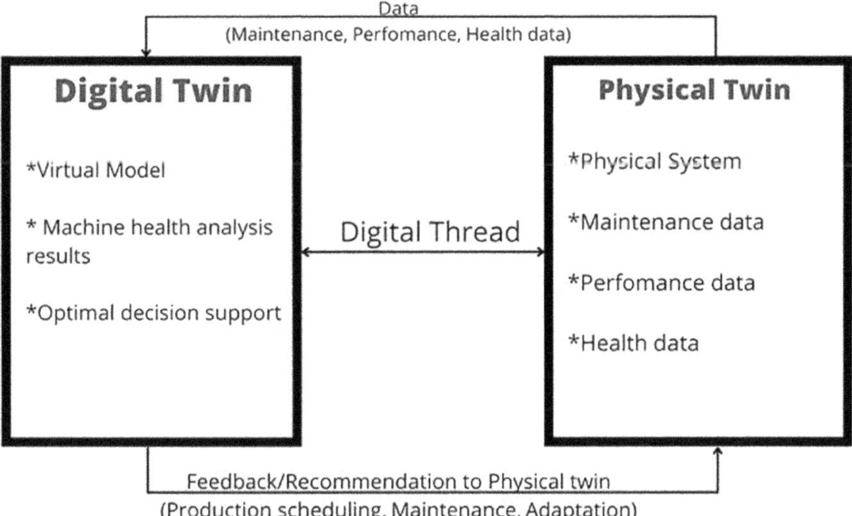


**FIGURE 1.1** Digital twin framework.

Digital twins, which cover the whole lifecycle of an asset or process and serve as the foundation for connected products and services, are predicted to become a commercial requirement. Companies who invest in digital twin technology are expected to enjoy a 30% increase in crucial process cycle times. It is estimated that the market for equivalent offerings might be worth $90 billion each year [5]. The digital twin concept will further make stimulation readily available, allowing for better decision-making across the whole product and process lifecycle.

The digital twin is a digital model that contains design and engineering requirements detailing the shape, materials, components, and component behaviors of a given item. More importantly, it also contains the operational data that are unique to its particular physical assets. For example, the digital twin includes a twin that is identifiable for the airplane as the identification number of the physical product unit. Data in an airplane's geometry from 3D aircraft models, aerodynamic models, technical modifications cut during manufacturing cycles, material qualities, inspections, operation maintenance data, aerodynamic models, and any deviations from the original design specifications approved due to issues and workarounds on the specific product unit [10].

## 1.4  A GLANCE OF IIOT

IoT has already revolutionized our understanding of applications across a broad spectrum of human endeavors. This trend is expected to accelerate in the near future as the future impact of IoT grows. IoT applications include smart energy, smart manufacturing, agriculture, health, security, and smart cities. The Internet of Things (IoT) is a complicated cyber-physical system that brings together a variety of devices with sensing, identification, processing, communication, and networking capabilities. Sensors and actuators, in particular, have become more powerful, less expensive, and smaller, making their use more widespread [11]. The development of the concept of IIoT has resulted from the use of IoT in the industry with the aim of enhancing productivity while lowering the cost of production [12, 13].

The term "industrial Internet of Things" (IIoT) refers to the widespread application of IoT in the industrial setting to achieve its goals. It was first implemented in 1999, and since then, many industries have used IIoT to enhance their production process. The things that separate it from IoT are the various technologies employed in an IIoT scenario, as well as the distinct goals and reasons for which these technologies are used [14].

"The IIoT vision of the world is one where smart connected assets (the things) operate as part of a larger system or systems of systems that make up the smart manufacturing enterprise"[15].

The IIoT is made up of a variety of devices that are linked together through communications software. IIoT devices' principal purpose is to monitor, collect, exchange, and analyze data and this data is further used by devices to update their behavior [14]. Data collection and analysis from a growing number of low-cost, intelligent sensors will improve corporate performance and asset reliability [15]. Due to the low cost of wireless sensors, the implementation of a large number of autonomous networks becomes easy and the full potential of sensor technology will be realized in a large-scale data flow. In [16] authors recommend a global sensor network to fulfill the idea of "sensor setwork." The Figure 1.2 gives the IIoT framework in Industry 4.0.

Manufacturing and factories aren't the only places where industrial technology is applied. Technology's maturity and cyber-physical control capabilities have expanded its application beyond typical factory contexts, and they now form a key portion of vital infrastructure on several fronts. Two such fields are energy generation and distribution infrastructure [12].

## 1.5  DIGITAL TWIN IN SMART CITIES

The academic research in this area is limited, but some case studies [17, 18] show that digital twins could make a huge difference in this modern period. As digital twins emerge as a new technology, the idea of creating parallel virtual versions of cities along with sharing of information and data

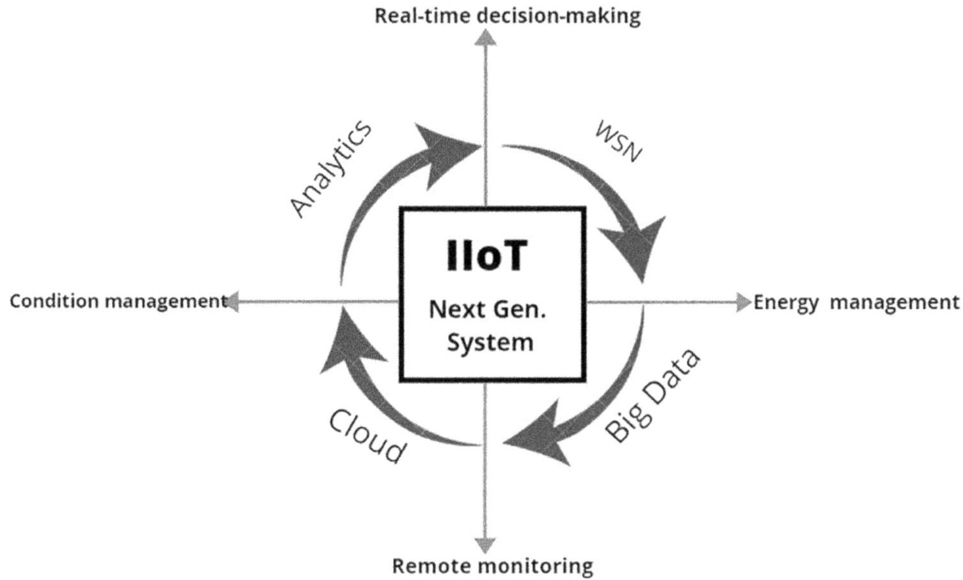


**FIGURE 1.2**  IIoT framework in Industry 4.0.

analytics through IoT devices is starting to take shape and making foundational development of smart city digital twins.

In cities, we need a higher understanding of how people interact with the environment and how information is exchanged. The case study in [17] depicts the digital twin of a city Atlanta (USA), which brings the connection between human infrastructures and technology in spatiotemporal dimensions (i.e., having both spatial extension and temporal duration). The rapid growth in magnitude, diversity, and entanglement of data generated by city infrastructures and human activities on a daily basis necessitates a major shift. The digital twin of Atlanta is a virtual reality (VR) platform built primarily on the Unity game engine (cross-platform). This platform incorporates Atlanta's 3-dimensional model, which covers nearly the whole city in virtual areas so that its human infrastructure systems are interactive and interoperable. The performance data for infrastructures (e.g., energy consumption) and human data (e.g., social network data) depends on their positions and their proximity. The data collected from the whole city allows the server system to gradually learn from the live digital simulation server system and provide analytical insights to examine the likely future situation, boosting decision-making.

The case study of [18] presents the creation of a digital twin of a city, an effective device in urban planning for this idea they chose a small town of Herrenberg, Germany, with a population of 30,000 people, and a town that is heavily affected by traffic and a certain degree of air pollution, presented opportunity to analyze several situations and solutions using a real-life case. The digital twin of the city enabled us to obtain a deeper knowledge of potential solutions for urban difficulties requiring public decision-making to attain unity. To make a virtual twin of an urban city, Herrenberg evaluated urban digital twins using techniques and procedures such as 3D modeling, wind flow simulation, people's mobility patterns, stationary activity data, and qualitative data regarding people's perspectives. The project also aims to support the strategy of software and data access by utilizing open-source software, such as COVISE, OpenCOVER, and OpenFOAM, to allow future research and create chances for planners and policymakers to adopt and promote these techniques. They also performed a survey with 39 people to see how the residents of this community reacted to the digital twin model. The urban digital twin, on the other hand, is unable to incorporate all of the information from the physical world. Furthermore, they proposed that there be information regarding other social, economic, and environmental variables that would aid in the future study for the advanced development of urban digital twins on a broad scale.

The Smart City Barcelona [19] program fosters and supports innovation, urban development, and improved quality of life for its residents. Different services are provided while collaborating with universities and businesses. Infrastructure plans, such as Wi-Fi and optical fiber, a mobility plan, heating, and cooling systems, and energy networks, are among the Smart City's primary projects. Smart districts, living labs, initiatives, e-services, infrastructures, and open data are all part of the Smart City plan. The Table 1.1 summarizes the research work done in field of digital twins in smart cities.

## 1.6  DIGITAL TWIN IN HEALTHCARE

Digital twins have many applications in Industries, but its main advantage is that it can replicate living things and so digital twins can have a huge impact on healthcare and well-being. The digital twin of humans helps to cure the illness, but it can also help improve the mental health of humans as today's daily life is so stressful.

By evaluating the real twin's previous illness and monitoring health on a regular basis, the digital twin can also help anticipate the emergence of the disease. Digital twins can also help to improve the psychological behavior of real twins by using artificial intelligence in which by analyzing the pattern of stressful situations to recommend avoiding or reducing stress [20]. In [21], the authors propose a cloud-based digital twin for elderly health services (CloudDTH), a cloud-based system for monitoring, diagnosing, and predicting health in human life. Digital twins can also improve the success rate of surgeries, it gives the ability to the doctor to perform pre-surgery checks remotely through digital twin which is another field of research "remote surgery."

Digital twins can be used in drug development to study medication to find the best one; we can test new potential drugs to predict which has more potential for success, reducing clinical trials if the first shoot is improved.

Digital twins also assist us in obtaining answers to if-then scenarios, knowing if any decision would lead to any improvement or deterioration of health [20, 22]. The use of this technology allows us to easily diagnose some diseases that are difficult to detect in the early stages, which aids in the proper cure of ailments. The future research of digital twins on healthcare industries is mainly focused on the virtual twin of a hospital, in which stakeholders can review the capacities and staffing and can apply analytics to predict actions to take for future challenges. For example, in COVID pandemic, thousands of people lost their lives because of bed shortage and oxygen shortage; here, a digital twin can assist in solving bed shortage and operating rooms. In [23] authors stated that "by comparing Digital Twins across large populations, we can gain a far clearer picture of health vs disease, and so sharpen the debate between therapy versus enhancement." Digital twins

---

**TABLE 1.1**
**Digital Twin in Smart Cities**

| Ref. No. | City | Concerns | Technology Used to Build Virtual City | Recommendations |
|---|---|---|---|---|
| [17] | Atlanta (USA) | Future scenarios | Unity (game engine) | Better data processing |
| [18] | Herrenberg (Germany) | Urban planning | COVISE, OpenCOVER | More social, economic data, and surveys |
| [19] | Barcelona (Spain) | Infrastructures and collaborative networks | FABLab, i2Cat LivingLab, LIVE | Collaborative system intelligent network technologies |

can replicate the hospital to create a better safe environment that will help optimize patient care and staff performance.

So it enhances strategic decisions to take in complex and sensitive environments.

## 1.7 DIGITAL TWIN IN SUPPLY CHAIN MANAGEMENT

The management of interconnected and dependent businesses is known as supply chain management that ensures the long-term availability of the products and services that customers require. It is a critical component in the effective transportation of products from suppliers to end customers through the distribution channel [24]. One of the primary difficulties in multinational organizations' rapid growth and market expansion is supply chain management. In a well-maintained society, supply chain management will increase employability; this will allow the bidirectional flow of information, production planning, and cash flow. Supply chain planning is vital in many processes, such as sourcing, production, and transportation. It also has an impact on the manufacturing process's cost, quality, and productivity. Supply chains are becoming more digitized, analytical, and automated as a result of information technologies and Industry 4.0[25]. Data exchange, data collection, and supply chain management have become more efficient with the help of digital twins and IIoT. DT also promotes faster action and response to reduce lead time.

DT in the supply chain has 3 components-real product, digital product, and data exchange. There is synchronization between RP and DP, having comprehensive data collection, quicker action, and response to shorten lead time [25]. Different DTs can communicate with each other and exchange data, allowing DTs to collect data from other systems. As a result, the massive data makes forecasting and planning more accurate over time, as well as comprehensive data collection, quicker action, and response to shortening lead time.

We know that Industry 4.0 comes with the combination of manufacturing with data management and communication technologies. The scope of digital twins is widely used in manufacturing industries and supply chains to give feedback for a physical environment for any modifications that will help the business or organizations to reach their goals. So the digital twin will play a key role in the product lifecycle management of an individual product. The authors in [26] propose "The Multitier Digital twin approach to collect information from the different management levels of the production company of small and medium enterprise (SME) into a novel multi-tier DT," which visualize and simulates the full digital model of company authors presents how goals of the company can be achieved by applying correct analytics and using software applications with the help of multi-tier digital twin approach [27, 28]. Another application of DT is improving the customer experience, the main goal for organizations is to provide customers the best experience and to get frequent feedback from customers that improves services.

In many firms, the manufacturing and supplying processes have become complex and, thus, less efficient and more costly, [29] but a digital twin can help you take a deep look at effective methods to identify where obstacles, time, waste, and errors are slowing down work and simulate the result of the particular target improvement plan.

For a better implementation of digital twin in industries, there should be some important changes one should be focusing on which involves changes in the production line, some alterations in product formula to make the product less expensive, and improving the usefulness of the product, this could increase efficiency, productivity and will reduce operational expenses [30, 31]. The authors in [32] presented a case study of the supply chain management of the aircraft landing gear. The supply chain of ALG includes complicated manufacturing and maintenance as its production and inventory units are distributed globally. The Table 1.2 summarizes the research done in the field of digital twins being used in supply chain management.

**TABLE 1.2**
**Digital Twin in Supply Chain Management**

| Ref | Type | Concern | Technology Used | Recommendation |
|---|---|---|---|---|
| [25] | Case study | Supply chain planning | Simulation | A comprehensive foundation for DT-driven SCP |
| [24] | Concept | Supply chain management | EDI, RFID, 3D printing | Reducing the time, it takes for a product to go from the manufacturer to the customer |
| [26] | Concept | Agile supply chain management | Software AG ARIS architect, Visual Components software | More case studies and research on data exchange |
| [27] | Concept | Product management | Big data, machine learning, and IoT | Research on data fusion |
| [29] | Review | Practical implementation of DT in manufacturing | MATLAB/Simulink and cloud interface for MEC | More research on manufacturing execution system (MEC) |

## 1.8  DIGITAL TWINS IN MANUFACTURING INDUSTRIES

A manufacturing digital twin allows both modeling and optimization of the production system, which also reviews potential problems as well as visualization of systems in the manufacturing process that begins with individual components and ends with the finished product [33]. As we all know, using digital twins are still in its infancy when it comes to implementation. However, several case studies and publications proposed innovative ideas to apply this technology in industries, especially in manufacturing. In this section, we are going to discuss several case studies in manufacturing industries and the status of the digital twin in manufacturing.

### 1.8.1  SMART MANUFACTURING BY DIGITAL TWINS

The cyber-physical integration of manufacturing is made easier with the use of a digital twin. Smart manufacturing optimizes the entire manufacturing business process and operating techniques, as well as assisting in the achievement of productivity targets. In the manufacturing system, a digital twin is defined as a data-oriented representation of all aspects of the manufacturing system. IIoT, big data, cloud computing, AI, digital twins, and other technologies are propelling the manufacturing industry toward smart manufacturing [31, 34].

The author in [34] divided into three stages in the case of smart production: unit level, system level, and SoS (system of the system) level. The unit-level digital twin is the equipment. The integration of several unit-level digital twins forms the system-level digital twin. The integration of digital twins at several system levels generates digital twins at the SoS level. A virtual plant model from the point of view of geometrical form, function, and operating conditions of equipment and production line was used to map the physical equipment. Basic qualities, real-time, status, and other data are transmitted to drive the simulation and prediction. Physical elements and virtual models co-evolve in the closed-loop interaction process.

The authors in [35] discuss the digital-twin-driven human-robot collaborative assembly system for industries; the software used by authors for simulation is Tecnomatix, which helped in three directions, (1) designing a digital twin as a 3D virtual representation of a human-robot working system, (2) calculating cycle time and establishing the robot's path, and (3) communication with function blocks for tasks execution. This approach result supports the concept of automation as well as the flexibility of assembly.

[36] presents a case study on ice cream machines, food sectors, and industrial or kitchen appliances, all of which are defined as e-gastronomic items since they are becoming increasingly networked. This paper gives a better insight into how a digital twin of e-gastronomic things would be better for monitoring and checking their performance, predicting potential usage, and the interaction and visualization between the digital twin and the physical twin via augmented reality or virtual reality. The authors suggested that such an approach like this requires a deeper study on more complex IoT security solutions, advanced artificial intelligence, and machine learning algorithms. The authors of [37, 32] examined the use of digital twins and big data in smart manufacturing. They concluded that when combined with big data's accurate analysis and prediction capabilities, digital twin-driven smart manufacturing will become more responsive and predictive, benefiting more reasonable and precise manufacturing management in a variety of ways.

MRO = maintenance, repair, and operations

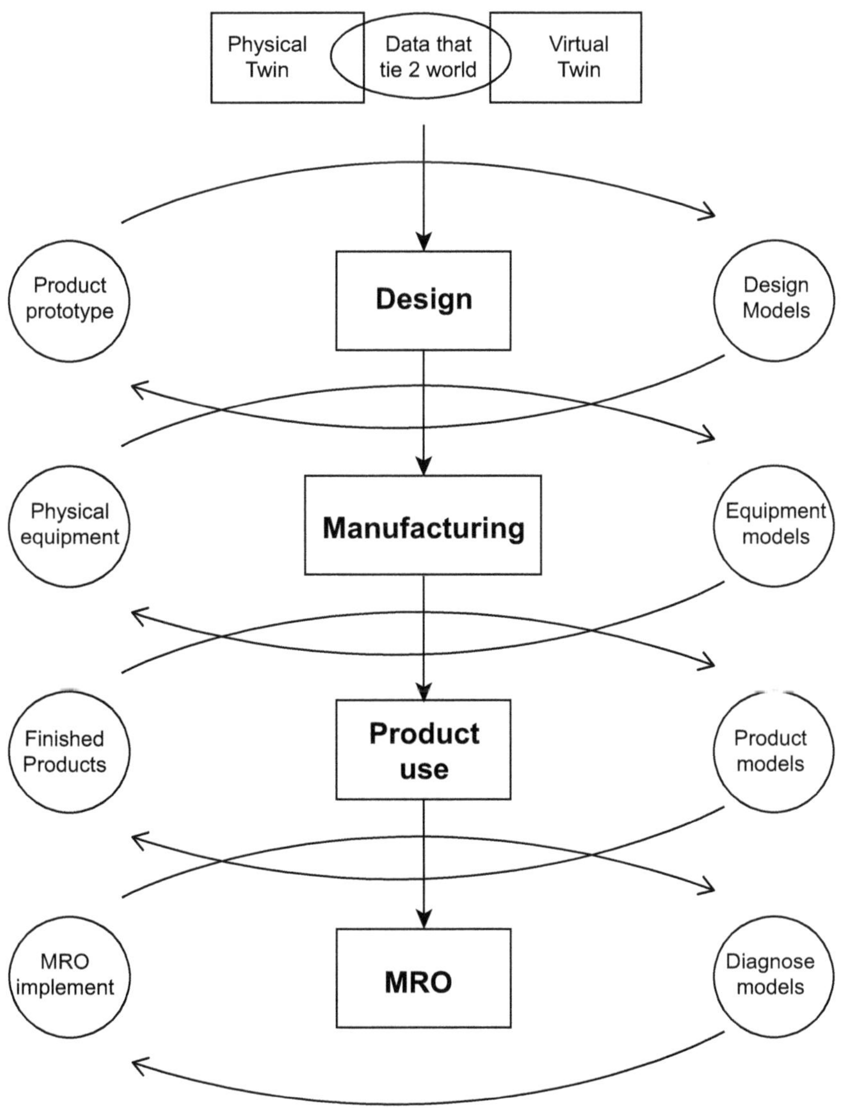


**FIGURE 1.3** Digital twin application in industries.

Figure 1.3 depicts the digital twins' applications in industries. IIoT technology will enable smart connected machines and smart connected manufacturing assets to be fully embedded with the rest of the organization. This will allow for more flexible and efficient manufacturing, which will be more profitable. The use of low-cost wireless sensors will boost asset performance. This aids in the collection of data and the use of that data to make better decisions [15]. The authors [38, 39] discuss the various challenges faced in IoT systems and propose possible solutions to them. The Table 1.3 summarizes the research done in the field of digital twins being used in smart manufacturing.

### 1.8.2 Production Management in Industries

Management of production concerns design and control systems responsible for the manufacturing of raw materials, human resources, equipment, and facilities for product or service development [50]. "The objective of production management is to produce goods and services of the right quality and quantity at the predetermined time and preestablished cost" [50].

---

**TABLE 1.3**

**Smart Manufacturing by Digital Twins**

| Ref | Type | Focused Area | Specific Area | Technology Used |
|---|---|---|---|---|
| [2] | Review | Manufacturing | CPS-based production system | Not available |
| [40] | Review | Digital twin | Challenges and open research | Simulation |
| [41] | Concept | Cyber-physical System | Methodology for data exchange between systems | Automation ML |
| [42] | Concept | Design and manufacturing | Product lifecycle | Not available |
| [43] | Concept | Manufacturing | Autonomous system in manufacturing | Simulation and automation |
| [29] | Review | Manufacturing | MES | Simulation |
| [34] | Concept | Smart manufacturing | Production optimization | Simulation |
| [44] | Case study | Manufacturing | Self-thinkable production | Simulation |
| [33] | Review | Manufacturing and DT, DM, DS | PPC, PLM | Simulation, CAD, optimization |
| [35] | Case study | Manufacturing technology | Human-robot collaborative system | Tecnomatix |
| [36] | Case study | Industrial technology | Food technologies | AR or VR |
| [45] | Case study | Manufacturing | Factory design | Simulation |
| [46] | Concept | Industry 4.0 | Smart IoT applications | SWeTI Platform |
| [47] | Concept | Production system | CPPS for Industry 4.0 | Simulation |
| [48] | Concept | Manufacturing | Smart CPPS system | Simulation |
| [49] | Concept | Smart product in manufacturing | Smart product lifecycle management | Graph database system Neo4j and SciGraph framework |
| [3] | Definition | Manufacturing | Proof of DT concept | CAD, web-based system |
| [23] | Concept | Industry | Healthcare | Simulation |
| [32] | Review | Manufacturing | DT and big data in smart manufacturing | API, cloud computing, IoT, big data |

DT = digital twin, DM = digital model, DS = digital shadow
PPC = production and planning control, PLM = product lifecycle management
MES = manufacturing execution systems

---

Rapid technological advancements in the manufacturing industry have paved the way for advanced manufacturing strategies. Because it incorporates technology such as IoT, digital twins, IIoT, big data, and AI, smart manufacturing has emerged as one of the routes for modern industrial development. Smart manufacturing utilizes methods such as digital modeling, simulation, and experimental verification to control product design, resource allocation, and production processes [51, 52].

Digital twin of the production system is a key component of Industry 4.0 that ensures adequate data quality and helps in optimizing the production process. Its goals are to increase production system transparency and enable real-time production control. A real-time locating system is used to track products and components in manufacturing processes. Sensor-based tracking systems are also used in industries. Simulation has been utilized to solve optimization challenges in manufacturing and logistics systems with great success [47]. Production management is critical for achieving industry goals, and as a result, it is being optimized more and more.

[47] deals with a concept of production management in small and medium enterprises, the contribution of digital twin in its development, and how different aspects of it affect the production process. Data acquisition and evaluation methods are discussed for optimizing solutions, leading to real-time production control. The separation of volatile and master data creates a secured system. The creation of a virtual production system generates data. Using the two data acquisition methods that have been developed, data collection hardware is implemented.

### 1.8.3 FUTURE OF MANUFACTURING INDUSTRY

Digital twins combine solutions such as machine learning, artificial intelligence, and software analytics to provide firms with unique opportunities. Also, in the Internet of Things (IoT) field, digital twins are very essential. Digital twin is in its early stages, and there is more need for research in industrial applications to find out the potential of the digital twin. Digital twins allow many applications in software design for complex smart cyber-physical systems as an online method that can utilize simulations and optimize system behavior. Hence, improves the software framework of a cyber-physical system. Various companies have already provided the applications of digital twins around us like General Electric. Digital twin aims to predict the health and performance of their product, SIEMENS focuses on increased production efficiency and quality. TESLA plans to produce digital twin for cars that enable information flow between car and factory [42, 53]. Microsoft delivers digital twin in its Azure Technology where companies can create spatial intelligence graphs represent how devices, places, and people interact, IBM uses digital twin technology where companies may build, test, monitor, and construct goods in a virtual manner, decreasing feedback delay between design and operation.

As advancement in technology increases, the products become smart and a new product generation evolved called "smart product (cyber-physical product)" and are intelligent products that can communicate with the other CPS for real-time synchronization. A lot of work has been done in the field of cyber-physical systems [54–56]. The smart product consists of three types of information (component information, architectural information, and smart product usage information). In [49] authors propose a new approach for smart product lifecycle management called semantic data management, which shows ways to manage all types of information that smart product has in a wide network, the outlook of SDM consists of five key concepts SP, SP instance, process, resources, and organization, and in order to implement, this they used graph database system. The authors in [57] discuss the digital twin in creating machine tools virtually for cyber-physical manufacturing by integrating sensory input and machine information. This approach can be used to integrate production and sensor data into them. The authors [41] aim in defining the digital twin in Industry 4.0 and how it is shaping the manufacturing world. The authors [58, 59] discuss distributed systems and solve the problem of fault prediction.

The overall aim of factories is to achieve their goal by the implementation of the digital twin. Factories become more dependent on DT to achieve their objectives. Besides implementation of digital twin, the autonomous system in industries should deal with some classes like self-organization, flexible manufacturing, and fault tolerance, as discussed in [46]. They also presented a new platform called SWeTI (Semantic Web of Things for Industry 4.0), which combines artificial intelligence technique with IoT and testing on real case scenarios to address Industry 4.0 challenges. Monitoring the performance of a fleet of airplanes is critical for ensuring optimal operation and detecting abnormalities that could increase fuel consumption or threaten flight safety [60]. Accurate Techniques for identifying failures and estimating life expectancy also produce Maintenance costs are decreased.

Digital twinning can enhance manufacturing productivity by providing consistent production data, allowing companies to remain competitive and meet client demand. This means that companies won't have to worry about their technology becoming outdated.

## 1.9   VERSATILE PRODUCTION SYSTEMS

Versatile production systems (VPS) are those systems being used for versatile jobs related to production. Nowadays, digital twins are being made for such VPS. Digital twins are able to make the analysis, design, evaluation, and optimization of the physical VPS quite easier. The digital twin can also be used for anomaly detection at a very early stage saving a lot on money and energy [52]. High rack storage system (or HRSS) was one of the experiments done under the project IMPROVE. It's a type of VPS. The main purpose of the project IMPROVE was to develop tools for Industrial IoT. The team of the project worked on various human machine interfaces. They developed the interfaces in such a way so that the optimization of the machines

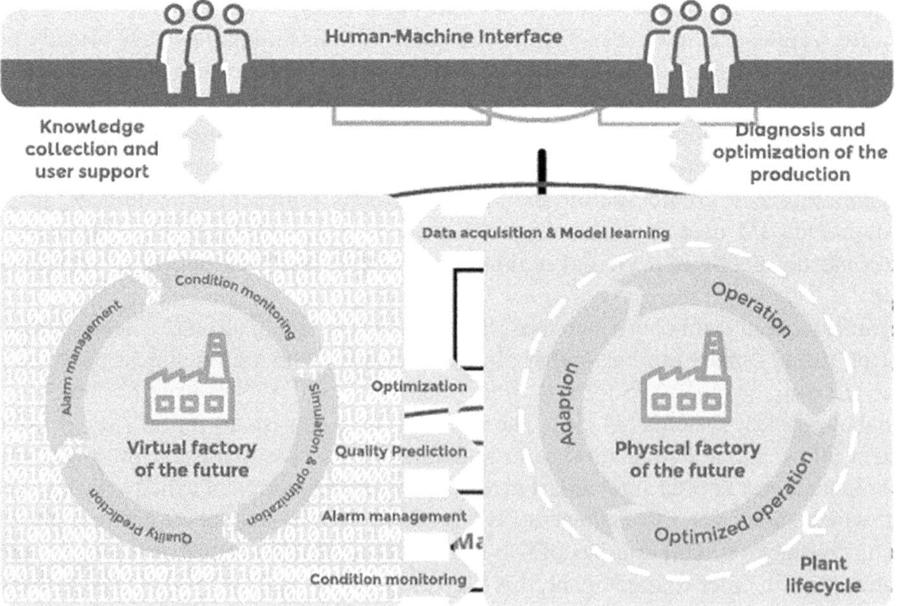


**FIGURE 1.4**   Human-machine interface system.

can be done in a better way. The diagram of such a human machine interface is given in the Figure 1.4. It clearly shows that alarm management, condition management, quality prediction and optimization can be very done with the help of digital twins providing human computer interface.

A high rack storage system is developed by the Improve project. It uses the human-machine interface in order to handle the cyber-physical system. Figure 1.5 shows a screenshot of the video shared by the Improve project.

The HRSS demonstrator takes the wares between different shelves. Intelligent energy management is depicted in the Figure 1.6.

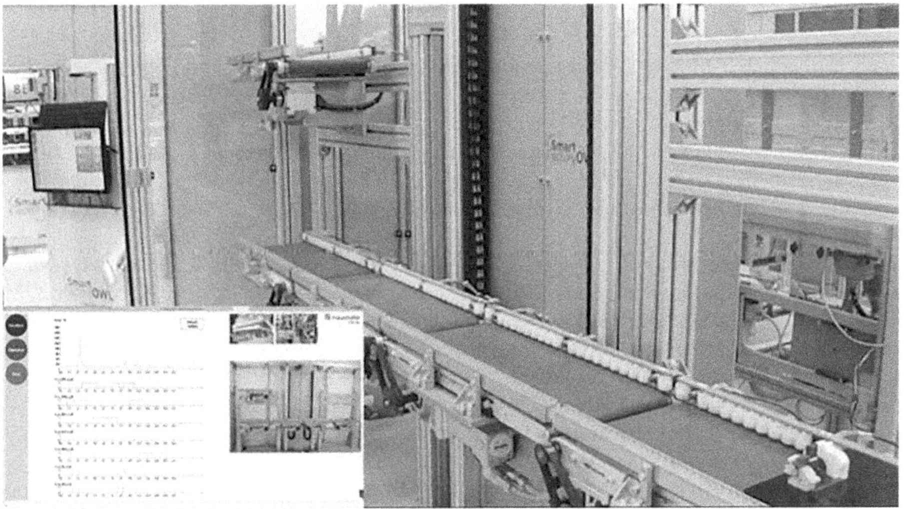

**FIGURE 1.5**  High rack storage system.

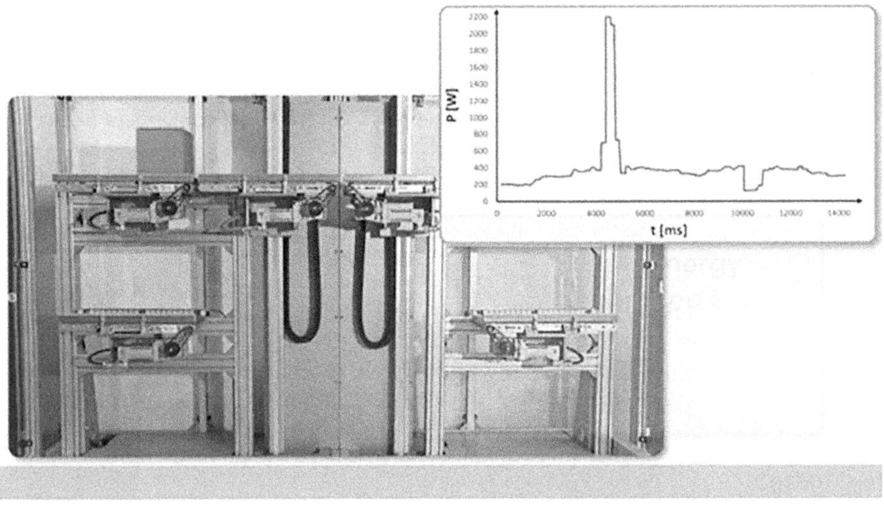

**FIGURE 1.6**  Intelligent energy management for the smart factory.

## 1.10 CONCLUSIONS

Digital twins are important instruments for dealing with today's industrial difficulties. In many cases, they provide a one-of-a-kind opportunity for increased efficiency and cost savings. Digital twins, which cover the whole lifecycle of an asset or process and serve as the foundation for connected products and services, are predicted to become a commercial requirement. The usage of digital twins in different domains like supply chain management, healthcare, and manufacturing industries was given in detail. The comparison of the work done by different researchers is also well presented in the form of various tables. In current pandemic times, healthcare domain is the one, which needs most of our attention. In future authors wish to develop a digital twin model to be used in healthcare domain.

## REFERENCES

[1] Vignesh Kamath, Jeff Morgan, Muhammad Intizar Ali, "Industrial IoT and Digital Twins for a Smart Factory", *2020 Global Internet of Things Summit (GIoTS)*, pp. 1–6, 2020. https://doi.org/10.1109/GIOTS49054.2020.9119497.

[2] Elisa Negri, Luca Fumagalli, Marco Macchi, "A Review of the Roles of Digital Twin in CPS-based Production Systems", in *Procedia Manufacturing 11 (2017). 27th International Conference on Flexible Automation and Intelligent Manufacturing, FAIM 2017*, 27–30 June 2017, Modena, Italy, pp. 939–948. ISSN 2351-9789.

[3] Sebastian Haag, Reiner Anderl, "Digital Twin—Proof of Concept", *2018 Society of Manufacturing Engineers (SME). Manufacturing Letters* 15 (2018): 64–66. https://doi.org/10.1016/j.mfglet.2018.02.006.

[4] N. Jazdi, "Cyber-Physical Systems in the Context of Industry 4.0", in *Automation, Quality and Testing, Robotics, 2014 IEEE International Conference*, pp. 1–4. https://doi.org/10.1109/AQTR.2014.6857843.

[5] Dirk Hartmann, Herman Van der Auweraer, "Digital Twins", *ArXiv*, abs/2001.09747. January 28, 2020.

[6] Werner Kritzinger, Matthias Karner, Georg Traar, Jan Henjes, Wilfried Sihn, "Digital Twin in Manufacturing: A Categorical Literature Review and Classification", *IFAC-PapersOnLine* 51, no. 11 (2018): 1016–1022. https://doi.org/10.1016/j.ifacol.2018.08.474.

[7] Kazi Masudul Alam, Abdulmotaleb El Saddik, "C2PS: A Digital Twin Architecture Reference Model for the Cloud-Based Cyber-Physical Systems", *IEEE Access* 5 (2017): 2050–2062. https://doi.org/10.1109/ACCESS.2017.2657006.

[8] Perin Unal, Özlem Albayrak, Moez Jomâa, Arne J. Berre. "Data-Driven Artificial Intelligence and Predictive Analytics for the Maintenance of Industrial Machinery with Hybrid and Cognitive Digital Twins", in *Technologies and Applications for Big Data Value*, pp. 299–319. Springer, Cham, 2022.

[9] E.H. Glaessgen, D.S. Stargel, "The Digital Twin Paradigm for Future NASA and U. S. Air Force Vehicles", in *53rd AIAA/ASME/ASCE/AHS/ASC Structures, Structural Dynamics and Materials Conference*, 2012, p. 1818. https://doi.org/10.2514/6.2012-1818.

[10] Milisavljevic-Syed, J., Allen, J. K., Commuri, S., Mistree, F., Milisavljevic-Syed, J., Allen, J. K., ...& Mistree, F., "Architecting networked engineered systems", *Architecting Networked Engineered Systems: Manufacturing Systems Design for Industry*, 4 (2020): 185–257.

[11] Christos Pylianidis, Sjoukje Osinga, and Ioannis N. Athanasiadis, "Introducing Digital Twins to Agriculture", *Computers and Electronics in Agriculture* 184 (2021): 105942.

[12] S. Ornes, "Core Concept: The Internet of Things and the Explosion of Interconnectivity", *Proceedings of the National Academy of Sciences* 113, no. 40 (2016): 11059–11060. https://doi.org/10.1073/pnas.1613921113.

[13] D. Serpanos, M. Wolf, *Internet-of-Things (IoT) Systems*, Chapter 5, pp. 55–76. Springer, Cham. https://doi.org/10.1007/978-3-319-69715-4.

[14] Hugh Boyes, Bil Hallaq, Joe Cunningham, Tim Watson, "The Industrial Internet of Things (IIoT): An Analysis Framework", *Computers in Industry* 101 (2018): 1–12. https://doi.org/10.1016/j.compind.2018.04.015.

[15] J. Conway, "The Industrial Internet of Things: An Evolution to a Smart Manufacturing Enterprise", *Schneider Electric Whitepaper*, 2015, p. 2. https://www.se.com/ww/en/download/document/998-2095-10-16-15BR0_EN/

[16] Karl Aberer, Manfred Hauswirth, Ali Salehi, "Infrastructure for Data Processing in Large-Scale Interconnected Sensor Networks", *International Conference on Mobile Data Management*, Mannheim, Germany, pp. 198–205, 2007. https://doi.org/10.1109/MDM.2007.36.

[17] Neda Mohammadi, John E. Taylor, "Smart City Digital Twins", *IEEE Symposium Series on Computational Intelligence (SSCI)*, Honolulu, HI, pp. 1–5, 2017. https://doi.org/10.1109/SSCI.2017.8285439.

[18] Fabian Dembski, Uwe Wössner, Mike Letzgus, Michael Ruddat, Claudia Yamu, "Urban Digital Twins for Smart Cities and Citizens: The Case Study of Herrenberg, Germany", *Sustainability* 12 (2020): 2307. https://doi.org/10.3390/su12062307.

[19] Tuba Bakıcı, Esteve Almirall, Jonathan Wareham, "A Smart City Initiative: The Case of Barcelona". *Journal of the Knowledge Economy* 4 (2013): 135–148. https://doi.org/10.1007/s13132-012-0084-9.

[20] Abdulmotaleb El Saddik, University of Ottawa, "Digital Twins The Convergence of Multimedia Technologies". *IEEE MultiMedia* 25, no. 2 (2018): 87–92. https://doi.org/10.1109/MMUL.2018.023121167.

[21] Ying Liu, Lin Zhang, Yuan Yang, Longfei Zhou, Lei Ren, Fei Wang, Rong Liu, Zhibo Pang, M. Jamal Deen, "A Novel Cloud-Based Framework for the Elderly Healthcare Services Using Digital Twin", *IEEE Access* 7 (2019): 49088–49101. https://doi.org/10.1109/ACCESS.2019.2909828.

[22] "Information Technology Virtual Reality", *Engineering & Technology*, IET May 2016. https://journals.scholarsportal.info/browse/17509637/v11i0004.

[23] Koen Bruynseels, Filippo Santoni de Sio, Jeroen van den Hoven, "Digital Twins in Health Care: Ethical Implications of an Emerging Engineering Paradigm", *Frontiers in Genetics* 9 (2018): 31. https://doi.org/10.3389/fgene.2018.00031.

[24] J. Singh, D.J. Raghuram, "Evolution of Supply Chain Management with Emerging Technologies", *International Journal of Mechanical Engineering and Technology* 8, no. 1 (2017).

[25] Yuchen Wang, Xingzhi Wang, Ang Liu, "Digital Twin-driven Supply Chain Planning", *Procedia CIRP* 93 (2020): 198–203. https://doi.org/10.1016/j.procir.2020.04.154.

[26] Eduard Shevtshenko, Kashif Mahmood, Tatyana Karaulova, Ibrahim Oluwole Raji, "Multitier Digital Twin Approach for Agile Supply Chain Management", *Proceedings of the ASME 2020 International Mechanical Engineering Congress and Exposition.* Vol. 2B: Advanced Manufacturing. Virtual, Online. November 16–19, 2020. V02BT02A012. ASME. https://doi.org/10.1115/IMECE2020-23760.

[27] Maninder Jeet Kaur, Ved P. Mishra, Piyush Maheshwari, "The Convergence of Digital Twin, IoT, and Machine Learning: Transforming Data into Action", *Digital Twin Technologies and Smart Cities. Internet of Things.* Springer, Cham. https://doi.org/10.1007/978-3-030-18732-3_1.

[28] Manolya Atalay, Pelin Angin, "A Digital Twins Approach to Smart Grid Security Testing and Standardization", in *2020 IEEE International Workshop on Metrology for Industry 4.0 & IoT*, pp. 435–440. IEEE, 2020.

[29] C. Cimino, E. Negri, L. Fumagalli, "Review of Digital Twin Applications in Manufacturing", *Computers in Industry* 113 (2019): 103130.

[30] B.S. De Ugarte, A. Artiba, R. Pellerin, "Manufacturing Execution System—A Literature Review", *Production Planning & Control* 20 (2009): 525–539.

[31] Martin Kunath, Herwig Winkler, "Integrating the Digital Twin of the Manufacturing System into a Decision Support System for Improving the Order Management Process", *Procedia CIRP* 72 (2018): 225–231. https://doi.org/10.1016/j.procir.2018.03.192.

[32] Valentina Zaccaria, Mikael Stenfelt, Ioanna Aslanidou, Konstantinos G. Kyprianidis, "Fleet Monitoring and Diagnostics Framework Based on Digital Twin of Aero-Engines", *Proceedings of ASME Turbo Expo 2018 Turbomachinery Technical Conference and Exposition GT2018 June 11–15*, 2018, Oslo, Norway.

[33] Werner Kritzinger, Matthias Karner, Georg Traar, Jan Henjes, Wilfried Sihn, "Digital Twin in Manufacturing: A Categorical Literature Review and Classification", 2018, IFAC (International Federation of Automatic Control) Hosting by Elsevier Ltd.

[34] Qinglin Qi, Fei Tao, Ying Zuo, "Digital Twin Service towards Smart Manufacturing", *Procedia CIRP* 72 (2018): 237–242. https://doi.org/10.1016/j.procir.2018.03.103.

[35] Arne Bilberg, Ali Ahmad Malik, "Digital Twin Driven Human-Robot Collaborative Assembly", 2019 Published by Elsevier Ltd on behalf of CIRP.

[36] Ahmet Mert Karadeniz, İbrahim Arif, Alper Kanak, Salih Ergün, "Digital Twin of eGastronomic Things: A Case Study for Ice Cream Machines", *2019 IEEE.*

[37] Nodirbek Yusupbekov, Fakhritdin Abdurasulov, Farukh Adilov, Arsen Ivanyan, "Concepts and Methods of 'Digital Twins' Models Creation in Industrial Asset Performance Management Systems", in *International Conference on Intelligent and Fuzzy Systems*, pp. 1589–1595. Springer, Cham, 2020.

[38] Qingfei Min, Yangguang Lu, Zhiyong Liu, Chao Su, Bo Wang, "Machine Learning Based Digital Twin Framework for Production Optimization in Petrochemical Industry", *International Journal of Information Management* 49 (2019): 502–519.

[39] Pooja Jain, Neha R. Kasture, Tapan Kumar, "Comparative Study of Speaker Recognition Techniques in IoT Devices for Text Independent Negative Recognition", *Scalable Computing: Practice and Experience* 21, no. 3 (2020): 359–368.

[40] Aidan Fuller, Zhong Fan, Charles Day, "Digital Twin: Enabling Technologies, Challenges and Open Research", IEEE Access Date of Publication May 28, 2020, Date of Current Version June 23, 2020.

[41] Greyce N. Schroeder, Charles Steinmetz, Carlos E. Pereira, Danubia B. Espindola, "Digital Twin Data Modeling with Automation ML and a Communication Methodology for Data Exchange", 2016, IFAC (International Federation of Automatic Control).

[42] Benjamin Schleich, Nabil Anwer, Luc Mathieu, Sandro Wartzack, "Shaping the Digital Twin for Design and Production Engineering", *CIRP Annals* 66, no. 1 (2017): 141–144. https://doi.org/10.1016/j.cirp.2017.04.040.

[43] Roland Rosen, Georg von Wichert, George Lo, Kurt D. Bettenhausen, "About the Importance of Autonomy and Digital Twins for the Future of Manufacturing", 2015, IFAC (International Federation of Automatic Control).

[44] E. Bottani, A. Cammardella, T. Murino, "From the Cyber-Physical System to the Digital Twin: The Process Development for Behavior Modeling of a Cyber Guided Vehicle in M2M Logic", *ELETTRONICO* (2017): 96–102. https://air.unipr.it/handle/11381/2837020.

[45] Jiapeng Guo, Ning Zhao, Lin Sun, Saipeng Zhang, "Modular Based Flexible Digital Twin for Factory Design", *Journal of Ambient Intelligence and Humanized Computing* 10 (2019): 1189–1200. https://doi.org/10.1007/s12652-018-0953-6.

[46] Pankesh Patel, Muhammad Intizar Ali, Amit Sheth, "From Raw Data to Smart Manufacturing", *IEEE Intelligent Systems* 33 (2018): 79–86. https://doi.org/10.1109/MIS.2018.043741325.

[47] H. Thomas, J. Uhlemanna, Christian Lehmanna, Rolf Steinhilpera, "The Digital Twin: Realizing the Cyber-Physical Production System for Industry 4.0", *Procedia CIRP* 61 (2017): 335–340. https://doi.org/10.1016/j.procir.2016.11.152.

[48] Thomas Gabor, Lenz Belzner, Marie Kiermeier, Michael Till Beck, Alexander Neitz, "A Simulation-Based Architecture for Smart Cyber-Physical System", *2016 IEEE International Conference on Autonomic Computing (ICAC)*, pp. 374–379. Wuerzburg, Germany, 2016. https://doi.org/10.1109/ICAC.2016.29.

[49] Michael Abramovici, Jens Christian Göbel, Hoang Bao Dang, "Semantic Data Management for the Development and Continuous Reconfiguration of Smart Products and Systems", *CIRP Annals* 65, no. 1(2016): 185–188. https://doi.org/10.1016/j.cirp.2016.04.051.

[50] Industrial Engineering and Production Management By Martand T. Telsang, p. 253, 259. S Chand Publishing, 2018. ISBN 9789352533794.

[51] Jinsong Bao, Dongsheng Guo, Jie Li, Jie Zhang, "The Modelling and Operations for the Digital Twin in the Context of Manufacturing", *Article in Enterprise Information Systems*, October 2018.

[52] Yutong Wang, Yansong Cao, Fei-Yue Wang, "Anomaly Detection in Digital Twin Model", in *2021 IEEE 1st International Conference on Digital Twins and Parallel Intelligence (DTPI)*, pp. 208–211. IEEE, 2021.

[53] Zhansheng Liu, Anshan Zhang, Wensi Wang, "A Framework for an Indoor Safety Management System Based on Digital Twin", *Sensors* 20, no. 20 (2020): 5771.

[54] A. Barthels, F. Ruf, G. Walla, J. Fröschl, H.-U. Michel, U. Baumgarten, "A Model for Sequence-Based Power Management in Cyber-Physical Systems", in *Information and Communication on Technology for the Fight against Global Warming*, pp. 87–101. Springer, 2011.

[55] Seppo Sierla, Mohammad Azangoo, Kari Rainio, Nikolaos Papakonstantinou, Alexander Fay, Petri Honkamaa, Valeriy Vyatkin, "Roadmap to Semi-Automatic Generation of Digital Twins for Brownfield Process Plants", *Journal of Industrial Information Integration* 27 (2022): 100282.

[56] Kung-Jeng Wang, Ying-Hao Lee, Septianda Angelica, "Digital Twin Design for Real-Time Monitoring–A Case Study of Die Cutting Machine", *International Journal of Production Research* 59, no. 21 (2021): 6471–6485.

[57] Yi Caia, Binil Starlya, Paul Cohena, Yuan-Shin Lee, "Sensor Data and Information Fusion to Construct Digital-Twins Virtual Machine Tools for Cyber-Physical Manufacturing", *Procedia Manufacturing* 10 (2017): 1031–1042. https://doi.org/10.1016/j.promfg.2017.07.094.

[58] Joey Pinto, Pooja Jain, Tapan Kumar, "Fault Prediction for Distributed Computing Hadoop Clusters Using Real-Time Higher Order Differential Inputs to SVM: Zedacross", *International Journal of Information and Computer Security* 12, no. 2–3 (2020): 181–198.

[59] Joey Pinto, Pooja Jain, Tapan Kumar, "Hadoop Distributed Computing Clusters for Fault Prediction", in *2016 International Computer Science and Engineering Conference (ICSEC)*, pp. 1–6. IEEE, 2016.

[60] Qinglin Qi, Fei Tao, Senior Member, "Digital Twin and Big Data Towards Smart Manufacturing and Industry 4.0: 360 Degree Comparison", *IEEE Access* 6 (2018): 3585–3593. doi: 10.1109/ACCESS.2018.2793265.

# 2 Delineating the Healthcare 5.0

*Nancy Deborah R, Gobinath A, Soundarya M,
and Manjula Devi C*

## 2.1 INTRODUCTION TO HEALTHCARE 5.0

The healthcare environment has been characterized by an unwavering pursuit of development and innovation, an unending quest toward enhancing the well-being of individuals and communities. We've seen tremendous developments in healthcare paradigms throughout the years, each driven by technical improvements, increasing social requirements, and a desire to enhance patient outcomes. We have made amazing progress from the primitive days of Healthcare 1.0, typified by manual record-keeping and limited medical expertise, to the digital revolution of Healthcare 4.0, when data and connection grabbed center stage.

However, as we stand on the brink of a new era, it is evident that we are not simply entering another stage of healthcare evolution; we are on the verge of a shift of historic proportions. This change, appropriately dubbed Healthcare 5.0, is a vision for healthcare's future that goes beyond incremental growth. It is a paradigm change, a reinvention of the very core of healthcare delivery, and a dedication to attaining the greatest levels of care, equity, and patient empowerment.

We are at the crossroads of cutting-edge technology, patient-centric philosophies, and data-driven decision-making in Healthcare 5.0. It is a healthcare ecosystem that prioritizes the individual, allowing patients to play an active part in their own health and well-being. It uses artificial intelligence, blockchain, telemedicine, and the Internet of Things to improve diagnosis, treatment, and prevention. Healthcare is no longer isolated to clinical settings but has permeated our daily lives, effortlessly blending with our routines (Arrow, 1963).

This chapter outlines the Healthcare 5.0 paradigm, including the concepts that underpin it, the technology that power it has, the ethical concerns it presents, and the problems it must overcome. We will begin on an exploration of the outlines of this transformational vision, obtaining insights into how it will impact the healthcare sector in the coming years. As we explore deeper into Healthcare 5.0, we encourage you to join us in imagining a future in which healthcare transcends boundaries, embraces innovation, and, most importantly, emphasizes the well-being of everyone. Welcome to Healthcare 5.0, a vision for a healthier, more connected future.

## 2.2 KEY CHARACTERISTICS OF HEALTHCARE 5.0

Healthcare 5.0 is a considerable change from previous versions, expressing a new vision for healthcare delivery. This paradigm is distinguished by many fundamental features that influence its identity and possible impact on the healthcare ecosystem:

1. Patient-Centric Treatment:
   Patient Empowerment: In Healthcare 5.0, patients are active participants rather than passive receivers of treatment. They have access to personal health data, may monitor their status using wearable devices, and are encouraged to collaborate with healthcare experts in shared decision-making.

Individualization: Healthcare planning and treatments are increasingly personalized. Patients are given care that is tailored to their specific genetic makeup, medical history, and lifestyle choices. This personalization leads to better and more efficient healthcare results (Brouwer et al., 2008).

2. Advanced Technology Integration:

Artificial Intelligence (AI) and Machine Learning: AI algorithms analyze large datasets to help with early illness identification, treatment suggestions, and patient outcome prediction. Based on real-world patient data, machine learning models are constantly improved.

Internet of Things (IoT): IoT has facilitated the growth of wearable health gadgets such as smartwatches and fitness trackers that monitor vital signs, activity levels, and even detect possible health concerns.

Telemedicine solutions enable patients to communicate with healthcare practitioners remotely. This is especially important for patients in rural or isolated places, individuals with limited mobility, and during public health emergencies such as pandemics.

3. Data-Informed Decision-Making:

Big Data Analytics: Healthcare organizations use big data analytics to uncover patterns and trends in patient data. Early illness identification, proactive treatments, and more effective resource allocation can all result from this.

Health Informatics: EHRs and health informatics systems guarantee that patient data is not only gathered but also available for clinical decision-making. These solutions help to reduce medical mistakes and increase patient safety.

4. Interoperability and Ecosystem Connectivity: Healthcare 5.0 envisions a continuous flow of information across all stakeholders, from patients to healthcare providers to researchers. This connection fosters teamwork and a more comprehensive approach to healthcare. Interoperability standards guarantee that diverse healthcare systems, such as EHRs and telemedicine platforms, may connect safely and share patient data as necessary. This lowers duplication while increasing efficiency.

5. Ethical and Regulatory Issues:

Data Privacy and Security: Strict standards control the privacy and security of patient data, such as HIPAA in the United States and GDPR in the European Union. The necessity of retaining patient confidence through comprehensive data protection procedures is emphasized in Healthcare 5.0.

Responsible AI Use: Guidelines and laws are being established to address ethical issues about artificial intelligence in healthcare, such as algorithm bias, openness in AI decision-making, and responsibility in AI-driven diagnosis and treatments.

6. Holistic Health Approach:

Preventive and Predictive Care: Healthcare 5.0 moves the emphasis from sickness treatment to illness prevention. It uses predictive analytics to identify those who are at risk and then implements actions to reduce those risks.

Integration of Mental Health: Mental health is given same weight as physical health. Integrated care approaches acknowledge the interdependence of mental and physical health, resulting in more complete patient treatment.

Global Reach: Telemedicine, mobile health units, and remote monitoring technology expand healthcare services to underserved and rural places. This worldwide presence contributes to closing the healthcare access gap.

Health Equity: Healthcare 5.0 prioritizes the reduction of health inequities across various communities. Its main premise is to give fair access to excellent care while addressing socioeconomic determinants of health and fostering health equity.

Healthcare 5.0 is defined as a patient-centered, technologically sophisticated, data-driven, networked, ethical, holistic, and internationally inclusive healthcare paradigm by these qualities. In the next sections of this chapter, we will look at how these qualities are driving innovation, revolutionizing healthcare delivery, and determining the healthcare industry's future.

## 2.3  TECHNOLOGICAL ADVANCEMENTS IN HEALTHCARE 5.0

Healthcare 5.0 is characterized by its heavy dependence on cutting-edge technology, which play a critical role in transforming healthcare delivery, improving patient outcomes, and redefining the healthcare environment. The following are some of the significant technology developments that constitute Healthcare 5.0 (Cunningham, 2011):

1. The intersection of Machine Learning (ML) and Artificial Intelligence (AI):
   Diagnosis and Disease Prognosis: AI-powered algorithms can evaluate medical pictures like X-rays and MRIs with amazing precision. They can detect minor irregularities, assisting in the early detection of illnesses like as cancer and offering predictive insights into patient outcomes.
   Treatment Personalization: Machine learning algorithms can scan large patient datasets to create treatment recommendations based on genetic composition, medical history, and response to medicines. Because of this personalization, therapies are more successful and have fewer negative effects.
   Administrative Efficiency: AI-powered chatbots and virtual assistants automate administrative activities like appointment scheduling and billing, allowing healthcare providers to focus on patient care.
2. IoT with Wearable Devices:
   Continuous Monitoring: IoT devices, such as wearable fitness trackers, smartwatches, and medical sensors, provide real-time monitoring of vital signs, physical activity, and chronic disorders. This information is beneficial to both people and healthcare practitioners.
   Early Warning Systems: IoT-enabled devices may identify deviations from typical health parameters and send notifications, allowing for early intervention in medical crises or worsening health.
   Healthcare 5.0 encourages the use of IoT devices for remote patient monitoring, which is especially useful for controlling chronic diseases and delivering care to homebound or geographically distant patients.
3. Telemedicine and Virtual Care:
   Remote Consultations: Telemedicine systems enable patients and healthcare practitioners to have secure video consultations. This technology improves patient access to care, decreases travel time and expenses, and increases patient convenience.
   Electronic Health Records (EHRs): Telemedicine is connected with EHRs, allowing healthcare clinicians to view and update patient information during virtual visits, guaranteeing continuity of treatment.
   Telehealth applications: Patients may use mobile applications and platforms to book virtual visits, view medical information, and receive remote monitoring services, all of which contribute to a more patient-centric approach.
4. Blockchain Technology:
   Data Security and Privacy: Blockchain technology provides safe and tamper-proof patient data storage. Patients have control over who has access to their health information, which protects data privacy and reduces the danger of data breaches.

Interoperability: Blockchain can promote the secure and smooth interchange of health data among various healthcare providers and institutions.

Drug Traceability: In the pharmaceutical industry, blockchain assists in tracing the origin and distribution of medications, improving drug safety and transparency across the supply chain.

5. 3D Printing:

Customized Prosthetics and Implants: 3D printing technology allows for the fabrication of personalized prosthetic limbs, dental implants, and orthopedic devices, which improves patient comfort and functionality.

Medical Models and Surgical Planning: Surgeons may plan difficult procedures using 3D-printed models of patients' anatomy, lowering surgical risks and increasing precision.

Drug Manufacturing: 3D printing may be used in drug manufacturing to create individualized drugs with precise doses and formulas.

These technology advances are not independent innovations; rather, they are profoundly woven into the fabric of Healthcare 5.0. They improve diagnosis accuracy, empower healthcare practitioners, and contribute to a more efficient and effective healthcare system. We may expect many more breakthroughs and synergies among these technologies as Healthcare 5.0 evolves, ushering in a new era of healthcare excellence.

## 2.4  PATIENT-CENTERED CARE IN HEALTHCARE 5.0

Patient-centered care in Healthcare 5.0 is a paradigm shift that transforms the traditional healthcare practice. It includes a major shift in the power dynamic, with patients no longer being passive recipients but active co-pilots of their health journeys. Patients have unparalleled access to their entire medical records, diagnostic data, and a multitude of educational materials, and this empowerment begins with information openness. They are encouraged to actively participate in shared decision-making in order to ensure that their own values and preferences are incorporated into their care plans (Driver, 2014).

Personalization is central to this approach, with treatment options tailored to the person. AI and genomics enable healthcare providers to build personalized regimens that take into consideration a patient's genetic composition, medical history, lifestyle, and even cultural views. Patients with chronic diseases, for example, receive tailored care regimens that take into account their daily habits and preferences, boosting adherence and improved health results.

Personalization is taken to the next level using patient-generated health data (PGHD). This data, collected via wearable devices and mobile apps, gives real-time insights into a patient's health state, ranging from vital signs to sleep habits and activity levels. Healthcare practitioners can use PGHD for continuous monitoring, detecting irregularities quickly and responding when required. A patient suffering from congestive heart failure, for example, can be remotely monitored, allowing physicians to alter prescriptions or prescribe lifestyle modifications as needed to avoid consequences.

Digital health solutions promote communication between patients and healthcare providers by allowing patients to plan appointments, obtain medication refills, and securely communicate their care teams. Telemedicine platforms increase accessibility by overcoming geographical barriers and improving patient convenience. Furthermore, electronic health records (EHRs) allow a continuous flow of information across healthcare professionals, increasing continuity of treatment and lowering the risk of mistakes caused by fragmented data.

Care coordination is an essential component of Healthcare 5.0. Complex patients, especially those with chronic illnesses, sometimes need the knowledge of many experts and healthcare professionals. Interdisciplinary teams work closely together in this paradigm to treat all aspects of a patient's health, guaranteeing a holistic approach that includes physical, mental, and social well-being.

The dedication of this paradigm to the patient experience is demonstrated through active solicitation of patient input. Patients' feedback is solicited on a regular basis by healthcare organizations in order to enhance care quality and the overall healthcare experience. Furthermore, healthcare personnel are educated to provide compassionate treatment, realizing that emotional and psychological support are just as important as clinical brilliance.

In summation, patient-centered care is more than a phrase in Healthcare 5.0; it is a significant revolution that places patients at the center of healthcare. It claims to raise care quality, enhance health outcomes, and construct a truly patient-centered and enjoyable healthcare environment through empowerment, customization, PGHD, sophisticated communication technologies, EHRs, care coordination, and a persistent focus on the patient experience (Gursoy et al., 2022).

1. Patient Empowerment:

    Informed Decision-Making: Patients in Healthcare 5.0 are knowledgeable partners in their healthcare journey. They may view their medical data, test findings, and treatment alternatives. This transparency allows them to actively engage in health-related choices.

    Shared Decision-Making: When making medical decisions, healthcare professionals cooperate with patients, taking their preferences and values into consideration. This collaborative decision-making approach ensures that care is consistent with patients' goals and beliefs.

2. Personalization of Care:

    Tailored Treatment Plans: Healthcare 5.0 makes use of new technology such as artificial intelligence (AI) and genetics to produce highly individualized treatment plans. These programs take into account a patient's individual genetic makeup, medical history, lifestyle, and preferences. Cancer therapies, for example, can be tailored to target specific genetic abnormalities, boosting efficacy.

    Preventive Care: Personalization also applies to preventive care. Patients are given advice and actions that are personalized to their specific health risks and requirements, allowing them to manage their health more effectively and avoid the emergence of chronic illnesses.

3. Patient-Generated Health Data (PGHD):

    Wearable Technology: Wearable gadgets, such as fitness trackers and smartwatches, allow patients to collect continuous health data. These gadgets track vital signs, physical activity, and sleep patterns, giving significant information on one's daily health and well-being.

    Remote Monitoring: Using PGHD, healthcare practitioners may remotely monitor patients with chronic illnesses. This proactive method enables early intervention in the event of abnormalities or deteriorating health, lowering hospital readmissions and increasing outcomes.

4. Improved Communication and Engagement:

    Digital Health Tools: Patients may use digital health tools and applications to communicate with healthcare professionals, schedule appointments, refill prescriptions, and access educational materials. These resources promote self-care and health management.

    Telehealth and Virtual Care: Telemedicine systems allow patients to consult with healthcare providers without leaving their homes. This accessibility eliminates geographic obstacles, increases access to care, and boosts patient happiness.

5. Continuity of Care:

    Electronic Health Records (EHRs): EHRs consolidate patient information, ensuring that healthcare practitioners have access to the entire medical history of a patient. This enhances continuity of care and lowers the possibility of medical mistakes.

Care Coordination: Care is coordinated across multiple healthcare professionals, specialists, and even community services in Healthcare 5.0 to ensure that patients receive holistic care that addresses their physical, emotional, and social requirements.
6. Emphasis on the Patient Experience:
Patient input is actively sought by healthcare institutions in order to enhance the quality of service and the patient experience. Surveys of patient satisfaction and feedback channels enable providers to make data-driven improvements.
Compassionate Care: Healthcare workers are taught to offer compassionate care, focusing on patients' emotional and psychological well-being as well as clinical outcomes.

The transition to patient-centered care in Healthcare 5.0 is more than simply a philosophical idea; it represents a fundamental revolution in healthcare delivery. It recognizes that each patient is unique and that their beliefs, preferences, and life circumstances have a significant impact on their health and well-being. Healthcare 5.0 aspires to increase the quality of treatment, improve health outcomes, and eventually lead to a more enjoyable and effective healthcare experience for all persons by adopting patient-centered care (Joshua, 2017).

## 2.5   DATA-DRIVEN HEALTHCARE IN HEALTHCARE 5.0

The widespread use of data and sophisticated analytics is critical in Healthcare 5.0, revolutionizing the healthcare environment by optimizing treatment delivery, improving patient outcomes, and promoting proactive health management. Several significant aspects highlight the importance of data in this new paradigm:

1. Detailed Patient Information:
Electronic Health Records (EHRs): EHRs act as central data repositories for patients, storing information such as medical history, diagnosis, treatments, prescriptions, and more. They give complete insights about a patient's health to healthcare providers, allowing for better informed decision-making.
Wearable gadgets, Internet of Things sensors, and mobile health apps capture real-time data on vital signs, physical activity, and chronic disease management. This constant stream of data allows healthcare personnel to remotely monitor patients, spot abnormalities quickly, and intervene as required.
2. Predictive Analytics:
Detection of Early Disease: Data analytics algorithms sift through vast datasets to find minor trends and abnormalities. These algorithms can detect early warning signals of illnesses like diabetes or heart disease, allowing for earlier intervention and prevention.
Predictive analytics are used in Healthcare 5.0 to stratify patients based on their risk indicators for certain illnesses. Identifying those at increased risk of stroke or difficulties following surgery, for example, allows for targeted preventative actions.
3. Personalized Medicine: Data-driven healthcare tailors treatment regimens to an individual's genetic makeup, reaction to medicines, and lifestyle. This tailored strategy reduces adverse effects while increasing therapeutic efficacy and patient adherence.
Drug Administration: Advanced analytics aid in the optimization of drug regimes. Algorithms can discover pharmaceutical interactions, monitor adherence, and change doses by evaluating patient data, therefore enhancing medication safety and efficacy.
4. Resource Allocation and Efficiency:
Resource Management: Hospitals and healthcare systems optimize resource allocation using data analytics. Predictive modeling can estimate patient admissions, allowing hospitals to staff effectively and efficiently utilize resources.

Administrative Burden Reduction: Automation and data analytics improve administrative procedures by eliminating paperwork and increasing billing accuracy. This efficiency allows healthcare workers to focus on patient care.

5. Research and Innovation:

Drug research: Data analytics speeds up drug research by analyzing massive databases to identify prospective medication candidates and forecast their efficacy.

Clinical research is aided by real-world data and electronic health records, which provide insights into treatment results and patient groups that may be used to drive future studies.

6. Population Health Management:

Public Health Treatments: Data analytics helps public health authorities track disease outbreaks, identify hotspots, and plan targeted treatments like vaccination programs.

Chronic Disease Management: Data-driven population health initiatives target at-risk groups for chronic illnesses, using preventative measures and lifestyle interventions to minimize disease burden.

Security Measures for Data Security and Privacy: To protect patient data, Healthcare 5.0 emphasizes the significance of comprehensive data security methods such as encryption, access restrictions, and compliance with legal frameworks like as HIPAA and GDPR.

Ethical Considerations: Ethical considerations drive appropriate data usage, ensuring that patient privacy is protected and data is utilized for legitimate medical objectives.

In summary, data-driven healthcare is a cornerstone of Healthcare 5.0, utilizing data and analytics to improve patient care, streamline operations, drive innovation, and improve overall health outcomes. This data-driven strategy has the potential to transform healthcare by ushering in an era of precision medicine, preventative care, and increased healthcare system efficiency.

## 2.6 ETHICAL AND REGULATORY CONSIDERATIONS IN HEALTHCARE 5.0

Healthcare 5.0, with its data-driven, patient-centered, and technologically enhanced approach, introduces a slew of ethical and regulatory concerns that must be addressed in order to ensure responsible and fair healthcare delivery. Here are some crucial points to consider (Kuhn, 2012):

1. Data Privacy and Security:

Ethical Concern: Healthcare 5.0 is highly reliant on patient data collecting and analysis. The privacy and security of this data are the focus of ethical issues. Patients must have confidence that their sensitive health information is safe from breaches or abuse. Regulations such as the Health Insurance Portability and Accountability Act (HIPAA) in the United States and the General Data Protection Regulation (GDPR) in the European Union establish high requirements for data privacy and security. It is critical to follow these requirements.

2. Ethical questions with Responsible AI Use: The use of artificial intelligence (AI) and machine learning in diagnosis, treatment planning, and predictive analytics raises ethical questions about algorithm transparency, accountability, and bias mitigation.

Regulatory Oversight: Regulatory bodies must develop standards and procedures for the ethical use of artificial intelligence in healthcare. Transparency in AI decision-making and the elimination of algorithmic bias are significant areas of emphasis.

3. Informed Consent and Patient Autonomy:

Ethical Concern: Patients are expected to actively engage in decision-making regarding their care in Healthcare 5.0. This necessitates a thorough awareness of the therapy alternatives, risks, and rewards. It is critical to ensure that patients have the ability to offer informed consent.

Regulatory Standards: Before providing therapy or participating in research, healthcare practitioners must get informed permission from patients. These guidelines strive to respect patients' autonomy while also ensuring that they understand the consequences of their decisions.

While Healthcare 5.0 has the potential to enhance healthcare access and outcomes, ethical problems arise if some communities, particularly vulnerable or underprivileged ones, are excluded or disadvantaged in the adoption of new technologies.

Mitigation of Regulatory Risks: Regulatory frameworks should address healthcare inequities and encourage fair access to modern healthcare services. Initiatives to bridge the digital gap and guarantee that technological improvements benefit everybody may be included in policies.

5. Data Transparency:

Ethical Concern: Patients and the general public should have access to information about how their health data is gathered, processed, and shared. Transparency can undermine faith in healthcare systems.

Requirements for Regulation: Regulations should require clear notification about data usage and sharing procedures. Patients should be informed about how their data will be used and given the choice to opt in or out as needed.

6. Ethical AI in Research:

Ethical Concern: Artificial intelligence and big data are being employed in medical research. Transparency of data sources, informed permission in research, and data ownership are all ethical issues.

Regulatory Oversight: Regulatory organizations must guarantee that AI research follows ethical standards and rules. This involves gaining informed permission, safeguarding vulnerable groups, and preserving data integrity (Pareto, 2014).

Ethical Concern: Accountability and Liability Determining accountability and culpability in situations of negative results from AI or data-driven judgments can be difficult. It is critical to hold responsible parties accountable.

Regulatory Clarity: In circumstances involving AI and data-driven healthcare, regulatory organizations should provide clear criteria for accountability and liability. Defining duties for healthcare providers, technology developers, and data custodians is part of this.

Addressing these ethical and regulatory issues is critical to the success of Healthcare 5.0 deployment. To guarantee that Healthcare 5.0 stays ethical, egalitarian, and trustworthy in its pursuit of improved healthcare outcomes, it is critical to strike the correct balance between innovation and maintaining patient rights, privacy, and well-being (Reisman, 1998).

1. Concerns about Data Security and Privacy:

Breach of Personal Information: As the dependence on digital health records and patient data grows, so does the potential of data breaches and cyberattacks. The security of patient information is of the utmost importance.

Compliance with regulations: Meeting severe data privacy standards, such as GDPR and HIPAA, necessitates substantial resources and can be complicated, particularly when data is shared across borders.

2. Interoperability Problems:

Fragmented Systems: Healthcare frequently involves a plethora of systems and software platforms that may not always connect easily. True interoperability is a substantial technological problem.

Standardization: It is critical yet difficult to establish common data standards and interoperability protocols across varied healthcare systems and devices.

3. Ethical Difficulties:

Algorithm Bias: Addressing biases in AI algorithms used in diagnosis and therapy is an ethical need. It is difficult to provide equal care for all patients when algorithms may inherit biases from training data.

Informed Consent: Obtaining informed consent for data gathering and AI-driven decision-making can be difficult, especially when patients are unfamiliar with the consequences of new technologies.

4. Allocation of Resources:

Costs and Investments: Healthcare 5.0 technology implementation necessitates considerable financial expenditures in infrastructure, training, and continuous maintenance. Many healthcare systems, particularly those with limited resources, may struggle with these expenditures.

Healthcare personnel require training to successfully utilize and comprehend data-driven technology. It is a significant problem to ensure that the healthcare personnel are sufficiently equipped.

5. Regulatory Difficulties:

Regulatory Lag: Regulatory frameworks frequently lag behind technical advances, causing uncertainty and limiting adoption.

Permission Procedures: Obtaining regulatory permission for novel AI-powered medical equipment and therapies can be time-consuming and difficult.

6. Data Quality and Reliability:

Data Accuracy: Data quality and reliability might vary. It is a constant struggle to ensure that data utilized for diagnosis and treatment is correct and up-to-date.

Data Integrity: It is critical for the reliability of AI and data-driven healthcare systems to maintain data integrity throughout its lifespan, which includes data collection, storage, and transfer.

7. Change Resistance:

Cultural and Organizational Barriers: Implementing Healthcare 5.0 frequently necessitates cultural and organizational changes. Change resistance can stymie development within healthcare institutions and among healthcare practitioners.

Patient Adoption: Patients, particularly the elderly or those with limited access to digital resources, may be hesitant to embrace new technology.

Issues of Equity and Access: The digital divide makes it difficult to provide fair access to healthcare technology, particularly in underserved or distant places with inadequate Internet connectivity.

Healthcare Disparities: While the advantages of Healthcare 5.0 should be given evenly, there is a risk that new technologies could worsen healthcare disparities if they are not applied with caution.

9. Data Overload and Clinical Workflow: Information overload can overburden healthcare practitioners due to the rush of data from wearable devices, sensors, and electronic health records. It is difficult to integrate this data into clinical workflows in a meaningful way.

Physician Burnout: Managing data-intensive healthcare systems may contribute to physician burnout due to increased administrative strain.

Changing Regulations: Regulatory Uncertainty: Healthcare rules are constantly changing, leaving healthcare organizations and technology suppliers in the dark.

To address these obstacles and barriers, healthcare professionals, technology developers, regulatory agencies, lawmakers, and patients will need to work together. Furthermore, continued research and innovation are required to find solutions that address these challenges and assure the seamless transition to Healthcare 5.0 (Thomason, 2022).

## 2.7 CONCLUSIONS

Furthermore, the shift to Healthcare 5.0 marks a watershed point in the evolution of healthcare, with an emphasis on patient-centered treatment, modern technology, data-driven decision-making, and ethical concerns. While the promises of enhanced patient outcomes, treatment personalization, and healthcare efficiency are enticing, this change is not without its own set of complicated problems and roadblocks. Among the key hurdles are data security and privacy concerns, interoperability issues, ethical quandaries about AI and patient autonomy, resource allocation, legal complications, and the requirement of equal access to treatment. To overcome these obstacles, healthcare stake-holders, legislators, technology developers, and academics must work together.

Additionally, addressing data integration, navigating evolving regulations, managing data ownership and control, overcoming resistance to change, ensuring comprehensive training, fostering interdisciplinary collaboration, and maintaining data quality are critical aspects of the Healthcare 5.0 transition. Ethical issues like as reducing algorithmic bias and guaranteeing AI explainability, as well as the scalability and long-term sustainability of healthcare systems, add to the complexity of this shift.

Despite these obstacles, the attractiveness of Healthcare 5.0 resides in its ability to greatly improve patient care, personalize treatments, prevent disease, and optimize healthcare operations. It is critical to retain a firm commitment to patient well-being, ethical standards, and inclusion while negotiating these difficulties. By addressing these problems and limitations jointly, we may usher in a new era of healthcare that utilizes the benefits of cutting-edge technologies while adhering to the values of ethics, equity, and patient-centric care.

## REFERENCES

Arrow, K. J. (1963). Uncertainty and the Welfare Economics of Medical Care. *Am. Econ. Rev.*, 53(5), 941–973.

Brouwer, W. B. F.; Culyer, A. J.; van Exel, N. J. A.; Rutten, F. F. H. (2008). Welfarism vs. Extra-Welfarism. *J. Health Econ.*, 27(2), 325–328.

Cunningham, S. (2011). Understanding Market Failures in an Economic Development Context. *Mesopartner*, 1, 1–69.

Driver, J. (2014). The History of Utilitarianism. *Stanford Encyclopedia of Philosophy*, September 22.

Gursoy, D.; Malodia, S.; Dhir, A. (2022). The Metaverse in the Hospitality and Tourism Industry: An Overview of Current Trends and Future Research Directions. *J. Hosp. Mark. Manag.*, 31, 527–534.

Joshua, J. (2017). Information Bodies: Computational Anxiety in Neal Stephenson's Snow Crash. *Interdiscip. Lit. Stud.*, 19, 17–47.

Kuhn, T. S. (2012). *The Structure of Scientific Revolutions* (4th ed.). The University of Chicago Press.

Pareto, V. (2014). *Manual of Political Economy: A Critical and Variorum Edition*. Oxford University Press.

Reisman, D. A. (1998). Adam Smith on Market and State. *J. Institutional Theor. Econ. (JITE)*, 154(2), 357–383.

Thomason, J. (2022). Metaverse, Token Economies, and Non-Communicable Diseases. *Glob. Health J.*, 6, 164–167.

# 3 Virus Dispersion in Environment

## *Fuzzy Approach for Infectious Diseases*

*Dilip Kumar Jaiswal and Sudhakar Kumar Chaubey*

## 3.1 INTRODUCTION

Since the COVID-19 pandemic, rapid global progress has been in the healthcare system. With or without actual data, various modeling problems for infectious diseases have been resolved and predictions made. Numerous techniques may be employed to solve mathematical model due to the unpredictability of health recovery or disease infection. In solving of mathematical modeling problems, artificial intelligence (AI) has played an important role. There have been concerns raised about the influence of various AI technologies on societal and personal issues as a result of their widespread disruption. In order to assure ethics, openness, and accountability, AI must be used responsibly. As a result, responsible AI was developed. Fuzzy theory, followed by various fuzzy membership functions, is one part of AI. Analytical and fuzzy form solutions differentiate deterministic and indeterministic solutions. The advection-diffusion equation, which describes the virus concentration distribution pattern with space and time in the deterministic model, is of the parabolic type. Dispersion is what spreads viruses in the environment, and as a flow velocity, advection aids in the rapid spread of viruses. This equation can be used to describe analogous processes in a variety of fields, including chemical engineering, biophysics, petroleum engineering, and soil physics.

It is possible to write the following as a one-dimensional linear advection-diffusion equation:

$$\frac{\partial}{\partial t} C(x,t) = \frac{\partial}{\partial x}\left( D_x(x,t)\frac{\partial}{\partial x} C(x,t) \right) - \frac{\partial}{\partial x}\left( u_x(x,t)C(x,t) \right) \tag{3.1}$$

where, if $D_x(x,t)$ and $u_x(x,t)$ are constants then are called dispersion coefficient and uniform velocity of the medium, respectively. $C(x,t)$ is the dispersing virus concentration at a position $x$ at a time $t$ (Banks and Jerasate, 1962;Rumer, 1962; Lin, 1977; Al-Niami and Rushton, 1979; Kumar, 1983). Under various initial and boundary conditions including effects on dispersion due to adsorption, first order decay, and zero order production, a number of analytical solutions to the advection-diffusion partial differential equations with constant coefficients have been compiled (Lindstrom and Boersma, 1989). Some works related with this assumption worth to mention include those of Aral and Liao (1996), Kumar and Kumar (1997), Li et al. (2007), Jaiswal et al. (2009, 2011, 2012, 2020, 2022), Jaiswal and Gulrana (2019), and Kumar et al. (2010).

The indeterminate models can be separated into stochastic and fuzzy (artificial intelligence) models, among others, in accordance with the variations in uncertainty theory (Zielinski, 1988; Loucks and Lynn, 1996; Hercules et al., 2001; Holger et al., 2001; Mujumdar and Sasikumar, 2002; Xu and Yin, 2003; Wang and Wang, 2005). Fuzzy models can be successfully used when there is limited knowledge or data available for the model parameters and boundary conditions. Triangular fuzzy numbers (Cheng, 1999; Chen, 2000), trapezoidal fuzzy numbers (Hsieh and Chen, 1999), and other new types of fuzzy numbers have all been introduced recently. The parameters of the model were described as symmetrical triangular fuzzy numbers by Li et al. (2007), and a two-dimensional fuzzy water model for sudden viral concentration/solute discharge was developed. By using the $\alpha$-cut technique and arithmetic operations on triangular fuzzy numbers, it is possible to derive from the fuzzy model the concentrations corresponding to the chosen confidence level of $\alpha$.

Artificial intelligence (AI) is a type of fuzzy theory/logic, or a subset of AI. The improvement of analytics and prediction models, as well as the detection of diagnostic trends, anomalies, and outliers, is all often accomplished using artificial intelligence (AI). As a result, AI applications in healthcare include disease prediction, image segmentation, and classification (Saraswat et al., 2022; Verma et al., 2022). Explainable artificial intelligence (EXAI) does, however, play a significant role in the medical field. It's used in healthcare sensor bias reduction, segmentation, management of medical data, and clinical diagnosis (Shaban-Nejad et al., 2020). The EXAI model divides the explanation's scope into local and global methods. Whereas the local approach just needs an explanation of each individual prediction, the global approach demands an explanation of the entire model (Mohseni et al., 2018). A huge number of datasets with very distinctive characteristics are being produced globally for use in healthcare applications. The majority of healthcare-related data is multidimensional, making it difficult and complex to use traditional machine learning models like decision trees and random forests.

A unique end-to-end architecture for ECG-based healthcare was developed by Raza et al. (2022) using explainable artificial intelligence and deep convolutional neural networks (CNNs). However, the latest generation of machine learning models, particularly those based on deep learning, can handle issues connected to multi-dimensional data issues due to their capacity for self-learning (Georgiou et al., 2020). Deep learning has been crucial in the healthcare sector, for example, in the diagnosis of life-threatening disorders (Miotto et al., 2018). AI will play a significant role in the deployment of 6G networks and related applications. According to Wang et al. (2023), AI can be used in 6G in a variety of methods, including the traditional ones of prescriptive, predictive, diagnostic, and descriptive analytics. Shelmerdine et al. (2021) examined and emphasized the important facts required for study evaluating AI systems in healthcare. Standard Protocol Items: Recommendations for Interventional Trials-AI (study protocols), Consolidated Standards of Reporting Trials-AI (randomized controlled trials), Standards for Reporting of Diagnostic Accuracy Studies-AI, and Transparent Reporting of a Multivariable Prediction Model for Individual Prognosis or Diagnosis-AI (prediction model studies) are a few examples of the commonly used reporting guidelines that have included revisions and updates in the past. AI is also taken into consideration for health interventions in some guidelines.

Fuhrman et al. (2022) looked at many traits of explainable and interpretable AI in relation to the assessment of infectious disease COVID-19 sickness and how it can restore faith in AI applications to this disease. The report claims that doing so will make it easier for COVID-19 AI system developers to quickly understand the basics of a variety of explainable AI techniques and to choose an approach that is both appropriate and effective for a given situation. Jaiswal et al. (2023) have been obtained analytical and fuzzy solutions for temporally dependent dispersion along uniform flow velocity. In the current study, solutions for the space-dependent virus dispersion in a semi-infinite medium under uniform input source conditions are found analytically, and also fuzzy solution is obtained based on fuzzy theory. The model is used to simulate the virus concentration for infectious diseases based on the analytical and fuzziness of the system.

## 3.2  SPATIALLY DEPENDENT DISPERSION ALONG THE NON-UNIFORM FLOW

The expression for the one-dimensional linear advection-diffusion partial differential equation is defined above as,

$$\frac{\partial}{\partial t}C(x,t) = \frac{\partial}{\partial x}\left(D_0\xi_1(x,t)\frac{\partial}{\partial x}C(x,t)\right) - \frac{\partial}{\partial x}\left(u_0\xi_2(x,t)C(x,t)\right) \tag{3.2}$$

where $D_0$ and $u_0$ are constants whose dimensions will depend upon the expressions for $\xi_1(x,t)$ and $\xi_2(x,t)$, respectively. The results of the experiment showed that the dispersion coefficient depends on the position along the column. This dependence might be brought on by the medium's inhomogeneity (Yates, 1990, 1992).

## 3.2.1 DETERMINISTIC (ANALYTICAL) SOLUTION

In the current investigation, the dispersion coefficient is thought to be proportional to the square of the advection coefficient. If so, such a function may be expressed as (Kumar et al., 2010),

$$\xi_1(x,t) = (1+ax)^2 \quad \text{and} \quad \xi_2(x,t) = (1+ax) \tag{3.3}$$

Then in Eq. (3.2) constants $D_0$ and $u_0$ have the dimensions which are inverse of the dimension of $t$. The continuous input concentration is introduced at the domain's origin, and the concentration gradient at the infinity is assumed to be zero. Let the semi-infinite domain begin with a solute-free state, where the concentration of virus or infectious solute particles is zero; hence, the conditions will are:

$$C(x,t) = 0,\ x \geq 0;\ t = 0 \tag{3.4}$$

$$C(x,t) = C_0,\ x = 0;\ t > 0, \tag{3.5}$$

$$\frac{\partial C}{\partial x} = 0,\ x \rightarrow \infty;\ t \geq 0 \tag{3.6}$$

With the Laplace transformation approach, the analytical solution might be obtained as (van Genuchten and Alves, 1982; Kumar et al., 2010):

$$C(x,t) = \frac{C_0}{2}\left[(1+ax)^{-1}\text{erfc}\left\{\frac{\log(1+ax)}{2a\sqrt{D_0 t}} - \eta\sqrt{t}\right\} + (1+ax)^{\frac{u_0}{aD_0}}\text{erfc}\left\{\frac{\log(1+ax)}{2a\sqrt{D_0 t}} + \eta\sqrt{t}\right\}\right] \tag{3.7}$$

where $\omega_0 = (au_0 - a^2 D_0),\ \eta = \sqrt{\dfrac{\omega_0^2}{4a^2 D_0} + au_0} = \dfrac{u_0 + aD_0}{2\sqrt{D_0}}.$

## 3.2.2 INDETERMINISTIC (FUZZY) SOLUTION

### 3.2.2.1 Principles of Triangular Fuzzy Numbers

The fuzzy theory states that the fuzzy number can use the uncertainty feature. Fuzzy numbers can assume many different shapes, including triangular, multilateral, trapezoidal, and Gaussian membership functions. In this chapter, triangular fuzzy numbers will be employed. The combination of triangular fuzzy number can be described as $(r,s,t)$, which are lower, middle, and upper values of a fuzzy variable or matter respectively, with $r \leq s \leq t$. Suppose that $\tilde{A} = (r,s,t)$ its membership function and is defined as (Cheng, 1999; Hsieh and Chen, 1999):

$$\tilde{A} = \begin{cases} 0, & if \ x < r \\ \dfrac{x-r}{s-r}, & if \ r \leq x \leq s \\ \dfrac{t-x}{t-s}, & if \ s \leq x \leq t \\ 0, & if \ x > t \end{cases} \tag{3.8}$$

A membership function can be used to estimate a triangular fuzzy number using an interval value. A range of numbers can be used to represent different membership gradations or confidence levels. Suppose that $\mu_{\tilde{A}}(x) = 1$ corresponds to most possible value, and $\mu_{\tilde{A}}(x) = 0$ corresponds to the extrems, namely, the lower and upper values. We assume that all the triangular fuzzy integers are positive due to the nonnegative nature of virus infectious data.

### 3.2.2.2  α-Cut Technique

A fuzzy set is defined on the universal set $X$ and any number $\alpha \in [0,1]$, the α-cut, $\tilde{A}^\alpha$, is defined as:

$$\tilde{A}^\alpha = \left\{ x : \mu_{\tilde{A}}(x) \geq 0 \right\} \tag{3.9}$$

That is, the α-cut of a fuzzy set $\tilde{A}$ is the crisp set $\tilde{A}^\alpha$ that contains all the elements of the universal set $X$ whose membership grades in $\tilde{A}$ are greater than or equal to the specified value of α (Chen, 2000; Kwiesielewicz, 1998).

### 3.2.2.3  Fuzzy Expected Value

Let $\tilde{C} = C_1, C_2, C_3$ be triangular fuzzy number, then the expected value of $\tilde{C}$ can be denoted as (Hojati, 2004):

$$E(\tilde{C}) = \frac{C_1 + C_2 + C_3}{3} \tag{3.10}$$

### 3.2.2.4  Fuzzy Solution for Uniform Input Source

Let $u_0, D_0$ be triangular fuzzy numbers and using α-cut technique, we convert such triangular fuzzy parameters as follows, namely, $\tilde{u}_0 = [u_L^\alpha, u_U^\alpha]$, $\tilde{D}_0 = [D_L^\alpha, D_U^\alpha]$, where $\alpha \in [0,1]$. Substituting these, we get fuzzy virus concentration model is:

$$\tilde{C}(x,t) = \frac{C_0}{2} \left[ (1+ax)^{-1} \, \mathrm{erfc} \left\{ \frac{\log(1+ax)}{2a\sqrt{\tilde{D}_0 t}} - \eta\sqrt{t} \right\} + (1+ax)^{\frac{\tilde{u}_0}{a\tilde{D}_0}} \, \mathrm{erfc} \left\{ \frac{\log(1+ax)}{2a\sqrt{\tilde{D}_0 t}} + \eta\sqrt{t} \right\} \right] \tag{3.11}$$

$$\text{where} \ \ \omega_0 = (a\tilde{u}_0 - a^2\tilde{D}_0), \ \eta = \sqrt{\frac{\omega_0^2}{4a^2\tilde{D}_0} + a\tilde{u}_0} = \frac{\tilde{u}_0 + a\tilde{D}_0}{2\sqrt{\tilde{D}_0}}.$$

## 3.3  NUMERICAL EXAMPLE AND DISCUSSIONS

Deterministic (analytical) solution Eq. (3.7) with space dependent dispersion and flow velocity (Kumar et al., 2010) and indeterministic solution Eq. (3.11) of that assumption are discussed in the present study. Let's assume the triangular fuzzy numbers representing the flow velocity and dispersion coefficients as follows: $\tilde{u}_0 = [0.01, 0.03, 0.05]$, $\tilde{D}_0 = [0.06, 0.21, 0.36]$ with the membership functions correspond to above triangular fuzzy parameters. We considered three control points $(1.0)km$, $(5.0)km$ and $(10.0)km$ at $t = 4 \ day$. By using α-cut technique, we may get,

$\tilde{u}_0 = [0.01 + 0.02\alpha, 0.05 - 0.02\alpha]$ and $\tilde{D}_0 = [0.06 + 0.15\alpha, 0.36 - 0.15\alpha]$. For three points, we may get the corresponding virus concentrations, namely, $\tilde{C}^\alpha_{1.0}$, $\tilde{C}^\alpha_{5.0}$, and $\tilde{C}^\alpha_{10.0}$. The input are plotted for a set of data $C_0 = 1.0, D_0 = 0.21, u_0 = 0.03$ at times $t\ (day) = 1, 4, 7$ for deterministic solution. The virus concentration values are plotted up to $x = 10.0$ km. The inhomogeneity parameter $a$ is assigned a value 1.0 and 0.1.

Figure 3.1 depicts the virus concentration ($C$) distribution behavior of uniform input. It is clear from figure that the virus concentration started from one point at origin and decreases along space domain at different time $t\ (day) = 1, 4, 7$ and $a = 0.1$. For Figure 3.2, the same patterned show for $a = 0.1$ at different time $t\ (day) = 1, 4, 7$.

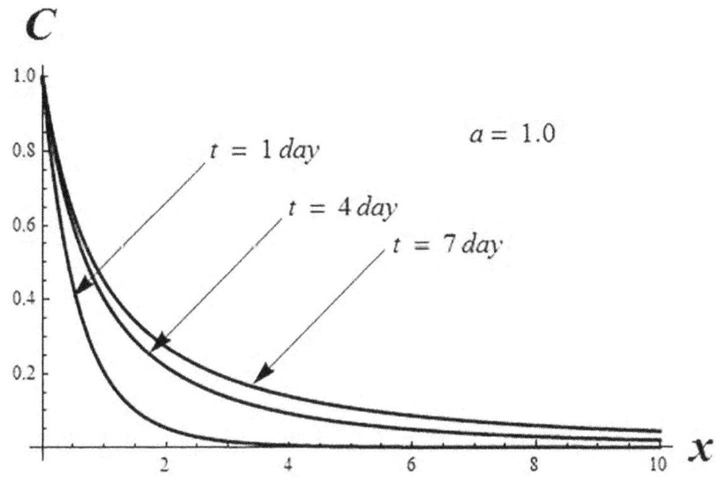


**FIGURE 3.1**    Distribution of virus concentration along position at various times $t(day) = 1, 4, 7$ with inhomogeneity parameter $a = 1.0$.

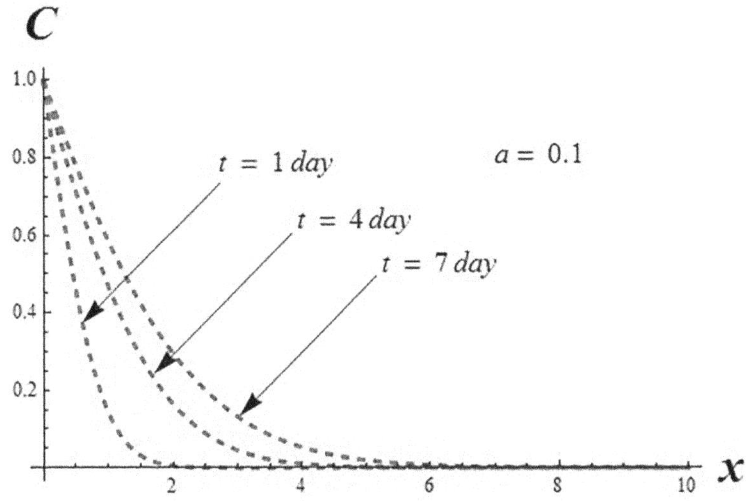


**FIGURE 3.2**    Distribution of virus concentration along position at various times $t(day) = 1, 4, 7$ with inhomogeneity parameter $a = 0.1$.

Figure 3.3 combined both the figures for visibility of inhomogeneity parameter at various time. The solid lines are show for $a = 1.0$ and dashed are show for $a = 0.1$. The inhomogeneity parameter $a$ is different for various species or various layers in environment.

For this situation, Figure 3.4 show pattern of inhomogeneity parameter $a = 0.3, 0.6, 0.9$ at one time $t\ (day) = 7$. In this figure, virus concentration distribution behavior decreases faster for higher inhomogeneity parameter than lower inhomogeneity parameter near to origin and converse farthest from origin.

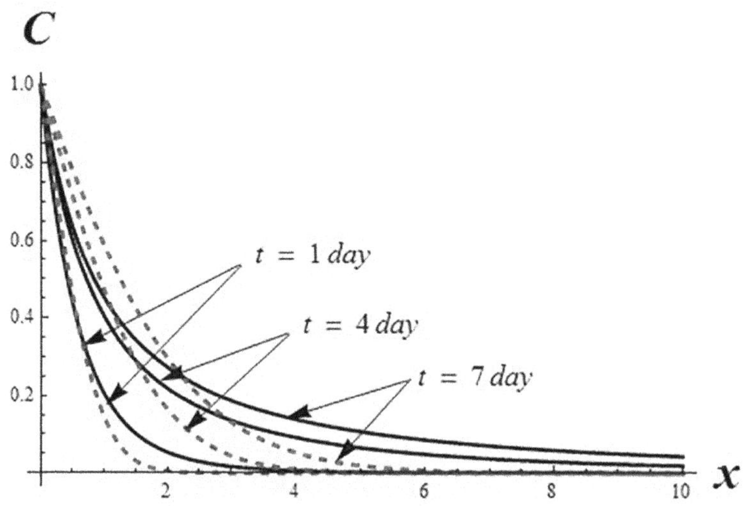


**FIGURE 3.3**   Comparison of virus concentrations along position at various times $t(day) = 1, 4, 7$ with inhomogeneity parameter $a = 1.0$ and $a = 0.1$.

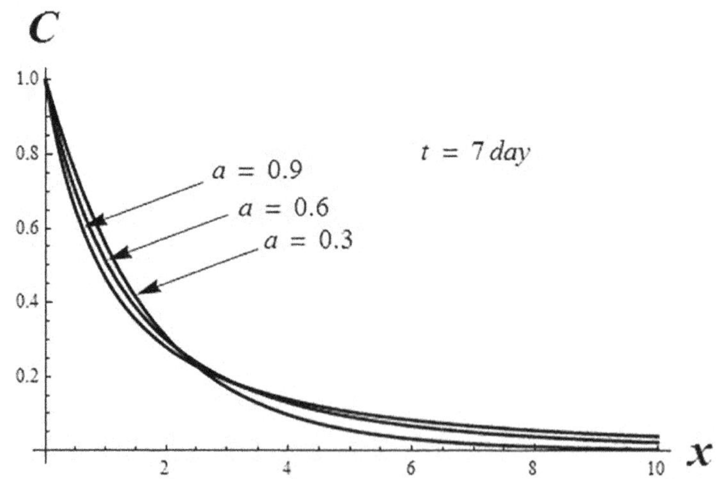


**FIGURE 3.4**   Distribution of virus concentration along position for various inhomogeneity parameter $a$ at one time $t = 7$.

The distribution of viral concentration for different positions over the time domain was shown in Figure 3.5. This demonstrates that the virus concentration at the point of genesis is quite high for a brief period of time and then declines as time passes. This situation was shown in the COVID-19 pandemic. Solutions Eq. (3.7) and Eq. (3.11) have the very close values for different set of velocity and dispersion coefficients, i.e., for lower and upper values of $u_0$ and $D_0$.

From the Table 3.1, at time $t = 4$ day, the values corresponding to $\alpha = 1$ are the most possible virus concentrations at each control point. Table 3.1 shows that when $\alpha$ goes to decrease, then the gap betweenlower and upper values of each triangular fuzzy virus concentration increases.

In actual circumstances, the virus concentrations for a species/environment drop along to space/position, that is, for away from the source of the virus. The definition of a triangular fuzzy parameter states that the maximum virus concentration is equivalent to the mean values for each parameter. In last two decades, a number of mathematical models have been put forth and examined analytically by Li et al. (2007), Jaiswal et al. (2020, 2022), and Kumar et al. (2010). The impact of global warming and environmental discharges has been studied with regard to the dynamics of carrier dependent diseases, and it has been demonstrated that the prevalence of carrier dependent diseases rises as either the temperature caused by global warming or the level of environmental discharges rises. Fuzzy and analytical solutions both have great advancement for the study of virus spreading in environment.

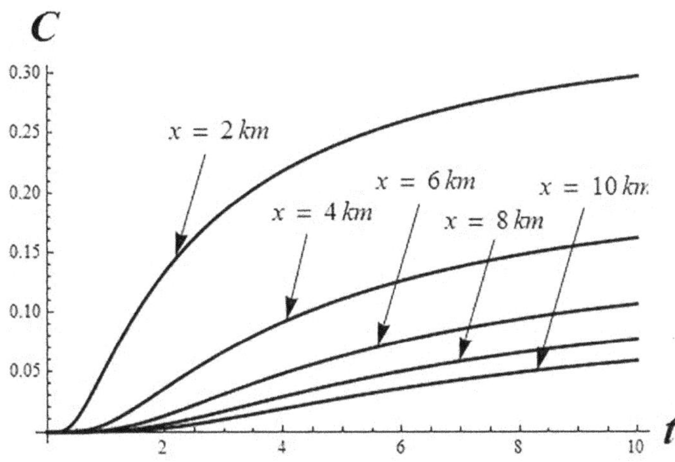


**FIGURE 3.5** Distribution of virus concentration along time at various positions $x(km) = 2,4,6,8,10$ with inhomogeneity parameter $a = 1.0$ .

**TABLE 3.1**

**For Different $\alpha$-Levels, the Interval (Lower and Upper) Values of Virus Concentrations**

| Control Point | (1.0) km | (5.0) km | (10.0) km |
|---|---|---|---|
| $\alpha = 1$ | 0.402379 | 0.06522 | 0.018895 |
| $\alpha = 0.95$ | 0.398565, 0.405978 | 0.0625223, 0.0678397 | 0.0176044, 0.0201825 |
| $\alpha = 0.90$ | 0.394516, 0.409379 | 0.0597461, 0.0703826 | 0.016314, 0.0214639 |
| $\alpha = 0.85$ | 0.390211, 0.412597 | 0.0568909, 0.0728501 | 0.0150277, 0.0227369 |
| $\alpha = 0.80$ | 0.385624, 0.415647 | 0.0539573, 0.0752439 | 0.0137499, 0.0239991 |
| $\alpha = 0.75$ | 0.385624, 0.418540 | 0.0509465, 0.0775656 | 0.0124856, 0.0252489 |

## 3.4 CONCLUSIONS

The current work investigated advection-dispersion equation (ADE) solutions that are deterministic (analytical) and indeterministic (fuzzy). Dispersion and advection both contribute to the spread of viruses within species and environments. In the COVID-19 pandemic, the virus concentration dispersed quickly from one species to another or in the environment. The number of casualties was therefore very high. For a semi-infinite inhomogeneous medium, the advection-dispersion equation is formulated analytically in one dimension. A fuzzy solution was also achieved by utilizing the triangle membership function principle and the α-cut approach. The virus transport equation's coefficients are based on spatially dependent functions where flow velocity is supposed to be directly proportional to dispersion. The validation of numerical solutions can benefit greatly from such solutions.

## REFERENCES

Al-Niami, A.N.S., Rushton, K.R., 1979. Dispersion in stratified porous media: Analytical solutions. *Water Resources Research* 15(5), 1044-1048.

Aral, M.M., Liao, B., 1996. Analytical solutions for two dimensional transport equation with time dependent dispersion coefficients. *Journal of Hydrologic Engineering ASCS* 1(1), 20-32.

Banks, R.B., Jerasate, S., 1962. Dispersion in unsteady porous media flow. *Journal of Hydraulics Division* 88(3), 1-21.

Chen, C.-T., 2000. Extensions of the TOPSIS for group decisionmaking under fuzzy environment. *Fuzzy Sets and Systems* 114(1), 1–9.

Cheng, C.-H., 1999. Evaluting weapon systems using ranking fuzzy numbers. *Fuzzy Sets and Systems* 107(1), 25–35.

Fuhrman, J.D., Gorre, N., Hu, Q., Li, H., El Naqa, I., Giger, M.L., 2022. A review of explainable and interpretable AI with applications in COVID-19 imaging. *Medical Physics* 49(1), 1–14.

Georgiou, T., Liu, Y., Chen, W., Lew, M., 2020. A survey of traditional and deep learning-based feature descriptors for high dimensional data in computer vision. *International Journal of Multimedia Information Retrieval* 9(3), 135–170.

Hercules, M., Petro, A., Jacques, G., 2001. Modelling of watr pollution in the Ther maios Gulf with fuzzy parameters. *Ecological Modelling* 142(1–2), 91–104.

Hojati, M., 2004. Bridging the gap between probabilistic and fuzzyparameter EOQ. *International Journal of Production Economics* 91(2), 215–221.

Holger, R.M., Tarek, S., Barbara, J.L., 2001. Forecasting cyanobacterium anabaenaspp. In the river Murray, South Australia, using Bspline nero-fuzzy models. *Ecological Modelling* 146(1–3), 85–96.

Hsieh, C.-H., Chen, S.-H., 1999. A model alogorithm of fuzzy product positioning. *Information Sciences* 121(1–2), 61–82.

Jaiswal, D.K., 2012. Temporally dependent solute dispersion in one-dimensional porous media. *ICMMSC 2012, CCIS* 283, 220–228.

Jaiswal, D.K., Dubey, A., Singh, V., Singh, P., 2023. Temporally dependent solute transport in one-dimensional porous medium: Analytical and fuzzy form solutions. *Mathematics in Engineering Science and Aerospace* 14(3), 711–719.

Jaiswal, D.K., Gulrana, 2019. Study of specially and temporally dependent adsorption coefficient in heterogeneous porous medium. *Application and Applied Mathematics: An International Journal (AMM)* 14(1), 485–496.

Jaiswal, D.K., Kumar, A., Kumar, N., 2020. Discussion on "Analytical solutions for advection- dispersion equations with time-dependent coefficients by Baoqing Deng, Fie Long, and Jing Gao, J. Hydrol. Eng. 2019, 24(8):06019006- 1-3", *Journal of Hydrologic Engineering (ASCE)* 24(8), 2020.

Jaiswal, D.K., Kumar, A., Kumar, N., Singh, M.K., 2011. Solute transport along temporally and spatial ly dependent flows through horizontal semi-infinite media: Dispersion being proportional to square of velocity. *Journal of Hydrologic Engineering (ASCE)* 16(3), 228–238.

Jaiswal, D.K., Kumar, A., Kumar, N., Yadav, R.R., 2009. Analytical solutions for temporally and spatially dependent solute dispersion of pulse type input concentration in one-dimensional semi- infinite media. *Journal of Hydro-environment Research* 2, 254–263.

Jaiswal, D.K., Kumar, N., Yadav, R.R., 2022. Analytical solution for transport of pollutant from time-dependent locations along groundwater. *Journal of Hydrology* 610, 127826.

Kumar, A., Jaiswal, D.K., Kumar, N., 2010. Analytical solutions to one-dimensional advection diffusion with variable coefficients in semi-infinite media. *Journal of Hydrology* 380(3–4), 330–337.

Kumar, N., 1983. Unsteady flow against dispersion in porous media. *Journal of Hydrology* 63, 345–356.

Kumar, N., Kumar, M., 1997. Solute dispersion along unsteady groundwater flow in a semi-infinite aquifer. *Hydrology and Earth System Sciences* 2(1), 93–100.

Kwiesielewicz, M., 1998. A note on the fuzzy extension of Saaty's priority theory [J]. *Fuzzy Sets and Systems* 95(2), 161–172.

Li, R.-Z., Shigeki, M., Hong, T.-Q., Qian, J.-Z., 2007. Fuzzy model for two-dimensional river water quality simulation under sudden pollutants discharged. *Journal of Hydrodynamics*19(4), 434–441.

Lin, S.H., 1977. Longitudinal dispersion in porous media with variable porosity. *Journal of Hydrology* 34, 13–19.

Lindstrom, F.T., Boersma, L., 1989. Analytical solutions for convective dispersive transport in confined aquifers with different initial and boundary conditions. *Water Resources Research* 25(2), 241–256.

Loucks, D.P., Lynn, W.R., 1996. Probabilistic models for prediction stream quality. *Water Resources Research* 32(3), 593–605.

Miotto, R., Wang, F., Wang, S., Jiang, X., Dudley, J.T., 2018. Deep learning for healthcare: Review, opportunities and challenges. *Briefings in Bioinformatics* 19(6), 1236–1246.

Mohseni, S., Zarei, N., Ragan, E.D., 2018. A multidisciplinary survey and framework for design and evaluation of explainable AI systems. *arXiv:1811.11839*.

Mujumdar, P.P., Sasikumar, K., 2002. A fuzzy risk approach for seasonal water quality management of a river system. *Water Resources Research* 38(1), 5–15.

Raza, A., Tran, K.P., Koehl, L., Li, S., 2022. Designing ECG monitoring healthcare system with federated transfer learning and explainable AI. *arXiv:2105.12497v2* [cs.LG].

Rumer, R.R., 1962. Longitudinal dispersion in steady and unsteady flow. *JournalHydraulics Division* 88(4), 147–172.

Saraswat, D., Bhattacharya, P., Verma, A., Prasad, K., Tanwar, S., Sharma, G., Bokoro, P.N., Sharma, R., 2022. Explainable AI for healthcare 5.0: Opportunities and challenges. *IEEE Access*. https://doi.org/10.1109/ACCESS.2022.3197671.

Shaban-Nejad, A., Michalowski, M., Buckeridge, D.L., 2020. Explainable AI in healthcare and medicine: Building a culture of transparency and accountability. *Proceedings AAAI International Workshop Health Intelligence (W3PHIAI)*, vol. 914. New York, NY: Springer. https://link.springer.com/book/10.1007/978-3-030-53352-6

Shelmerdine, S.C., Arthurs, O.J., Denniston, A., Sebire, N.J., 2021. Review of study reporting guidelines for clinical studies using artificial intelligence in healthcare. *BMJ Health Care Inform*, 28, e100385.

van Genuchten, M.T., Alves, W.J., 1982. Analytical solutions of the one dimensional convective-disper sive solute transport equation. *Technical Bulletin*, No. 1661. US Department of Agriculture.

Verma, A., Bhattacharya, P., Patel, Y., Shah, K., Tanwar, S., Khan, B., 2022. Data localization and privacy-preserving healthcare for big data applications. *Architecture and Future Directions, Emerging Technologies for Computing, Communication and Smart Cities*, 233–244.

Wang, C., Wang, P.-F., 2005. Model of calculating water quantity needed to di lute and purify pollutants in river network and its applications. *Journal of Hydrodynamics Series B* 17(4), 418 428.

Wang, S., Qureshi, M.A., Miralles-Pechuan, L., Huynh-The, T., Gadekallu, T.R., Liyanage, M., 2023. Applications of explainable AI for 6G: Technical aspects, use cases, and research challenges. *arXiv:2112.04698v2* [cs.NI].

Xu, Z.-X., Yin, H.-L., 2003. Development of two-dimensional hydrodynamics and water quailty model for Huangpu River. *Journal of Hydrodynamics, Series B* 15(2), 1–11.

Yates, S.R., 1990. An analytical solution for one—dimensional transport in heterogeneous porous media. *Water Resources Research* 26(10), 2331-2338.

Yates, S.R., 1992. An analytical solution for one—dimensional transport in porous media with an exponential dispersion function. *Water Resources Research* 28(8), 2149-2154.

Zielinski, A.P., 1988. Stochastic dissolved oxygen model. *Journal of Environmental Enginering* 114(1), 74–90.

# 4 Revolutionizing COVID-19 Diagnosis

## *A Hybrid Quantum Neural Network-Based Framework for Accurate Detection of Lung Abnormalities from CT Scans Using Custom Computer Vision Model and AI Edge Device*

*Senthilkumar Vijayakumar*

## Introduction

The timely identification of diseases is crucial not only for expeditious medical intervention, but also for the isolation of patients, efficient monitoring, containment measures, and an effective public health response. X-ray imaging is widely employed as a prevalent diagnostic modality for COVID-19, yet its efficacy in detecting the many phases of pulmonary engagement is deemed unreliable. Consequently, health experts from the World Health Organization (WHO) have advised placing primary reliance on clinical and chest CT findings for the purpose of detecting the different phases of lung involvement and ascertaining the suitable treatment protocols. Radiologists are currently facing significant challenges because to the unique characteristics of COVID-19. They are under immense pressure to minimize both false negatives and false positives in their diagnostic process. Additionally, there is a pressing need to streamline their workload by providing accurate diagnosis within shorter timeframes. Nevertheless, government officials face a challenge in implementing patient isolation and transmission control measures at diagnostic and healthcare centers, emergency rooms, and hospitals, mostly due to the significant population density in these facilities. During a pandemic epidemic, diagnostic centers can serve as a potential vector for the transmission of infectious diseases. The aforementioned statement highlights the driving force for the creation of a unique Transfer Learning for Computer Vision model. This model is specifically designed to train hybrid quantum neural network (QNN) models, with the aim of detecting and classifying novel COVID-19 at different stages. The utilization of transfer learning in Computer Vision models is employed to support radiologists in real-time analysis of CT images, consequently augmenting the accuracy and efficiency of COVID-19 diagnosis.

This research introduces a unique framework for the diagnosis of COVID-19, utilizing transfer learning and hybrid QNNs. Transfer learning is a technique that effectively decreases the training time of deep learning models for image analysis tasks by using pre-trained models and transferring knowledge to new tasks. This approach yields enhanced accuracy and precision in



DOI: 10.1201/9781003442066-4

the resulting models. The incorporation of hybrid QNNs into the training procedure not only expedites the training process but also enhances the precision of the models. This paper suggests the incorporation of hardware and software accelerators onto AI edge devices integrated with CT scanners. This integration aims to enhance the speed of inferencing, presenting a potential solution for creating an effective diagnostic tool that aids radiologists in diagnosing mild to severe cases. This study employs research approaches that enable swift analysis and categorization of lung lesions linked with COVID-19 at different stages, potentially alleviating the impact of COVID-19-related lung disease. The aforementioned technology has promising capabilities in enhancing the efficiency and precision of many stages involved in the detection and diagnosis of COVID-19, thereby leading to a transformative impact on the field of lung disease diagnosis and therapy. The aforementioned technology possesses the capacity to significantly transform COVID-19 diagnostics and enhance patient outcomes through expedited identification and intervention.

The necessity for precise and timely identification of COVID-19 through lung CT scans has stimulated the creation of an innovative methodology that employs transfer learning for computer vision and a hybrid QNN for model training. The utilization of classical layers facilitates the effective transfer of features to the deepest layers of the hybrid QNN, leading to enhanced model accuracy via the implementation of transfer learning techniques. The application of this method has promise in assisting radiologists and analysts in efficiently and precisely identifying different phases of COVID-19 biomarkers in real time within a CT scanning, facilitating accurate identification of the disease across its multiple stages. The system framework that has been suggested has three primary subsystems. (1) The collection and organization of CT scan data pertains to lung conditions of varying severity in the medical field. (2) This study presents a training framework that demonstrates the process of transfer learning in computer vision for the purpose of detecting COVID-19. The focus is on utilizing a hybrid QNN model to identify noticeable ground-glass opacity lesions and crazy-paving patterns in the peripheral and posterior lungs, as observed in chest CT scan pictures. (3) The implementation and live inference of the model on an AI Edge device, which can be seamlessly linked with a CT scanner, offers assistance to radiologists in diagnosing different levels of lung involvement in COVID-19 cases.

## 4.1  MOTIVATION AND SOLUTION OVERVIEW

AI and data science computational techniques, from hardware to software to systems, become more sophisticated as data grows and complexity, yet traditional computing is linear by design, particularly in deep learning. This is because of the following requirements:

### 4.1.1  MODEL TRAINING PIPELINE

Building an efficient COVID-19 detection model training pipeline that is scalable and can learn high-dimensional features from multiple lung CT scans datasets is the first obstacle to overcome. Therefore, a hybrid accelerated training pipeline is formed by combining pre-trained computer vision model architecture with scalable quantum layers in order to attain improved model accuracies without initially training the network from scratch (Killoran et al., 2008; Mari et al., 2020).

### 4.1.2  LESSER TRAINING TIME

Amid a pandemic of considerable scale, there exists a pressing imperative to expeditiously construct computer vision models at an unparalleled pace. These models play a crucial role in aiding radiologists in the prompt and precise identification of lung anomalies associated with COVID-19 at different stages. In order to efficiently manage the extensive quantity of lung CT scans, it is imperative to employ sophisticated artificial intelligence models that possess the capability to swiftly process and interpret numerous images with optimal efficacy. The utilization of a transfer learning pipeline on quantum circuits is a powerful technique that can significantly contribute to the attainment of this goal. By harnessing the computational capabilities of concurrent calculations at the hardware level, the pipeline has the potential to greatly enhance processing capacity, resulting in a substantial reduction in training time. This, in turn, can contribute to the creation of very sophisticated benchmark models.

Moreover, the utilization of hybrid QNN models, which possess the capability to effectively incorporate dense features into deep layers, renders them exceptionally proficient for competitive implementations in the identification of COVID-19. The integration of sophisticated technologies has the potential to significantly aid radiologists in delivering prompt and efficient interventions for individuals exhibiting lung abnormalities associated with COVID-19 (Houssein et al., 2022).

### 4.1.3   Real-Time Inferencing for Real-World Deployments

The utilization of a quantum hardware transfer learning model for the detection of different stages of anomalies in COVID-19 will be implemented on an AI edge device that is embedded into a CT scanner. This methodology empowers radiologists to efficiently and accurately render diagnoses, as the AI edge gadget possesses the capability to analyze CT images in real time, hence facilitating prompt delivery of outcomes. The utilization of embedded artificial intelligence (AI) technology exhibits the capability to identify and analyze various patterns, including ground glass opacities (GGO), the crazy-paving pattern (GGO with superimposed inter- and intralobular septal thickening), and consolidation. This ability to accurately detect such patterns plays a crucial role in diagnosing lung abnormalities associated with COVID-19.

Furthermore, the implementation of the AI edge devices on the CT scanner enables a more efficient diagnostic procedure, as it eliminates the requirement for distinct processing and interpretation of CT scans. The implementation of this technology has the potential to substantially alleviate the burden on radiologists and other healthcare practitioners, allowing them to allocate their attention toward other essential facets of patient care. The integration of CT scanning and AI edge technology has the potential to better patient outcomes and optimize the efficiency of medical services (Vijayakumar et al., 2023).

## 4.2   SYSTEM DESIGN AND FRAMEWORK

The system design and framework are shown in Figure 4.1, it comprises three major subsystems: (1) medical mild to severe lung CT scan data collection and orchestration, (2) design and development of transfer learning framework, and (3) deployment and real-time inferencing on AI edge device.

### 4.2.1   Medical Mild to Severe Lung CT Scan Data Collection and Orchestration

COVID-19 patients undergo multiple pulmonary CT scans to provide reliable radiological dynamic pattern data, and from the point of symptoms and before recovery from COVID-19 pneumonia, four stages of lung involvement CT scans are recorded. Typically, mild COVID-19 pneumonia (1) begins as small subpleural, unilateral, or bilateral GGOs most predominantly in the lower lobes, (2) which then progresses into the crazy-paving pattern and (3) subsequent consolidation. (4) After more than two weeks, lesions are slowly replaced by residual GGOs and subpleural parenchymal bands. Since COVID-19 is a novel virus pandemic and data is very limited, we collected these four-stage CT scan images and biomarkers from open-source, research journals, and publications (Bernheim et al., 2019; Chung et al., 2019) related to COVID-19 chest CT scan images for Computer Vision model training.

## 4.2.2 DESIGN AND DEVELOPMENT OF TRANSFER LEARNING FRAMEWORK

### A. Motivation for Transfer Learning

Conventional learning methods are limited to training models on specific tasks, datasets, and isolated models that lack the ability to transfer knowledge from one model to another. Transfer learning, on the other hand, allows for the utilization of pre-trained weights from an already trained model, which has been exposed to numerous images of various classes and has undergone training for several days, to predict new classes. Transfer learning is beneficial in cases where there is less data for the new task, reduces training time, and improves the performance of the model for image classification. The objective of this chapter is to showcase the efficacy of transfer learning through the adaptation of established image classifiers, namely, VGG, ResNet, and Faster RCNN Inception-V3. The focus is on utilizing these classifiers to identify abnormalities in lung scans, specifically early-stage subpleural, unilateral, or bilateral ground-glass opacities (GGOs) primarily located in the lower lobes. Furthermore, the classifiers are employed to detect the progression of these abnormalities into the severe "crazy-paving" pattern observed in CT scans of patients diagnosed with COVID-19 (Ng et al., 2019; Palmer, 2019; Pan et al., 2019).

### B. Data Collection and Augmentation

The initial stage of each classification task involves data preparation. In the case of COVID-19, data is limited in open source with biomarkers indicating various stage abnormalities in lungs, on conspicuous ground-glass opacity lesions (mild) and crazy-paving pattern (severe). Therefore, data augmentation techniques need to utilized, and we collected CT scan images and biomarkers from open-source databases, research journals, and publications related to COVID-19 CT scan images for use in transfer learning (Amin et al., 2022).

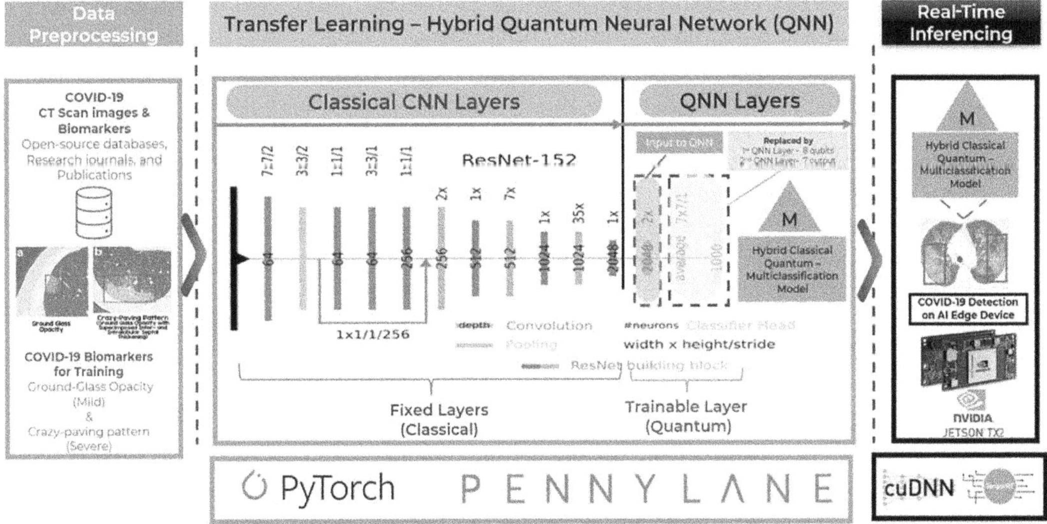


FIGURE 4.1 System design and framework for transfer learning computer vision modeling on hybrid quantum neural network (QNN) for COVID-19 biomarker detection.

In deep learning, data augmentation is a popular technique to increase the dataset's size and enhance the model's generalizability. This technique involves transforming the original data by rotating, flipping, cropping, stretching, or applying lens correction. To implement this technique, the open-source neural-network library Keras provides the ImageDataGenerator() class, which can be customized to perform several transformations on the dataset. Once the data is generated, it is important to adjust the data values to the intended network range values, which is done by setting the Keras.applications.inception V3 preprocess_input module's parameter. The next step is to customize the parameters for rotation, shifting, shearing, zooming, and flipping transformations. This process results in a variety of examples, which helps the deep learning model to learn from a diverse set of data. As a result, the model's accuracy, precision, and robustness are improved, making it suitable for various testing conditions during inferencing.

**C.  Data Preparation for Transfer Learning**

   i.  *train_images:* Images that are in DICOM format will be used to train the model. In this folder, the annotated classes (Normal/ COVID-19 CT scan images) and the actual bounding boxes coordinates for every class is placed.
   ii.  *test_images:* Images in this folder are used to predict with the trained model. The classes and bounding boxes for those classes are absent in this collection to calculate the loss and accuracy during cross validation.
   iii.  *train.csv:* An XML file contains the annotated label data that will be generated for each image and stored in train and test folders, respectively. Later the XML file will be converted to a CSV file that contains the annotated information like name, class, and the bounding box coordinates for each image.

**D.  Custom Transfer Learning of Hybrid Quantum Neural Network (QNN) in the Detection of Various Stages of COVID-19**

VGG, ResNet, and Faster RCNN Inception-V3 are prominent convolutional neural network (CNN) architectures that have been extensively pre-trained on the large-scale ImageNet dataset, comprising over a million images, for generic image classification tasks. The models' depth, reaching 48 layers, allows them to capture complex features in images and classify them into one of 1000 object categories, such as animals, people, flowers, computers, and pens. As a result, these models have developed a high-level understanding of the visual world and can generalize well to novel images through transfer learning. In this research paper, the performance of VGG, ResNet, and Faster RCNN Inception-V3 CNN architectures will be evaluated and compared to identify the best-performing model for classifying various stages of COVID-19 in CT scan DICOM format images (Jing et al., 2022).

Due to the limited size of the dataset consisting of CT scan images and biomarkers related to various stages of COVID-19, obtained from open-source databases, research journals, and publications, the use of pre-trained deep neural network models is essential. However, the similarity between this dataset and the well-known ImageNet dataset is quite low, which renders direct application of a pre-trained model on this dataset ineffective. In this context, transfer learning can be employed to leverage the pre-trained model's learned features for a different but related task. In particular, the initial layers (let's assume k) of the pre-trained model can be frozen, and only the remaining (n-k) layers can be fine-tuned with respect to the new dataset. The idea behind freezing the initial layers is to avoid losing the generic features that the pre-trained model has learned, which can be useful for the new task. By fine-tuning the top layers according to the new data collection, the model can be optimized to recognize specific features and patterns present in the COVID-19 related CT scan images in DICOM format and biomarkers. This way, the resulting model can achieve better performance despite the limited size and low similarity of the dataset, since the initial layers' weights are preserved and adapted to the new dataset.

i. *Preparing the Pre-Trained Model:* Deep neural network models, namely, VGG, ResNet, and Faster RCNN, which were pre-trained on the ImageNet dataset for generic tasks, were utilized in this chapter to perform image classification on a new dataset. To accomplish transfer learning, only the final layer, specifically the FC-layer, was modified, and was retrained with a quantum simulator. The training dataset utilized in this study consisted of lung abnormalities, such as conspicuous ground-glass opacity lesions (mild) and crazy-paving pattern (severe). This resulted in a specific task of multiclass image classification that the resulting model (M) can perform with high accuracy.

ii. *Retrain:* Hyperparameters of quantum layer (last layer): In this study, CNN layers running on PyTorch framework are employed as a feature extractor to extract features from CT scan images related to COVID-19. These features are then passed to dense layers that are trained using the COVID-19 CT scan image dataset. The hyperparameters of the last CNN layer, i.e., the FC-layer, are trained using a quantum simulator with a new dataset. To achieve this, all hyperparameters of the previous CNN layers remain unchanged, and only the FC-layer (trainable layer) is updated to accommodate the replacement of the quantum 8 qubit and 7 output layers, respectively, for multiclass classification bounding box output, to detect Normal and various stages of COVID-19 abnormalities in lung, such as conspicuous ground-glass opacity lesions (mild) and crazy-paving pattern (severe). The weights are preserved without any changes, and the focus of the network is shifted toward learning the specific features in the new dataset in subsequent quantum layers.

   The quantum component of the model is based on the variational quantum circuit designed on PennyLane, is an open-source software framework for quantum machine learning (QML). Training an end-to-end hybrid QNN from scratch on a noisy intermediate-scale quantum (NISQ) device is not an effective approach. Instead, quantum layers are used in conjunction with classical layers to enhance the learnable contextual parameters and spatial correlations, thereby accelerating the training process. The classical layers assist in learning and transferring features efficiently to the deepest layers of the hybrid QNN, resulting in increased model accuracy through transfer learning (Bergholm et al., 2018).

iii. *Freeze the weights of the first few layers:* During this phase, the weights of the initial layers of the Faster RCNN Inception-V3 network are kept frozen, and only the subsequent layers are retrained. This is due to the fact that the first few layers typically capture fundamental features that are applicable to new specific problems, such as curves and edges. Therefore, these weights are preserved while the network is trained to focus on learning the specific features in the new COVID-19 dataset using subsequent quantum 8 qubit and 7 output layers. Once the layers are trained, the checkpoint with the highest accuracy and lowest loss obtained during the training process is used to generate the frozen inference graph in the form of a .pt file.

**TABLE 4.1**
**Model Performance Metrices**

| Pretrained CNN Architecture | Training Time (Mins) | | Validation Loss (%) | | Validation Accuracy (%) | | Inferencing Rate on AI Edge Device (fps) |
| --- | --- | --- | --- | --- | --- | --- | --- |
| | Classical CNN | Hybrid QNN | Classical CNN | Hybrid QNN | Classical CNN | Hybrid QNN | |
| VGG16 | 160 | 110 | 19.25 | 14.7 | 80.75 | 85.3 | 0.06 |
| VGG16BN | 160 | 120 | 16.75 | 12 | 83.25 | 88 | 0.07 |
| ResNet50 | 175 | 135 | 10.25 | 5.5 | 89.75 | 94.5 | 0.040 |
| ResNet152 | 210 | 140 | 7.25 | 4.15 | 92.75 | 95.85 | 0.030 |
| Faster RCNN Inception-V3 | 225 | 150 | 6.25 | 2.18 | 93.75 | 97.82 | 0.037 |

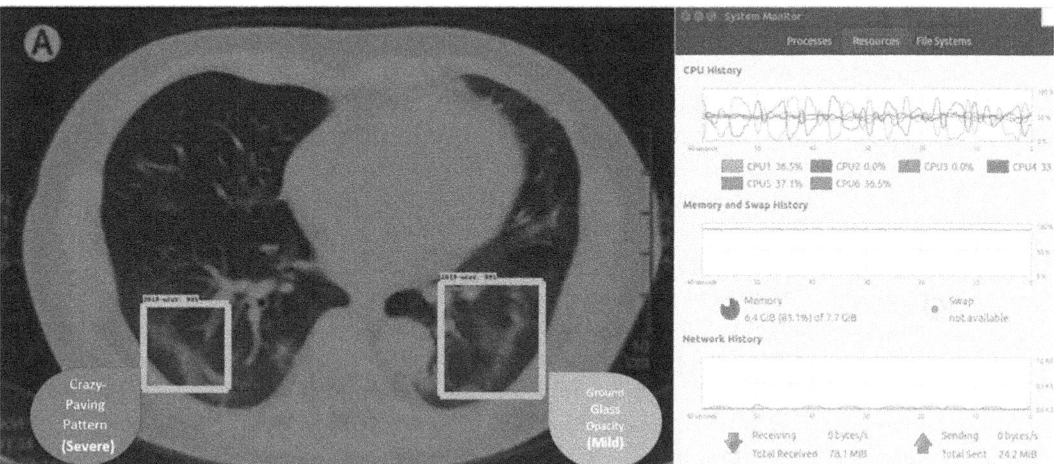


**FIGURE 4.2**   COVID-19 mild and severe biomarker detection model trained on transfer learning with hybrid QNN layers and real-time model inferencing on AI edge device (NVIDIA Jetson TX2).

### 4.2.3   DEPLOYMENT AND REAL-TIME INFERENCING ON AI EDGE DEVICE

Transfer learning with various CNN architectures like VGG16, VGG16 with Batch Normalization, ResNet50, ResNet152, and Faster RCNN Inception-V3 with the last layer replaced by a two-layered QNN was performed and the results obtained are tabulated in Table 4.1.

The research paper utilizes a transfer learning framework with hybrid QNN for detecting scan various stages of COVID-19 abnormalities in lung on CT, such as conspicuous ground-glass opacity lesions (mild) and crazy-paving pattern (severe) The utilization of Faster R-CNN Inception-V3 in the proposed approach enables rapid and accurate object detection in images with significantly reduced training time compared to classical CNN architecture. In addition, this approach outperforms Faster RCNN Inception-V3 with Hybrid QNN benchmarks in terms of accuracy and reduced training time. The presented results show that the model outperforms classical CNN architecture benchmarks for training on conventional computer systems and has 98% (Faster RCNN Inception-V3 with Hybrid QNN) bounding box accuracy in detecting lung abnormalities, such as conspicuous ground-glass opacity lesions (mild) and crazy-paving pattern (severe) on CT scan with inferencing rate of 0.037 fps on AI edge device shown in Table 4.1, making it suitable for production deployments to inference lung CT scan images in DICOM format and video formats in real-time onboard CT scanners.

## 4.3  CONCLUSION

The research presented in this chapter introduces innovative methodologies in the fields of medical imaging, quantum computing, and artificial intelligence. These methodologies were utilized to develop a model that has the ability to detect different phases of COVID-19 anomalies in the lungs. Furthermore, the model incorporates real-time biomarker inference on AI edge devices. Figure 4.2 demonstrates the effective implementation of the model on an AI edge device, namely, the NVIDIA Jetson TX2. This achievement represents a notable advancement in the timely identification of COVID-19 associated lung irregularities using biomarker detection. The model demonstrated improved efficiency and accuracy in identifying biomarkers associated with different phases of COVID-19 with the implementation of a transfer learning architecture incorporating hybrid QNN layers. Furthermore, the model achieved high inferencing rates when integrated into the CT scanner due to the utilization of NVIDIA's software (CUDA, CuDNN, Jetpack, TensorRT) and hardware (NVIDIA Jetson TX2- Pascal™-family GPU) accelerators. These accomplishments underscore the capacity of AI, quantum, and edge computing to revolutionize medical diagnosis and improve patient outcomes.

"AI could help identify early onset of COVID-19 on chest CT, particularly in health care settings without access to many radiologists," according to Eric Stern, MD, chair of the ACR DSI Thoracic Panel. "Such an AI solution may prove to be a very useful application towards COVID-19 diagnosis and containment," he said (Stern et al., 2022).

The combination of transfer learning and hybrid QNNs in conjunction with the implementation of AI edge technology on CT scanners presents a new comprehensive framework for the precise and effective detection of lung anomalies associated with COVID-19. The suggested methodology effectively decreases the duration necessary for training deep learning models, resulting in enhanced accuracy and precision of the resultant models. The AI edge gadget integrated into the CT scanner exhibits a notable capability to identify and analyze patterns with a remarkable level of precision, hence playing a crucial role in the accurate diagnosis of COVID-19. The implementation of this technology has the potential to optimize the diagnostic procedure, alleviate the burden on healthcare practitioners, and ultimately enhance patient outcomes. The findings highlight the potential of AI technology in transforming the landscape of lung disease diagnosis and treatment, inspiring future research in this area.

## REFERENCES

Amin, Javaria, Muhammad Sharif, Nadia Gul, et al. Quantum Machine Learning Architecture for COVID-19 Classification Based on Synthetic Data Generation Using Conditional Adversarial Neural Network (2022). https://doi.org/10.1007%2Fs12559-021-09926-6

Bergholm, Ville, Josh Izaac, Maria Schuld, et al. PennyLane: Automatic Differentiation of Hybrid Quantum-Classical Computations, 2018. https://arxiv.org/abs/1811.04968

Bernheim, Adam, Xueyan Mei, Mingqian Huang, et al. Chest CT Findings in Coronavirus Disease-19 (COVID-19): Relationship to Duration of Infection. https://pubs.rsna.org/doi/10.1148/radiol.2020200463

Chung, Michael, Adam Bernheim, Xueyan Mei, et al. CT Imaging Features of 2019 Novel Coronavirus (2019-nCoV). https://pubs.rsna.org/doi/full/10.1148/radiol.2020200230

Houssein, Essam H., Zainab Abohashima, Mohamed Elhoseny, et al. Hybrid Quantum-Classical Convolutional Neural Network Model for COVID-19 Prediction Using Chest X-Ray Images. *Journal of Computational Design and Engineering* 9(2), 343–363 (2022). https://doi.org/10.1093/jcde/qwac003

Jing, Yu, Xiaogang Li, Yang Yang, et al. RGB Image Classification with Quantum Convolutional Ansatz (2022). https://arxiv.org/abs/2107.11099

Killoran, Nathan, Thomas R. Bromley, Juan Miguel Arrazola, et al. Continuous-Variable Quantum Neural Networks. https://arxiv.org/pdf/1806.06871.pdf

Mari, Andrea, Thomas R. Bromley, Josh Izaac, et al. Transfer Learning in Hybrid Classical-Quantum Neural Networks. *Quantum* 4, 340 (2020). https://arxiv.org/abs/1912.08278

Ng, Ming-Yen, Elaine Y. P. Lee, Jin Yang, et al. Imaging Profile of the COVID-19 Infection: Radiologic Findings and Literature Review (2019). https://pubs.rsna.org/doi/full/10.1148/ryct.2020200034

Palmer, Whitney J. Chest CT Findings Reflect Time of Coronavirus 19 (COVID-19) Disease Course (2019). https://www.diagnosticimaging.com/ct/chest-ct-findings-reflect-time-coronavirus-19-covid-19-disease-course

Pan, Feng, Tianhe Ye, Peng Sun et al. Time Course of Lung Changes on Chest CT During Recovery from 2019 Novel Coronavirus (COVID-19) Pneumonia (2019). https://pubs.rsna.org/doi/10.1148/radiol.2020200370

Stern, Eric J., Adam Bernheim, Michael Chung. ACR DSI Publishes AI Use Case on COVID-19. https://www.acr.org/Advocacy-and-Economics/Advocacy-News/Advocacy-News-Issues/In-the-March-14-2020-Issue/ACR-DSI-Publishes-AI-Use-Case-on-COVID-19

Vijayakumar, S., et al. A Hybrid QNN-Based Framework for Accurate Early Detection of HCV Liver Abnormalities from CT Scans Using Custom Transfer Learning and AI Edge Device (2023), IEEE Region 10 Symposium (TENSYMP). https://ieeexplore.ieee.org/abstract/document/10223624

# 5 The Role of Explainable AI for Healthcare 5.0
## Best Practices, Challenges, and Opportunities

*Srija Chattopadhyay, Subhadeep Barman, and Lakshmi D*

## 5.1 INTRODUCTION

In recent years, the need for transparency and accountability in AI decision-making has increased as AI has become increasingly common in many industries. This need is met through XAI approaches that provide insight into the inner workings of an AI model, including how it processes incoming data, generates predictions, and makes decisions. Some XAI techniques use visualization tools like decision trees or heatmaps to show how the AI model works for humans. Other methods include AI models that are inherently easier to understand, such as decision rule-based systems or training models for less complex and more readable data representations. In critical sectors such as healthcare, finance, and autonomous cars, where transparency and accountability are essential for the safety and well-being of users, the importance of XAI is particularly evident. Healthcare 5.0 can be developed and implemented using XAI. It is important to ensure that healthcare systems are open, reliable, and trustworthy as they increasingly rely on AI-based technology to diagnose and treat patients. The need for interpretability and explainability is one of the biggest obstacles to the adoption of artificial intelligence in the healthcare sector. Patients, doctors, and regulators need to understand the decision-making process and the criteria considered in an AI system. This is crucial for critical applications such as medical diagnosis or treatment planning, as the stakes are high, and mistakes can have catastrophic consequences. Integrating cutting-edge technologies such as artificial intelligence (AI), Internet of Things (IoT), big data analytics, blockchain and 5G, next-generation healthcare systems to enhance efficiency, improve patient outcomes, and revolutionize the healthcare landscape. It is also known as Healthcare 5.0. The patient-centered Healthcare 5.0 paradigm is characterized by a greater focus on preventive healthcare and personalized medicine. Leveraging data from multiple sources, such as wearables, electronic health records, and social media, is key to understanding patient health and delivering proactive, personalized care. XAI can provide the necessary transparency and explainability to help build trust in AI-based healthcare systems. XAI techniques can be used to visualize and explain how an AI model processes patient data and makes decisions, allowing clinicians to better understand and interpret results. This can help clinics diagnose and treat patients more effectively and increase patients' trust in the healthcare system. XAI can also help identify biases in AI systems that can lead to discriminatory results. By providing a transparent and interpretable view of how an AI model works, XAI enables stakeholders to identify and address distortions in data or algorithms.

To achieve reliable analysis in healthcare operations, XAI has been implemented in several clinical decision models. It is used for segmentation, classification, and management of medical data, clinical diagnosis, and reduction of bias in health sensors (Shaban-Nejad et al., 2020). The XAI model divides the explanation into local and global methods. While the local approach requires clarification of each prediction, the global approach requires clarification of the entire model (Mohseni et al., 2018).

### 5.1.1 REVIEW OF LITERATURE

XAI has witnessed substantial growth and exploration, fostering a deeper understanding of the significance, challenges, and strategies involved in making machine learning models interpretable. Ribeiro et al. (2016a) introduced a pivotal contribution by delineating a comprehensive taxonomy of interpretability methods tailored to the diverse nature of the interpretability concept, stressing that the appropriateness of different methods varies across tasks and scenarios (Ribeiro et al., 2016b). Building upon this foundation, Molnar (2019) offered a panoramic view of the expansive XAI landscape, elucidating the rapid progression of the field and the multifarious techniques available for rendering AI models more transparent and interpretable (Molnar, 2019). Guidotti et al. (2020) undertook a comprehensive survey of the state-of-the-art in XAI, emphasizing its potential to bolster trust and transparency in AI systems, thereby catalyzing the development of more reliable and ethically responsible AI (Guidotti et al., 2020).

In the context of human-computer collaboration, Singh and Ribeiro (2020) highlighted how explainability serves as a crucial bridge, facilitating human understanding, trust-building, and effective interaction with AI systems (Singh & Ribeiro, 2020). Adadi and Berrada (2018) proposed a systematic framework to guide the design and evaluation of XAI systems, offering a structured approach to ensuring the efficacy of explanations in enhancing user comprehension and decision-making (Adadi & Berrada, 2018). Montavon et al. (2018a) provided further validation of the rapid proliferation of techniques in the XAI domain, reinforcing the notion that the field is witnessing significant advancements and attracting considerable attention due to its potential to make AI systems more transparent and accountable (Montavon et al., 2018a). Lipton (2018) added a pragmatic dimension to the discourse by suggesting that while the quest for perfectly comprehensive explanations may be elusive, the focus should be on generating explanations that are "good enough" to be useful for humans with varying levels of expertise (Lipton, 2018). To underscore the complexity of the challenge, Molnar (2017) surveyed the intricacies of interpretability in machine learning, revealing the manifold dimensions of the problem, ranging from algorithmic transparency to the understandability of complex models (Molnar, 2017). Collectively, these seminal works collectively shape the narrative around XAI, illuminating its central role in fostering transparency, accountability, and collaboration between humans and AI systems.

## 5.2 RATIONALE OF THE STUDY

This chapter provides an overview of the XAI design process and the XAI analysis methodology. This chapter also aims to provide insights into the types of XAIs, XAI use cases, mechanisms of action, disease management and decision-making processes, case studies, comparisons, challenges, and future directions. The overview of the chapter is shown in Figure 5.1.

*CI = computational intelligence

## 5.3 TYPES OF XAI

XAI refers to artificial intelligence that can provide meaningful and meaningful explanations for their decisions and actions. There are several ways and means of working in XAI.

The major three types of XAI are shown in Figure 5.2.

Here are some of the prominent types:

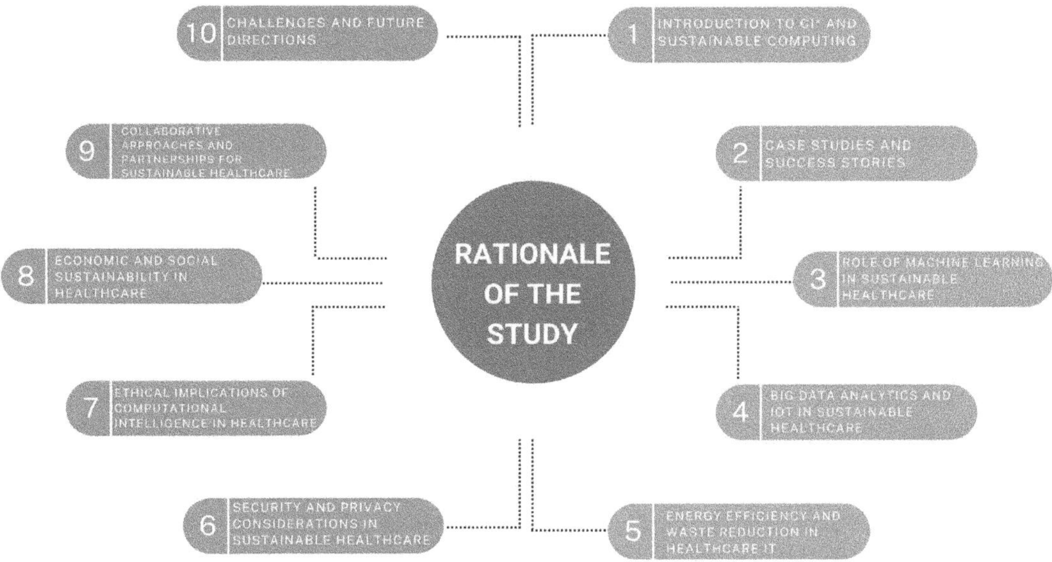


**FIGURE 5.1**    Rationale of the study.

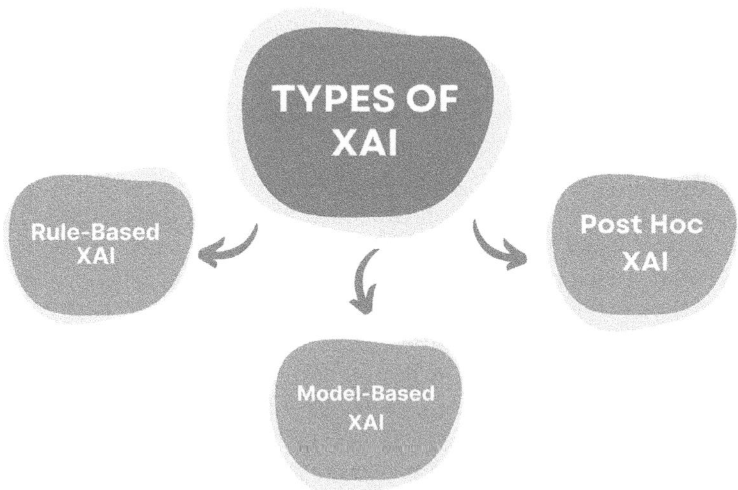


**FIGURE 5.2**    Types of XAI.

## 1.  Rule-Based XAI

Rule-based interpretation is particularly useful in areas where clarity and interpretation are needed. In the expert system for medical research, the rule-based approach offers several distinct advantages. The main advantage is the traceability of decisions. As the system follows predetermined rules, each decision can be further linked to a specific situational characteristic. This transparency is extremely valuable for physicians who not only need to rely on AI recommendations but also need to understand the theory behind. Furthermore, the potential of rule-based modeling human-readable descriptions unite AI with medical experts. Health professionals can examine the legality and rationale of the policy and provide feedback. This iterative process allows codes to be refined and improved over time, resulting in more accurate and reliable diagnostic tools. A rule-based approach to complex clinical situations enables the incorporation of domain expertise. Medical knowledge can be translated into explicit codes, taking into account the implicit relationships between symptoms, conditions, and medical history. This ensures that the AI system is consistent with established medical policies and guidelines, increases system credibility among healthcare professionals and, furthermore, transparency of code-based interpretations for patients understanding and participation. When patients experience a disease with a clear explanation based on recognizable symptoms, they are more likely to believe in the diagnosis and adhere to the recommended treatment. This empowerment of patients through meaningful explanation is helpful improve health outcomes.

However, it's essential to acknowledge the limitations of rule-based models. They might struggle with handling uncertainties, exceptions, or complex interactions among symptoms. Some medical conditions could present with atypical combinations of symptoms, which might not be adequately covered by predefined rules. As a result, the rule-based system might not provide accurate diagnoses in every case. In conclusion, the rule-based approach to generating explanations in expert systems, especially for medical diagnosis, strikes a balance between transparency, interpretability, and domain expertise. By leveraging explicit rules and logical statements, these systems offer medical professionals and patients alike the opportunity to comprehend and trust the decision-making process of AI. While challenges exist, the collaboration between AI and human experts can refine these rule-based models, making them valuable tools in the medical field.

## 2. Model-Based XAI

Model-based explanations bridge the gap between the accuracy of complex AI models and the need for transparency and interpretability, especially in critical areas such as medical imaging. It involves neural networks benefits

The accuracy of deep veins in disease classification in clinical imaging has changed the diagnostic approach. But the "black box" nature of these networks in which decisions are made using complex combinations of factors learned from large amounts of data raises concerns about reliability and traceability of results. The approach describing complex AI decisions requires trade-offs between accuracy intervals and definitions in a simplified model building process. Methods such as decision trees, linear regression, or simple neural network architecture aim to simulate the behavior of complex underlying models. In medical imaging, these simplified models serve as a road map tangible and imaginative how AI can reach conclusions. Each decision node in the decision tree corresponds to an image feature, and the path through the tree identifies the various factors that contribute to the final diagnosis This method allows physicians to validate that AI's diagnosis, and any errors or biases are detected. If the description of the decision tree indicates that a particular region or part of the image has a significant effect on AI detection, physicians should investigate this with their expertise to ensure that the interpretation is consistent with known medical practice.

Model-based explanations also facilitate collaboration between AI and medical experts. These explanations provide a common basis for thinking about the reasoning behind AI decisions. As the practitioner gains insight into how his AI model predicts, it can provide valuable information that improves the overall accuracy and relevance of the AI system, but it is important to understand as a description-based model, it does not capture the connection patterns of all complex tissues. Simplifying an inherently complex model can result in some loss of detail and accuracy, and some nuances learned from the deep web may not be adequately represented in the simplified version therefore need to find an appropriate balance between robustness and accuracy to develop and define these models -based specification. In summary, model-based explanations provide a valuable perspective for clarifying and understanding AI-driven medical research. These techniques allow physicians to gain confidence, acceptance, and efficiency in their AI systems through simplified models that reflect complex decision-making neural networks, which ultimately drive patients better care and better outcomes.

## 3. Post Hoc XAI

Post hoc annotation represents an important step forward in addressing the annotation challenges posed by complex AI models, especially in areas such as healthcare where the obvious statistics are paramount and the core of the presentations lies in their retrospective nature—reflecting the "black box" decisions of AI models delivering their results. Next, feature-importance methods such as LIME and SHAP are key features of ad hoc translation methods. These approaches seek to shed light on the decision-making process by quantifying the contribution of individual factors or inputs to the sample output. This analysis helps to identify factors that play an important role in AI model decision-making, and elucidate the logic behind forecasting. By perturbing the input data and monitoring the resulting changes in the predictions, LIME gains insight into feature importance. This "model-agnostic" approach ensures that the semantic approach can be applied to any AI model, regardless of its architecture, without requiring knowledge of the model's inner workings while SHAP extends the concept of essential features about to capture connections and dependencies between objects. It draws inspiration from collaborative game theory, where the contribution of each aspect to the final prediction is evaluated by considering all possible combinations of factors. This holistic approach provides comprehensive understanding on how factors together influence the output of an AI model.

In the context of medical applications, post hoc explanations offer tremendous value. Imagine a scenario where a deep learning model diagnoses diseases from medical images. While the model's accuracy might be impressive, medical professionals rightfully demand insight into the rationale behind each diagnosis. Post hoc explanations can provide a breakdown of which image characteristics—like shapes, textures, or structures—contributed to the model's decision. This empowers medical experts to validate the model's predictions, correct any potential biases, and potentially identify novel insights for medical research. Additionally, post hoc explanations encourage collaboration between AI experts and domain specialists. When medical professionals can see the specific features that influenced an AI diagnosis, they can provide domain-specific insights and verify the clinical relevance of the AI's conclusions. This collaboration enriches the overall decision-making process and leads to more accurate and reliable diagnoses. However, it's important to recognize that post hoc explanations have their limitations. While they provide valuable insights into feature importance, they might not fully capture the intricate internal representations of deep neural networks. Furthermore, the explanations they provide are localized, focusing on specific instances, which may not generalize to the entire model's behavior.

In conclusion, post hoc explanations serve as a critical tool for enhancing the interpretability of AI models in medical applications. By retrospectively analyzing model decisions and quantifying feature importance, these techniques bridge the gap between complex AI outputs and human understanding. This transparency not only fosters trust but also encourages collaboration and refinement in the pursuit of accurate and responsible healthcare AI.

### 5.3.1 METHODS

XAI encompasses various methods and techniques designed to make the decision-making process of artificial intelligence models more transparent and understandable to humans. Here are some key methods in the field of XAI shown in Figure 5.3:

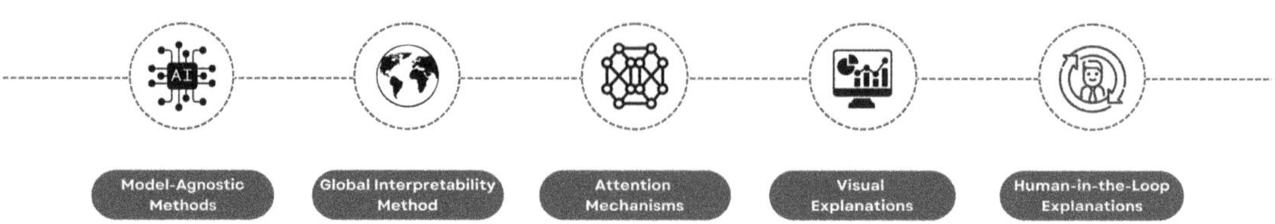



**FIGURE 5.3**　XAI methods.

### 5.3.2　Model-Agnostic Methods

The process of generating explanations through perturbation involves manipulating the input data to derive insights into a black-box model's decision-making (Zolanvari et al., 2021). This approach entails the training of an interpretable model, such as linear regression or decision trees, using the perturbed instances of the input data (Gianfagna & Di Cecco, 2021). This interpretable surrogate model serves the purpose of approximating the intricate behaviors of the underlying black-box model in a localized context (Darias et al., 2021). This nuanced technique enhances transparency by offering a comprehensible representation of how the black-box model arrives at its decisions.

The perturbation-driven explanation begins by creating variants of the input data, each with slight alterations (Bobek et al., 2021). These perturbed instances serve as training data for the interpretable model (Gianfagna & Di Cecco, 2021). The interpretable model learns from this perturbed dataset, aligning itself to mirror the decision trends observed within the black-box model, albeit in a simplified and transparent form (Zolanvari et al., 2021). This surrogate model functions as a local explainer, shedding light on the critical facets influencing the black-box model's predictions within a specific context (Darias et al., 2021). The concept of "anchors" emerges as a pivotal component in this methodology. Anchors are succinct if-then rules that act as powerful elucidators of decision logic. They carry a dual attribute of sufficiency (being valid) and necessity (being irreplaceable) concerning a particular prediction (Zolanvari et al., 2021). Anchors effectively unveil the minimal conditions under which the black-box model's prediction can be reliably anticipated.

The journey toward discovering anchors involves generating perturbations of the input data and observing how the black-box model responds (Zolanvari et al., 2021). Perturbed instances are systematically presented to the model, and their resulting predictions are assessed (Darias et al., 2021). This iterative process encapsulates the essence of how anchors materialize—by isolating specific combinations of perturbed features that consistently drive the black-box model to a particular prediction (Zolanvari et al., 2021). The perturbation-driven explanation methodology operates on the premise of local interpretability, providing a contextualized perspective on how the black-box model behaves with respect to specific input instances (Gianfagna & Di Cecco, 2021). This approach is particularly valuable in domains where accurate explanations are essential, such as medical diagnostics or financial risk assessment. The interpretable surrogate model created through perturbation acts as a bridge, connecting the complexity of black-box models to human graspable insights (Zolanvari et al., 2021).

### 5.3.3　Global Interpretability Method

Global interpretability methods aim to provide insights into the overall behavior and decision-making process of a machine learning model across its entire input space. These methods focus on understanding the model's general tendencies, relationships between features, and how different inputs contribute to its predictions on a larger scale. Here are some common global interpretability methods:

This approach encompasses various sophisticated techniques, including partial dependence plots (PDPs), accumulated local effects (ALE) plots, and the utilization of global surrogate models. The essence of this method lies in its endeavor to transcend local insights, unveiling the holistic relationship between features and model output. Central to this methodology, PDPs unravel the interplay between a specific feature and the AI model's output, while neutralizing the influence of other features. This is achieved by systematically altering the values of the chosen feature while keeping other features constant. Through this orchestrated variation, the average prediction for each value is computed and graphically represented. PDPs offer an illustrative panorama of how the chosen feature's manipulation impacts the model's predictions across various scenarios. Complementing the insights garnered from PDPs, ALE plots delve into quantifying the cumulative impact of a feature. ALE plots encapsulate the overarching behavior of a feature by integrating the partial dependence function over a specified range of feature values. This technique transcends individual instances, shedding light on how changes in a feature impact the model's predictions across a spectrum of scenarios. This quantitative insight contributes to a comprehensive grasp of feature contributions. Global surrogate models serve as the pinnacle of the global interpretability method. These models operate by creating interpretable approximations of the intricate black-box model's behavior. This is achieved by training an interpretable model using the original features as inputs and the predictions of the black-box model as targets. The resultant surrogate model stands as a transparent intermediary, reflecting the essence of the black-box model's decisions in a comprehensible form.

The global interpretability method encapsulates a panoramic view of AI model behavior. The tandem of PDPs and ALE plots, bolstered by global surrogate models, empowers analysts to unearth intricate relationships between features and predictions. This method's application is diverse, spanning domains like medical diagnostics and financial risk assessment, where understanding holistic relationships is paramount.

## 5.3.4 Attention Mechanism

The attention mechanism is a critical component in XAI especially in the context of neural network architectures like transformers. Originally developed to improve the performance of machine translation tasks, attention mechanisms have found application in various fields, including natural language processing and computer vision, and they also contribute to making AI models more interpretable. Here's how attention mechanisms are used in XAI: Attention mechanisms, a cornerstone of deep learning models such as recurrent neural networks (RNNs) and transformer models, serve as a pivotal facet of XAI. These mechanisms assume the role of spotlight bearers, assigning weights to input features or intermediary representations, thereby illuminating their pivotal significance. The bedrock of attention mechanisms lies in their capacity to capture feature interactions and dependencies, rendering them indispensable instruments in unraveling complex decision-making processes. The orchestration of attention mechanisms involves the deployment of techniques like dot-product attention and self-attention. Dot-product attention scrutinizes the relationship between input features by computing dot products, culminating in a comprehensive depiction of their interconnectedness. Self-attention, on the other hand, allocates weight to each feature while considering its own relevance within the context of the entire input sequence. These mechanisms interlink features, discerning their roles in generating predictions. Attention mechanisms excel in capturing intricate feature interactions and dependencies that underpin the AI model's decision-making. By varying levels of importance to input features, attention mechanisms discern their roles in shaping the model's output. This nuanced approach is particularly adept at capturing non-linear relationships and contextual dependencies that may elude traditional analytical methodologies. An exemplary facet of attention mechanisms is their capacity to generate attention weights, representing the saliency of input features. These weights provide a visual manifestation of the model's focus, revealing which features significantly influenced its decision. By visualizing attention weights, practitioners gain a deep understanding of feature relevance, enabling them to corroborate AI predictions with domain knowledge. Attention mechanisms resonate across domains where feature significance is pivotal. In medical image analysis, these mechanisms can spotlight regions within images that contribute to diagnostic predictions. Similarly, in natural language processing, attention mechanisms can unveil the crucial words or phrases that influence sentiment analysis outcomes.

### 5.3.5 Visual Explanations

Saliency maps are generated by computing the gradient of the model's output with respect to the input features. The magnitude of these gradients indicates the importance of each feature in influencing the prediction, and saliency maps visualize this information by overlaying it on the input data. Heatmaps represent feature importance by assigning color gradients to different regions of the input based on their contribution to the output. Gradient-based visualizations use the gradients to highlight important regions or patterns in the input data that contribute to the model's decision. The essence of saliency maps lies in their genesis through gradient computation. Specifically, gradients of the model's output are computed with respect to the input features. These gradients act as torchbearers of importance, capturing the extent to which each feature influences the model's prediction. The magnitude of these gradients assumes a pivotal role—higher magnitudes signify greater influence. The distinctive attribute of saliency maps lies in their transformative ability to overlay the computed gradients onto the input data. This overlay visually manifests the influence of each feature, demarcating regions that carry substantial influence from those that play a lesser role. By rendering this overlay on the input data, saliency maps create a tangible linkage between model behaviors and input attributes. Expanding the repertoire of visual explanations, heatmaps offer a compelling rendition of feature importance. Heatmaps employ a gradient-based approach to assign distinct color gradients to different regions within the input data. The intensity of these colors corresponds to the feature's contribution to the model's output. Thus, heatmaps bestow a panoramic view of where the model's attention is focused, effectively highlighting significant regions.

At the heart of this methodology lies gradient-based visualizations, which ingeniously spotlight influential patterns within the input data. By leveraging the gradients, these visualizations identify critical regions that decisively sway the model's prediction. This approach extends its utility across domains such as medical image analysis or language processing, where discerning patterns can unlock vital insights. The application of visual explanations is fortified by their technical underpinnings. In domains like medical diagnostics, saliency maps can unveil regions within medical images that contribute to predictions. In natural language processing, they can spotlight pivotal phrases that influence sentiment analysis.

### 5.3.6 Human-in-the-Loop Explanations

Human-in-the-loop approaches can incorporate various techniques, such as active learning, interactive visualization, or natural language interfaces. Active learning allows users to label specific instances to improve the model's performance and generate explanations tailored to their preferences. Interactive visualization tools enable users to explore the model's behavior, modify inputs, and observe the resulting changes in predictions and explanations. Natural language interfaces allow users to ask specific questions about the model's decisions and receive explanations in human-readable form, facilitating better understanding and trust. Active learning, a central tenet of HITL explanations, manifests as a reciprocal enrichment process. It empowers users to judiciously label specific instances, thereby augmenting the model's proficiency. Through this interactive annotation, the model absorbs valuable insights, enhancing its predictive accuracy. The explanations resulting from active learning are tailored to user preferences, providing a more nuanced and customized understanding. Within the HITL framework, interactive visualization tools serve as instrumental aids in deciphering the model's behavior. These tools facilitate an immersive exploration, enabling users to manipulate inputs, observe resultant changes in predictions, and concurrently witness explanations evolving in response. This interactivity empowers users to grasp the cause-and-effect dynamics, fostering a tactile understanding of the model's decision-making.

Central to HITL explanations is the inclusion of natural language interfaces, a conduit that bridges the gap between users and the model's insights. These interfaces allow users to pose targeted queries about the model's decisions in human-readable language. The ensuing explanations are crafted in a linguistic format, rendering intricate AI rationale comprehensible to human experts. This conversational interaction cultivates understanding and nurtures trust. The technical underpinnings of HITL explanations are underscored by their capacity to synergize human cognition with AI complexities. In medical diagnostics, HITL techniques empower clinicians to fine-tune models by providing expert annotations. In financial risk assessment, users can manipulate input variables to comprehend the impact on predictions, bolstering decision-making. A summarized diagram (Figure 5.4) illustrates the key points of methods used by XAI.

## 5.4  USE CASES

XAI techniques provide methods and tools to enhance transparency, trustworthiness, and accountability in the use of AI systems. Here are some potential use cases for each of the XAI techniques in Healthcare 5.0, explained in more technical terms:

### 5.4.1  RULE-BASED SYSTEMS

**Clinical decision support:** Rule-based systems in clinical decision support provide a systematic framework to incorporate medical knowledge and guidelines into practical tools that aid healthcare practitioners in making informed decisions. These systems utilize explicit rules that are carefully crafted based on a combination of expert insights, established medical guidelines, evidence-based practices, and domain-specific heuristics. The process begins with identifying and formalizing the rules that encapsulate various medical scenarios and conditions. These rules serve as the foundation for generating recommendations, offering a structured approach to address different clinical situations. When a healthcare practitioner interacts with the system, the patient's data is inputted, and the rules are applied to analyze the data and generate relevant guidance. Rule-based clinical decision support systems offer a structured and standardized approach to medical decision-making. They

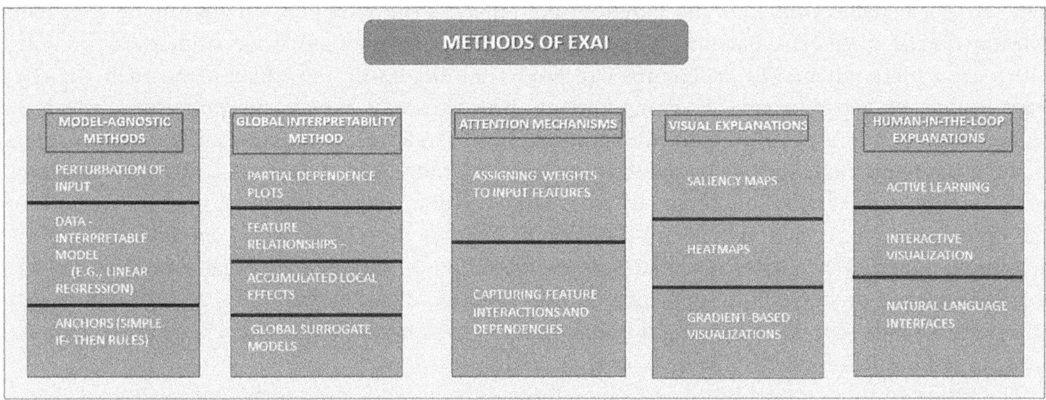


**FIGURE 5.4**  Methods of XAI.

help healthcare professionals navigate through the complexity of medical knowledge by providing context-specific recommendations that adhere to current medical standards. This ensures that best practices are consistently applied across different clinical scenarios. Moreover, these systems can contribute to reducing variability in clinical decision-making, enhancing patient safety, and optimizing resource utilization. They can be particularly valuable in scenarios where rapid decision-making is crucial, such as in emergency situations or when dealing with complex medical cases. Rule-based systems in clinical decision support provide a transparent and structured approach to integrating medical knowledge into practice. By offering clear explanations for their recommendations, these systems empower healthcare practitioners to make informed decisions while adhering to established medical guidelines.

**Adverse event detection:** Rule-based systems prove invaluable in the context of adverse event detection, where they can be designed to identify potential issues such as adverse drug reactions or medication interactions. These rules are constructed using a foundation of known risk factors, clinical evidence, and safety guidelines. When patient data is analyzed, the system applies these explicit rules to flag potential adverse events, thereby enhancing patient safety. The strength of rule-based systems lies in their capacity to offer precise explanations for detected adverse events. When an adverse event is highlighted, the system can elucidate the specific rules that were triggered by the patient's data. This granular explanation assists healthcare professionals in comprehending the rationale behind the flagged event and deciding on the appropriate interventions. In both clinical decision support and adverse event detection, the use of rule-based systems streamlines the integration of medical expertise and evidence into automated processes. Moreover, their explanatory nature enhances trust and confidence in the AI-generated insights among healthcare practitioners. These systems not only enhance clinical efficiency but also contribute to patient safety by offering transparent and understandable explanations for their recommendations.

### 5.4.2 Model Introspection Techniques

**Image analysis:** In the evolving landscape of healthcare imaging, the integration of model introspection techniques has brought unprecedented clarity and understanding to AI-driven decisions. Among these techniques, saliency maps and gradient-based methods stand out as powerful tools that illuminate the decision-making process within healthcare imaging models. By applying these techniques, we can visually uncover and emphasize the pivotal regions within medical images that significantly influence the model's predictions, thus providing a tangible means of comprehending the intricacies of AI's reasoning (Selvaraju et al., 2017). Saliency maps, a prominent model introspection technique, serve as a guiding light by revealing the areas of an image that capture the AI model's attention during decision-making. Through the visual enhancement of these regions, saliency maps enable clinicians and radiologists to discern the visual cues the AI model considers essential for its diagnostic insights. This capability holds exceptional value in medical imaging, where even subtle anomalies or features can hold vital diagnostic information. As such, saliency maps bridge the gap between AI's computational processes and human interpretation, fostering a deeper understanding of AI's contributions to medical diagnoses. Complementing saliency maps, gradient-based methods such as the widely recognized Grad-CAM technique, add a layer of granularity to the interpretability landscape. By leveraging the gradients of the model's output concerning the input image, these methods unveil the specific regions that drive the AI model's predictions. In doing so, they offer a more nuanced perspective on the visual elements that influence the AI's decision-making process. This sophisticated introspection enriches the dialogue between healthcare professionals and AI, nurturing a collaborative environment that values both computational prowess and clinical expertise (Montavon et al., 2018b).

The utility of these model introspection techniques transcends their technical intricacies, yielding profound benefits for healthcare imaging. By providing clear visual explanations for AI-driven decisions, these techniques empower medical practitioners to validate and comprehend the rationale underpinning AI-generated recommendations. Furthermore, these insights bolster education within the medical field, enabling clinicians to effectively communicate diagnostic findings to patients by illustrating the specific features or patterns that guided the AI's conclusions. In the grand scheme of things, the integration of saliency maps, gradient-based methods, and analogous model introspection techniques holds the potential to revolutionize medical decision-making. Through enhanced transparency, collaboration, and a mutual appreciation of each entity's strengths, these techniques are steering healthcare toward a future where AI augments human expertise while ensuring decisions remain transparent, accessible, and in accordance with established medical standards.

**Feature importance:** Model introspection techniques encompass a variety of methods, including permutation importance and SHAP (Shapley additive explanations) values, which provide invaluable insights into the significance of input features within predictive models (Altmann et al., 2010; Lundberg, 2017). These techniques quantify the relative importance of each feature, facilitating a deeper understanding of the model's decision-making process and enabling researchers and clinicians to identify key variables with implications for disease mechanisms and clinical investigations. Permutation importance entails systematically shuffling the values of a specific feature while observing its impact on the model's performance. The extent to which the model's performance deteriorates after permuting a feature reflects its importance. This technique offers a straightforward yet powerful means of ranking features based on their influence, aiding in the identification of critical factors that underlie the model's predictions. SHAP values, on the other hand, leverage game theory principles to attribute contributions to each feature in a prediction. These values provide a unified framework for understanding the impact of features on individual predictions and model behavior. SHAP values offer a holistic perspective, allowing researchers and clinicians to explore how combinations of features interact to influence outcomes.

By leveraging these introspection techniques, healthcare professionals can uncover hidden relationships between variables and disease mechanisms. For instance, in a medical context, these techniques could reveal which patient characteristics, biomarkers, or clinical measurements contribute most significantly to a disease prediction. This knowledge is instrumental in not only building more robust and accurate models but also guiding further research and clinical decision-making. Moreover, feature importance insights derived from these techniques play a pivotal role in healthcare, where the identification of critical variables can inform treatment strategies, disease prevention efforts, and patient management protocols. By prioritizing important features, medical practitioners can focus resources on interventions that are likely to yield the most substantial impact. In essence, the application of model introspection techniques like permutation importance and SHAP values reveals the intricate relationships between features and outcomes within predictive models. These insights empower healthcare professionals to make informed decisions, drive targeted research initiatives, and advance the understanding of complex diseases and medical conditions.

### 5.4.3　Local Interpretable Model-Agnostic Explanations (LIME)

**Predictive models in personalized medicine:** Predictive models have an impact on medicine as they help customize treatments for patients by considering their distinctive traits and medical backgrounds. However, the intricate nature of machine learning models used in this field can sometimes make them difficult to interpret. That's where approaches like LIME (local interpretable model-agnostic explanations) come into play aiming to bridge the divide, between effectiveness and comprehensibility.

LIME offers a revolutionary approach to generating explanations for individual predictions made by machine learning models. It achieves this by approximating the decision boundary of the model within a localized region surrounding a specific instance. By creating a simplified and interpretable surrogate model within this localized region, LIME effectively captures the essence of the original model's behavior in a comprehensible manner. This surrogate model, while being much simpler than the original model, accurately emulates its decision-making process within the specific context of interest (Ribeiro et al., 2016a). The significance of LIME's contributions becomes especially evident when applied to personalized medicine. In this context, understanding the rationale behind a model's prediction for a particular patient is not only beneficial but often critical for making informed treatment decisions. LIME's explanations shed light on which features or variables of the patient's profile influenced the model's prediction and to what extent. This empowers medical practitioners to comprehend the underlying factors that drive the model's recommendation, effectively bridging the gap between AI-driven insights and human expertise.

By providing interpretable insights into individual predictions, LIME enhances the collaboration between machine learning models and healthcare professionals. Doctors can leverage these explanations to better grasp the basis of a model's recommendation and evaluate its alignment with their clinical intuition. This transparent decision-making process, facilitated by LIME, is particularly valuable in personalized medicine, where tailoring treatments based on an accurate understanding of the patient's condition is essential. In a broader sense, LIME's application in predictive models for personalized medicine holds the potential to revolutionize healthcare practices. The ability to interpret and trust AI-generated predictions facilitates more informed treatment planning, ultimately leading to improved patient outcomes. The seamless integration of AI's predictive prowess with human understanding through LIME exemplifies the synergy between technology and medicine, paving the way for a more effective and efficient healthcare system.

**Adverse drug event prediction:** In the field of predicting drug events, where patient safety is of utmost importance the use of LIME is seen as a significant breakthrough. Adverse drug events can greatly impact health making it crucial, for healthcare providers to understand the contributing factors behind incidents. LIME provides an approach to unravel the complexity of models in this specific context. LIMEs methodology involves approximating how a predictive model behaves within a localized setting that is tailored to each patients records and prescribed medications. By creating an understandable model within this setting LIME effectively captures the core decision-making process of the original model. Even though this surrogate model is much simpler it mimics the behavior of the model. Highlights key features that influence predictions regarding adverse drug events. The application of LIME in predicting drug events brings benefits to both healthcare providers and patients alike.

The application of LIME in adverse drug event prediction yields tangible benefits for healthcare providers and patients alike. The explanations generated by LIME serve as a beacon of transparency, enabling healthcare professionals to comprehend the intricate interplay between patient characteristics, prescribed medications, and the likelihood of adverse events. These explanations effectively bridge the gap between machine-generated predictions and human understanding, empowering healthcare providers to make well-informed decisions.

By pinpointing the influential features contributing to the prediction of adverse drug events, LIME assists healthcare professionals in evaluating the risks associated with specific medications for individual patients. This personalized insight into potential adverse events fosters more informed treatment decisions, where healthcare providers can adjust prescriptions or treatment plans based on a comprehensive understanding of the underlying factors. Moreover, the integration of LIME's explanations into the clinical decision-making process instills an additional layer of accountability and trust. Patients can receive clearer explanations regarding the potential risks of prescribed medications, enabling them to actively participate in treatment discussions and make informed choices about their healthcare journey. In the broader landscape of healthcare, where precision and patient well-being are paramount, LIME's role in adverse drug event prediction stands as a testament to the harmonious fusion of advanced technology and human-centered care. The synergy between predictive models and interpretable explanations paves the way for safer and more effective medication management, ultimately enhancing patient outcomes and fostering a more resilient healthcare system. The application of LIME in adverse drug event prediction offers a transformative approach to enhancing patient safety. By generating explanations that demystify the intricate relationships between patient profiles and medication risks, LIME empowers healthcare providers with the knowledge needed to make informed treatment decisions. This holistic understanding enriches the patient-provider partnership and exemplifies the potential of XAI in revolutionizing healthcare practices.

### 5.4.4 Counterfactual Explanations

**Treatment planning:** The integration of counterfactual explanations offers a dynamic approach to guide healthcare providers. Counterfactual explanations involve generating alternative treatment plans and simulating patient outcomes by manipulating input factors or considering different treatment alternatives. This technique holds immense potential for revolutionizing treatment planning and decision-making processes, enabling healthcare providers to navigate a multitude of scenarios and assess the potential effects of various therapeutic options (Emanuel & Wachter, 2019). Counterfactual explanations empower healthcare professionals by presenting a range of plausible treatment pathways and their corresponding outcomes. By altering input factors or introducing alternative treatments, providers can explore the intricate web of cause-and-effect relationships that shape patient responses. This approach goes beyond static predictions and fosters a deeper understanding of how different interventions could influence the course of treatment and patient well-being. The application of counterfactual explanations in treatment planning addresses the inherent uncertainty that often accompanies medical decisions. Healthcare providers can quantify the potential benefits, risks, and trade-offs associated with different treatments, facilitating more nuanced and informed decision-making. This approach is particularly valuable in cases where the optimal treatment path isn't immediately clear or where patient-specific factors necessitate personalized approaches.

Furthermore, counterfactual explanations empower patients to actively participate in their treatment journey. By presenting a range of potential outcomes based on different interventions, patients gain insights into the potential trajectories of their health under various scenarios. This transparency fosters collaborative discussions between patients and healthcare providers, where treatment decisions are made with a comprehensive understanding of the potential effects. In the broader context of healthcare, the integration of counterfactual explanations aligns with the goals of personalized medicine and evidence-based practice. The ability to explore multiple treatment avenues, simulate outcomes, and quantify uncertainties empowers healthcare providers to make choices that align with patient preferences, medical best practices, and the available evidence. Counterfactual explanations represent a transformative approach to treatment planning and decision-making in healthcare. By simulating alternative treatment scenarios and outcomes, this technique equips healthcare providers with the tools needed to navigate complex medical decisions. Through enhanced transparency, patient involvement, and evidence-based choices, counterfactual explanations hold the potential to elevate the standard of care, leading to improved patient outcomes and a more patient-centric healthcare ecosystem.

The integration of counterfactual explanations introduces a powerful tool for identifying factors that significantly elevate a patient's susceptibility to specific diseases. Counterfactual explanations facilitate the pinpointing of causative elements that contribute to a heightened risk of contracting a particular disease. Healthcare providers can leverage this approach to unravel the complex web of interactions that influence disease susceptibility and evaluate potential interventions aimed at mitigating such risks. Counterfactual explanations empower healthcare providers by enabling them to understand the causal relationships between various risk factors and disease outcomes. By simulating hypothetical scenarios where specific risk factors are adjusted, providers can gain insights into how these modifications might impact a patient's risk profile. This approach transcends mere risk estimation by delving into the underlying mechanisms driving disease susceptibility, offering a deeper level of understanding. The applicants have collaborative discussions. Patients become active participants in their healthcare journey, making informed choices based on a clear understanding of their risk factors and potential interventions.

In the broader landscape of healthcare, the application of counterfactual explanations in risk assessment is particularly valuable when evaluating the potential efficacy of interventions. Healthcare providers can model scenarios where interventions are introduced to modify certain risk factors, allowing them to gauge the potential impact on reducing the patient's risk of developing the disease. This proactive approach equips providers with a comprehensive view of the potential benefits and limitations of different interventions, aiding in informed decision-making. Furthermore, counterfactual explanations provide a pathway for patient engagement and shared decision-making. By presenting patients with understandable explanations of their disease risks and the potential effects of interventions, providers foster the principles of personalized medicine and preventive care. By uncovering the intricate relationships between risk factors and disease outcomes, healthcare providers can tailor interventions to address individual patient profiles. This approach holds the potential to not only enhance patient outcomes but also contribute to the broader goal of public health and disease prevention. In conclusion, counterfactual explanations offer a novel and impactful approach to risk assessment within healthcare. By dissecting the causal links between risk factors and disease susceptibility, healthcare providers gain actionable insights into potential interventions for reducing patient risk. Through transparency, patient engagement, and informed decision-making, counterfactual explanations pave the way for more targeted and effective healthcare strategies, ultimately advancing patient well-being and population health.

### 5.4.5    Interactive Visualizations

**Patient education:** Interactive visualizations have revolutionized the way medical concepts, conditions, and procedures are presented to patients. Traditional methods of patient education often relied on verbal explanations, static images, or complex medical jargon that could be overwhelming and confusing for individuals without a medical background. However, with the advent of technology, healthcare providers now have the means to leverage interactive visualizations to convey information in a more accessible and engaging manner. Anatomical models, for instance, offer patients a three-dimensional representation of their own bodies or specific body parts. These models can be manipulated digitally, allowing patients to zoom in, rotate, and explore different angles, enhancing their understanding of their anatomy and the areas of concern. For patients diagnosed with conditions such as heart disease or joint problems, interactive anatomical models can illustrate the exact location and nature of the issue, helping patients grasp the significance of their diagnosis.

Interactive diagrams take patient education a step further by breaking down complex medical processes into manageable steps. These diagrams can show the progression of diseases, the effects of certain treatments, or the mechanisms behind medical procedures. Patients can interact with these diagrams to see cause-and-effect relationships, which is particularly useful for visual learners or those who prefer a more hands-on approach to learning. Multimedia presentations, including videos, animations, and audio explanations, engage patients on multiple sensory levels. These presentations can take patients on a virtual tour of their body, showcasing the inner workings, potential problem areas, and treatment options. Hearing a medical professional's voice explaining procedures or seeing a visual representation of a surgical intervention can alleviate anxiety and make patients feel more informed and prepared (Saravanan et al., 2023). The impact of interactive visualizations on patient empowerment and participation in decision-making cannot be overstated. When patients have a clearer understanding of their health conditions, they are more likely to ask informed questions, express their preferences, and actively collaborate with their healthcare providers to formulate treatment plans. This shift from a passive recipient of care to an engaged participant fosters a sense of ownership over one's health, leading to improved treatment adherence and overall health outcomes. Moreover, interactive visualizations can bridge language barriers and health literacy gaps. By presenting information visually and interactively, healthcare providers can convey important concepts without relying solely on written or spoken language (Madlon-Kay & Mosch, 2000; Bhattacharya et al., 2022). This inclusivity ensures that all patients, regardless of their language proficiency or educational background, can access and comprehend critical medical information. Interactive visualizations in patient education have revolutionized the way medical information is conveyed. These visualizations, whether they involve anatomical models, interactive diagrams, or multimedia presentations, empower patients by making complex information understandable and engaging. This, in turn, enhances patient participation in decision-making, improves treatment adherence, and ultimately contributes to better health outcomes. As technology continues to evolve, the potential for even more immersive and personalized patient education experiences becomes increasingly promising.

Comparative utilization of textual, visual, and example-based explanations has been demonstrated in Figure 5.5.

**Training and education:** These tools are reshaping how medical students, residents, and even experienced professionals learn and refine their skills. By harnessing the power of technology, interactive visualizations offer dynamic and engaging learning experiences that significantly enhance the training process. One of the most significant advantages of interactive visualizations is their ability to simulate complex medical scenarios. Medical professionals can immerse themselves in virtual patient cases that replicate real-world situations, allowing them to practice critical decision-making skills in a risk-free environment. For instance, a surgical trainee can use interactive simulations to perform virtual surgeries, evaluate different techniques, and understand potential complications before they encounter these scenarios in an actual operating room (Bhattacharya et al., 2022). Moreover, interactive visualizations are adept at demonstrating the effects of various interventions. Healthcare professionals can witness the outcomes of different treatment approaches in real time, observing how their choices impact patient well-being. This not only fosters a deeper understanding of medical procedures but also encourages evidence-based decision-making. Trainees can experiment with different interventions, observe the consequences, and refine their strategies accordingly (Frank et al., 2017).

The interactive nature of these visualizations is particularly beneficial in unraveling complex medical concepts. Abstract ideas and intricate anatomical structures can be challenging to comprehend through traditional methods alone. However, interactive models allow learners to manipulate and explore these concepts in three dimensions, providing a tactile and visual understanding that

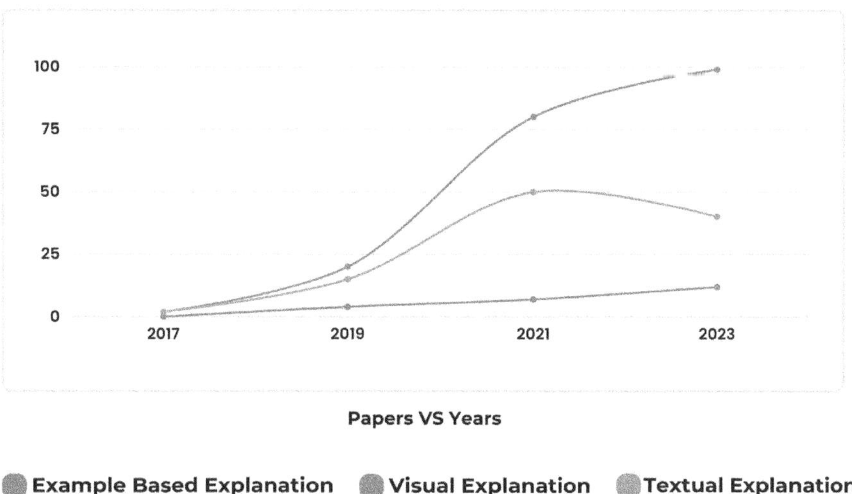


**FIGURE 5.5**  Use of textual, visual, and example-based explanations.

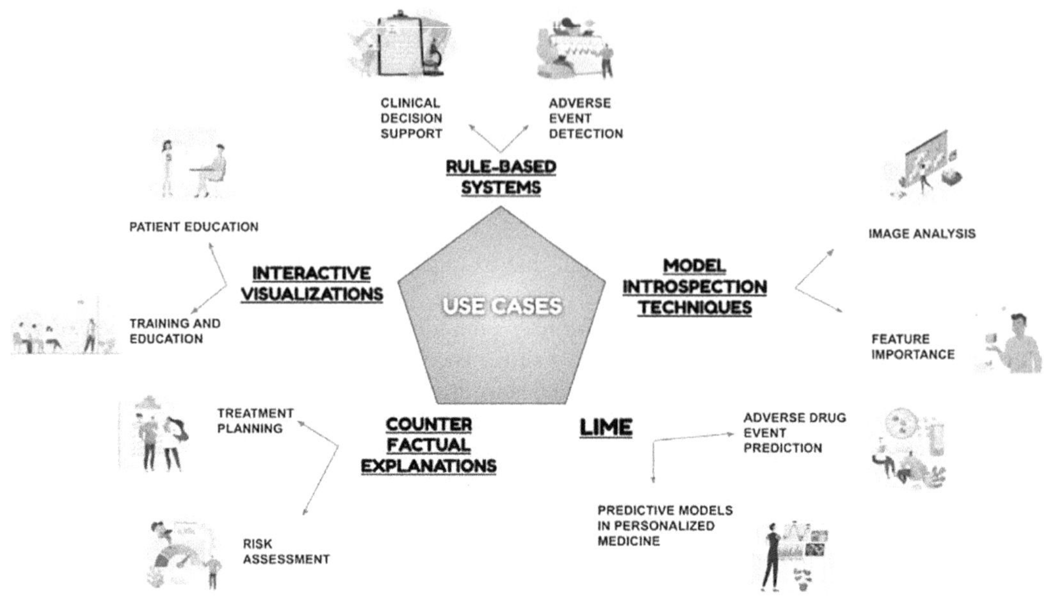


**FIGURE 5.6**   Use cases of different models of XAI.

surpasses what textbooks and lectures can offer. This hands-on engagement enhances both comprehension and knowledge retention, making learning more effective and enjoyable. Collaborative learning is another facet where interactive visualizations excel. Healthcare professionals can use these tools to collaboratively explore medical cases, discuss diagnoses, and brainstorm treatment plans. Virtual rounds or case discussions can be conducted, even across different physical locations, fostering a sense of teamwork and shared learning experiences. As technology continues to evolve, the potential for personalized and adaptive learning experiences using interactive visualizations grows. Machine learning and artificial intelligence can analyze learners' interactions and responses to tailor the educational content to their individual needs. This level of customization ensures that each healthcare professional receives the targeted training required to address their specific learning gaps. Interactive visualizations are revolutionizing healthcare professionals' training and education. These tools offer the ability to simulate scenarios, demonstrate interventions, and enhance the understanding of intricate concepts. The hands-on and immersive nature of these visualizations fosters better comprehension, critical thinking, and knowledge retention, ultimately resulting in well-prepared and skilled healthcare practitioners who can deliver high-quality patient care (Morton, 1966; Saravanan et al., 2022; Finegold, 2017).

A summarized depiction of the use cases is displayed in Figure 5.6.

## 5.5 SUCCESSFUL CASE STUDY

### 5.5.1 DeepPatient

One of the notable successful case studies showcasing the application of XAI techniques in healthcare is the DeepPatient project conducted by Columbia University.

The project DeepPatient undergoes the following steps:

1. In the healthcare sector, the utilization of deep learning models for predicting patient outcomes and diseases through electronic health records (EHRs) has gained considerable attention due to their potential to offer accurate insights into patient health. A significant

challenge that researchers have grappled with in this endeavor is the inherent complexity and opacity of deep learning algorithms, often referred to as the "black-box" nature of these models (Lipton, 2018). This opacity arises from the intricate relationships and non-linear transformations that occur within deep neural networks, making it difficult to decipher how the model arrives at its predictions (Montavon et al., 2018b). As the research community pushes the boundaries of AI applications in healthcare, the need to understand the decision-making process of these models becomes paramount, especially in critical scenarios like patient care. While deep learning models excel at pattern recognition and prediction, the lack of transparency can hinder their acceptance and adoption by healthcare professionals and regulatory bodies (Caruana et al., 2015). The black-box challenge becomes particularly pronounced when considering the ethical and regulatory aspects of deploying AI in healthcare settings, where explanations for predictions are crucial for accountability and trust (Guidotti et al., 2018). The DeepPatient project conducted by Columbia University is an illustrative example of how this challenge was acknowledged and addressed (Rajkomar et al., 2018). By initially creating a deep learning model that utilizes EHRs to predict patient outcomes, the researchers highlighted the potential of AI in healthcare. However, the inherent opacity of the model's decision-making process presented a significant roadblock in translating these predictions into actionable insights. The difficulty in comprehending and interpreting the model's predictions stems from the intricate network of connections formed during the training phase. The model learns patterns and features from the data, and these patterns are not always easily interpretable by humans. The result is a trade-off between model complexity and interpretability—the deeper and more complex the model, the harder it is to understand its internal workings (Zhang et al., 2018). To overcome this challenge, the researchers turned to XAI techniques. These techniques aim to provide insights into how a model arrives at its decisions, effectively bridging the gap between the model's complexity and human understanding (Doshi-Velez and Kim, 2017). In the case of the DeepPatient project, the application of local interpretable model-agnostic explanations (LIME) was pivotal. LIME generates explanations for individual predictions by approximating the model's behavior around specific instances, enabling healthcare professionals to gain insights into the factors contributing to the model's predictions (Ribeiro et al., 2016a). By using LIME to shed light on the model's predictions, the DeepPatient project not only made the predictions more understandable but also demonstrated a commitment to transparency and accountability in AI-driven healthcare. The incorporation of XAI techniques like LIME showcased a path forward in making AI models accessible and useful for real-world medical decision-making, enhancing the prospects of widespread AI adoption in healthcare. In conclusion, the black-box nature of deep learning algorithms presents a significant challenge in their application to healthcare, where interpretability and transparency are paramount. The DeepPatient project's recognition of this challenge and subsequent incorporation of XAI techniques exemplify the ongoing efforts to make AI-driven predictions comprehensible and actionable for healthcare professionals. This endeavor not only contributes to the responsible use of AI but also paves the way for the integration of advanced AI technologies into the medical field.

2. A deep learning model was employed to forecast patient outcomes and diseases using EHRs, the researchers confronted a common hurdle in deploying complex machine learning models in real-world scenarios: the black-box nature of these models. The inability to comprehend and interpret the rationale behind a model's predictions can limit its adoption, especially in critical domains like healthcare. To surmount this challenge, the research team turned to XAI techniques, a critical approach to bridge the gap between complex models and human understanding. Among the XAI techniques available, they selected LIME to provide insight into the model's predictions (Rajkomar et al., 2018). LIME's core idea lies in creating simpler, interpretable surrogate models that approximate the behavior

of the underlying complex model. This surrogate model is trained to mimic the black-box model's predictions within a localized region of the feature space—hence the term "local" interpretable explanations. By perturbing the input data and observing the changes in predictions, LIME constructs a model that provides explanations for the complex model's outputs on specific instances. In the case of the DeepPatient project, LIME operated by generating explanations for individual patient predictions. For each prediction made by the deep learning model, LIME created a locally faithful surrogate model that could approximate the model's behavior around that specific patient's data. The surrogate model, being more interpretable, provided insights into the factors and features within the patient's health record that significantly influenced the deep learning model's prediction. These insights, presented in a human-understandable format, included variables such as medical history, test results, and other relevant EHR data. The key impact of using LIME was the transformation of the deep learning model's outputs from cryptic numerical predictions to intelligible and actionable insights. Healthcare professionals were able to comprehend the reasons behind the model's decisions on a case-by-case basis. This not only engendered trust in the AI-driven predictions but also empowered medical practitioners to confidently apply these predictions to patient care. For instance, if the model predicted a certain outcome, LIME's explanations could highlight specific clinical indicators or historical data points that contributed to that prognosis. By incorporating LIME as part of the DeepPatient project, the research team effectively demonstrated how XAI techniques can act as a bridge between advanced, complex machine learning models and human understanding. This process is crucial for deploying AI technologies in domains where informed, responsible decision-making is paramount, such as healthcare. In conclusion, the application of LIME in the DeepPatient project showcases the potential of XAI techniques to enhance the interpretability of complex machine learning models. LIME's ability to generate local, human-understandable explanations serves as a pivotal step toward building trust, transparency, and collaboration between AI systems and healthcare professionals.

3. Absolutely, the use of LIME in the DeepPatient project had profound implications for healthcare professionals' ability to interpret and utilize the deep learning model's predictions. Here's an expanded discussion of its impact: By integrating LIME into the DeepPatient project, researchers successfully unlocked the intricate decision-making process of the deep learning model for each patient. This achievement marked a significant breakthrough in addressing the opacity of complex machine-learning models in healthcare (Rajkomar et al., 2018). With LIME in place, healthcare professionals gained unprecedented insights into the factors that underpinned the model's predictions for individual patients. In essence, LIME acted as a translation mechanism, transforming the numerical outputs of the deep learning model into a comprehensible narrative. Clinicians were provided with clear and understandable explanations detailing the specific features, variables, or historical data within the patient's EHRs that had the most significant influence on the model's prognosis. These explanations held transformative value for healthcare professionals. By peering into the inner workings of the model, clinicians were equipped with a deeper understanding of the logic driving its predictions. This understanding, in turn, enabled them to make more informed and rational decisions concerning patient care. For instance, if the model predicted a high likelihood of a specific medical condition, LIME's explanations could highlight the relevant medical history, test results, or risk factors that contributed to that prediction. Perhaps the most noteworthy impact of LIME's explanations was their role in fostering personalized treatment plans. Armed with a clear grasp of the model's decision factors, clinicians could tailor interventions and treatments to address the unique needs of each patient. This bespoke approach to healthcare delivery is a significant departure from traditional one-size-fits-all methodologies. The nuanced insights provided by LIME allowed clinicians to identify specific areas of concern and allocate

resources accordingly, leading to more effective and patient-centric treatment strategies. The integration of LIME's explanations also established a productive synergy between human expertise and AI-driven insights. Clinicians were no longer passive recipients of model predictions but active participants in the decision-making process. Their medical judgment was bolstered by the interpretability provided by LIME, leading to a harmonious collaboration between human intuition and machine-derived insights. In conclusion, the application of LIME within the DeepPatient project bore witness to the transformative potential of XAI in healthcare. The transparency achieved through LIME's explanations not only demystified complex machine learning predictions but also empowered healthcare professionals with the knowledge needed to make well-informed decisions and craft-tailored treatment plans. This harmonization of advanced technology and human expertise exemplifies the promise of AI in enhancing healthcare outcomes and patient well-being.

4. By enhancing the interpretability and transparency of deep learning models, the project exemplified the vital role of XAI in bridging the gap between advanced AI systems and effective clinical decision-making (Rajkomar et al., 2018). Through the integration of XAI techniques like LIME, the project illuminated the previously opaque decision-making process of the deep learning model. This interpretability was a cornerstone in building trust and fostering understanding among healthcare professionals who needed to rely on AI-generated predictions for patient care. The traditional black-box nature of deep learning models had, at times, hindered the full acceptance of AI systems in critical healthcare scenarios. The insights provided by XAI techniques, as showcased in the DeepPatient project, were instrumental in reversing this trend. One of the pivotal challenges in implementing AI in healthcare is establishing trust between clinicians and AI systems. Healthcare professionals are accustomed to making decisions based on well-understood, evidence-based information. The complex predictions of deep learning models, though accurate, were initially met with skepticism due to their lack of interpretability. The introduction of XAI techniques addressed this issue directly. By offering clear and localized explanations for the model's predictions, LIME enabled healthcare professionals to "peek under the hood" of the AI system, comprehending the reasoning behind its conclusions. This newfound transparency brought about a paradigm shift in how healthcare professionals approached AI-driven predictions. The confidence fostered by XAI made it possible for clinicians to embrace AI recommendations, treating them as valuable insights rather than enigmatic outputs. This, in turn, accelerated the adoption of AI in clinical decision-making processes. Healthcare professionals could now understand the factors that influenced the model's predictions and could correlate these factors with their medical expertise to develop well-informed treatment plans. In the broader context, the success of the DeepPatient project established a precedent for the responsible integration of AI in healthcare. It showcased that advanced machine learning models need not be treated as inscrutable "black boxes." Instead, by leveraging XAI techniques like LIME, AI predictions could be made intelligible, actionable, and seamlessly integrated into the clinical workflow. In conclusion, the DeepPatient project exemplified the transformative power of XAI in healthcare by enhancing the interpretability and transparency of deep learning models. Through the application of techniques like LIME, healthcare professionals were empowered to trust and understand AI-generated predictions, paving the way for their incorporation into clinical decision-making. This shift not only signifies a new era of collaboration between AI systems and human experts but also sets a precedent for the ethical, transparent, and impactful use of AI in healthcare settings.

This case study highlights the significance of XAI in bridging the gap between complex AI models and human understanding in healthcare, ultimately leading to improved patient care and outcomes.

### 5.5.2 Predicting Diabetic Retinopathy and Its Progression Using XAI and Deep Learning

Researchers from Google AI, Verily Life Sciences, and Stanford University collaborated on a study published in JAMA Ophthalmology in 2019. The study aimed to develop an AI system that could accurately predict diabetic retinopathy and its progression using deep learning techniques while also providing explanations for its predictions. The following are some of the XAI techniques:

### 1. Grad-CAM (Gradient-Weighted Class Activation Mapping)

Grad-CAM is a technique used to generate visual explanations for the predictions made by a deep learning model, particularly in image classification tasks. It helps highlight the regions or areas in an input image that were most influential in the model's decision-making process.

The process of Grad-CAM involves the following steps:

a. **Forward Pass:** The input image is fed into the trained deep learning model, which propagates the image through its layers, performing a forward pass to compute activations at different layers.

b. **Gradient Computation:** The gradients of the target class (i.e., the class for which we want to explain the prediction) with respect to the final convolutional layer's feature maps are computed. These gradients represent the importance of each feature map for the target class prediction.

c. **Global Average Pooling:** The gradients are then globally average-pooled, obtaining the importance of each feature map across all spatial locations.

d. **Weighted Sum:** The feature maps are linearly combined, with the computed importance weights as the coefficients. This produces a weighted combination that highlights the regions that contributed most to the target class prediction.

e. **Activation Map Visualization:** Finally, the weighted combination is used to produce a heatmap that visually represents the regions in the input image that were most relevant to the model's decision.

In the case of diabetic retinopathy prediction, Grad-CAM helped identify and visualize the specific regions in the retinal images that the deep learning model focused on when making predictions related to the presence or severity of diabetic retinopathy.

### 2. Salient Features Visualization

Salient feature visualization is another technique used to gain insights into the decision-making process of a deep learning model. It aims to identify and visualize the most important features or patterns in the input data that influenced the model's predictions.

The process of salient feature visualization involves the following steps:

a. **Model Activation:** Similar to Grad-CAM, the input image is passed through the deep learning model, and activations are computed at different layers.

b. **Activation Analysis:** Researchers analyze the activations to understand which neurons or channels were most activated for a particular input image. High activations indicate that specific features or patterns in the image strongly influenced the model's decision.

c. **Visualization:** To visualize the salient features, the model's activations can be overlaid on top of the input image. This overlay highlights the regions where the most important features were detected by the model.

By visualizing the salient features in retinal images related to diabetic retinopathy, researchers were able to gain a better understanding of the features that the model relied on when making predictions. This enhanced interpretability helped build trust in the model's predictions and facilitated its adoption in clinical settings.

## 3.  Results

The developed deep learning model demonstrated excellent performance in diagnosing diabetic retinopathy and predicting its progression. The accuracy metrics used to evaluate the model's performance, such as precision, recall, F1 score, and area under the receiver operating characteristic curve (AUC-ROC), indicated that the model achieved high discriminative ability and generalization on the test dataset.

The model's precision, which measures the proportion of true positive predictions among all positive predictions, was high, indicating that it had a low false positive rate. The recall, which measures the proportion of true positive predictions among all actual positive instances, was also high, suggesting that the model effectively captured most positive cases of diabetic retinopathy. The F1 score, a harmonic mean of precision and recall, was close to one, indicating a balanced trade-off between precision and recall.

The AUC-ROC metric, which measures the model's ability to distinguish between positive and negative cases, showed a value close to one, indicating that the model's predictions were well-separated and had a high discriminatory power. This has been demonstrated in Figure 5.7.

## 4.  Impact

The explanations provided by the model through Grad-CAM and salient features visualization played a crucial role in the model's successful adoption and acceptance in the healthcare domain. The interpretability and transparency offered by these techniques empowered ophthalmologists and healthcare professionals to understand the model's decision-making process, leading to the following impactful outcomes:

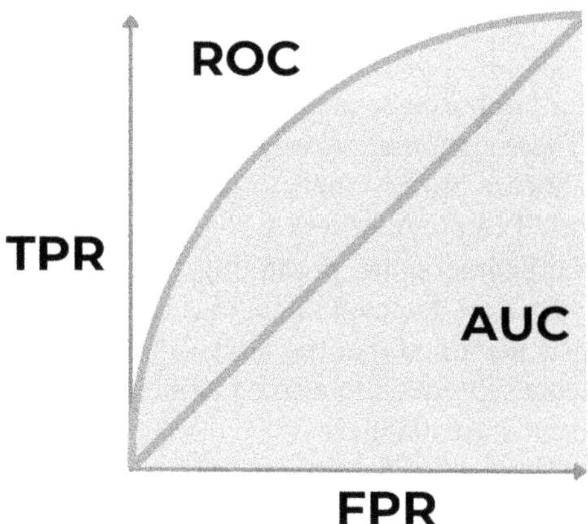


**FIGURE 5.7**   AUC–ROC graph.

1. **Increased Trust:** By understanding the regions and features that influenced the model's predictions, medical experts gained confidence in the model's capabilities. The ability to explain how the model arrived at its decisions helped alleviate concerns about black-box AI systems and fostered trust in the model's outputs.
2. **Enhanced Clinical Decisions:** With a clear understanding of the model's decision rationale, healthcare professionals were better equipped to interpret the model's predictions in the context of patient care. This interpretability enabled them to make more informed clinical decisions, such as determining appropriate treatment plans or referrals for patients with diabetic retinopathy.
3. **Error Analysis and Model Improvement:** The visual explanations provided by Grad-CAM and salient features visualization also facilitated error analysis. By identifying the specific regions where the model might have misclassified or made uncertain predictions, researchers could identify potential limitations and improve the model's performance in challenging cases.
4. **Knowledge Discovery:** The visualization of salient features allowed researchers to gain insights into the important image features associated with diabetic retinopathy. This knowledge could contribute to a better understanding of the disease and potentially lead to the discovery of new biomarkers or disease characteristics.

## 5.6 HOW XAI REDEFINES HEALTHCARE AI LANDSCAPE

### 5.6.1 Bias and Fairness

One significant challenge in the application of artificial intelligence (AI) within the healthcare sector is the potential for bias and fairness issues. AI algorithms trained on biased or unrepresentative datasets may produce unfair outcomes, particularly impacting underrepresented groups in healthcare. This bias can lead to misdiagnoses, inadequate treatments, and unequal access to healthcare resources. Researchers have recognized the critical need to address this challenge to ensure equitable healthcare provision. For instance, a study by Obermeyer et al. (2019) investigated the presence of racial bias in an algorithm used for managing population health, highlighting the importance of scrutinizing and mitigating biases in AI systems (Obermeyer et al., 2019).

### Solution Using XAI

XAI techniques, such as feature importance analysis and causal reasoning, can identify and mitigate bias in AI algorithms. These methods provide insights into which features contribute most to AI decisions, allowing healthcare professionals to understand and rectify biased outcomes. For example, if an AI system is used to predict disease risk, XAI can reveal which features led to a biased outcome for a particular demographic, prompting adjustments to the model's training data. In radiology, an AI system using XAI detected racial bias in its diagnostic predictions. By analyzing the explanation, radiologists identified that the model's bias was attributed to a lack of diverse training data. The radiology team subsequently worked to include a broader range of patient images, leading to more equitable and accurate diagnoses.

For example, In the field of diagnostic AI systems, such as those employed to identify skin diseases from images, XAI plays a crucial role. By furnishing explanations for the decisions made by the model, medical professionals can gain insight into the factors influencing a particular diagnosis. If bias is detected, XAI can pinpoint the specific features contributing to this bias, enabling data collection efforts to rectify imbalances in datasets.

### 5.6.2 Lack of Transparency

The lack of transparency in AI models, often referred to as black-box AI, poses a significant hurdle in healthcare. Many AI algorithms, especially deep learning models, make decisions that are difficult to understand or explain, hindering trust and acceptance among healthcare professionals. This opacity can impede collaboration between human experts and AI systems. To address this challenge, efforts have been made to develop intelligible models that offer insights into AI decisions. Caruana et al. (2015) explored methods for creating intelligible models in healthcare, aiming to predict pneumonia risk and hospital readmission rates (Caruana et al., 2015).

### Solution Using XAI

XAI methods offer transparent insights into AI decision-making, making complex models more understandable for healthcare professionals. Techniques like LIME can create simpler, interpretable models that approximate the behavior of the AI model for specific instances.

A deep learning application: Radiology imaging model for disease classification produced accurate results but lacked transparency. By using LIME, doctors gained explanations for individual diagnoses, highlighting which visual features led to the AI's conclusions. This transparency improved trust among medical professionals and led to more informed clinical decisions.

For example, in radiology, AI assists in detecting anomalies in medical images. XAI can generate heatmaps showing which regions of an image were most relevant for a diagnosis. Radiologists can then see the evidence supporting the AI's decision, enhancing their trust in the technology.

### 5.6.3 SAFETY AND RELIABILITY

Ensuring the safety and reliability of AI-driven healthcare interventions is a paramount concern. Incorrect or unexplained decisions made by AI systems can have serious implications for patient outcomes. Therefore, the ability to understand and validate the reasoning behind AI decisions is crucial. A study by Miotto et al. (2016) introduced an approach known as DeepPatient, which utilized unsupervised representation learning to predict future patient conditions from electronic health records. This research underscores the importance of building robust and reliable AI models in healthcare (Miotto et al., 2016).

### Solution Using XAI

XAI can provide explanations for AI predictions, allowing healthcare providers to validate the rationale behind recommendations. When an AI system suggests a treatment plan, XAI can reveal the specific patient data and medical evidence that influenced the decision. An AI-powered patient monitoring system alerted medical staff to a critical condition. By analyzing the XAI explanation, doctors verified that the AI detected an unusual combination of vital signs that indicated a potential crisis. This verification ensured timely intervention and avoided unnecessary alarms.

For example, in intensive care units, AI monitors patients' vital signs. XAI can generate explanations for alarms triggered by the AI system. If the AI suggests intervention, the medical team can assess the reasoning and determine if the proposed action aligns with the patient's condition.

### 5.6.4 DATA PRIVACY AND SECURITY

AI's integration in healthcare brings about transformative possibilities, but it also introduces complex challenges, particularly concerning data privacy and security. The sensitive nature of healthcare data underscores the critical importance of stringent privacy standards to prevent breaches and unauthorized access that could lead to misuse or compromise of patient information. Protecting the privacy of individuals while harnessing the power of AI requires a delicate balance. Choi et al. (2016) shed light on this issue through their exploration of recurrent neural network (RNN) models for the early detection of heart failure onset. This study exemplifies how AI can leverage health data to generate valuable insights while still upholding privacy safeguards. By employing techniques that allow analysis and prediction without directly exposing personal data, researchers can navigate the fine line between utilizing patient information and maintaining privacy. In the study by Choi et al. (2016), the utilization of RNN models demonstrates the potential of AI to glean meaningful patterns from health data without compromising individual privacy. These models can operate on encrypted or anonymized data, enabling the extraction of predictive insights without the need to access specific patient identifiers. This approach aligns with the principles of privacy-preserving machine learning, which seeks to develop AI algorithms that can learn from data while minimizing exposure to sensitive information.

However, it's essential to note that even with privacy-preserving measures, there's still a possibility of re-identification attacks or unintended privacy leaks. Thus, researchers and practitioners in the field of healthcare AI must continuously stay informed about the latest advancements in privacy-enhancing technologies and ensure that their AI systems undergo rigorous security audits.

## Solution Using XAI

XAI techniques offer a powerful solution to address the challenge of harnessing the benefits of AI in healthcare while safeguarding patient data privacy. One such approach involves the utilization of model distillation, a process where a simplified model approximates the behavior of a more complex AI model. This enables the extraction of meaningful insights from sensitive health data without compromising the confidentiality of individual patient records. Consider the scenario where wearable devices collect health data from numerous patients. By employing XAI techniques, a distilled model can be trained to analyze this data and predict potential health events, such as cardiac anomalies. The distilled model encapsulates the essential patterns and trends from the original AI model, while being interpretable and significantly smaller in size. This approach ensures that the analysis of health data occurs without directly exposing individual patient information.

For instance, the distilled model could identify increased heart rate variability, which might indicate the potential onset of a health issue. These insights provide valuable information to healthcare professionals for timely intervention. Importantly, the use of the distilled model means that patient-specific data remains concealed, thus upholding the principle of data privacy. This integration of XAI with model distillation demonstrates a remarkable synergy between technological advancement and ethical considerations. Healthcare stakeholders can benefit from predictive insights derived from AI while preserving patient privacy rights. As the field of XAI continues to evolve, such strategies hold the potential to transform healthcare by striking a harmonious balance between innovation and individual data protection.

For example, the integration of XAI in patient health monitoring holds significant promise for revolutionizing continuous health data analysis and early detection of health events (Smith et al., 2020). Wearable devices have emerged as indispensable tools for real-time patient data collection, furnishing valuable insights into individual well-being. XAI techniques play a pivotal role in scrutinizing this data, recognizing patterns, and forecasting potential health incidents, all the while prioritizing patient privacy. Within the domain of patient health monitoring, XAI distinguishes itself by not only providing predictive capabilities but also by rendering these predictions comprehensible (Ribeiro et al., 2016b). Instead of presenting complex algorithmic outputs or raw data, XAI distills insights into explanations that are easily understandable. This approach ensures that healthcare professionals and patients can grasp the rationale behind predictions without requiring specialized technical expertise.

An essential consideration when employing XAI for patient health monitoring is the imperative of safeguarding patient privacy (Goodman & Flaxman, 2017). Given the continuous data collection from wearable devices, concerns about data security and confidentiality are valid. XAI addresses this challenge by working with aggregated, anonymized, or encrypted data, assuring that individual patient identities and sensitive information remain undisclosed. Explanations generated by XAI focus on identified patterns, trends, and potential health risks, refraining from divulging specific patient particulars. Imagine a scenario where a wearable device tracks a patient's vital signs and activity levels over time. XAI algorithms can scrutinize this data and identify anomalies, such as a sudden spike in heart rate. The XAI system can subsequently produce an explanation that underscores the detected irregularity and its possible implications. Armed with this information, healthcare professionals can make informed choices about further steps or interventions, all the while respecting patient privacy. In summation, the fusion of XAI into patient health monitoring presents a transformative approach to harnessing wearable device data for proactive healthcare. By offering lucid explanations while upholding patient privacy, XAI empowers healthcare providers and patients to collaborate more effectively in managing health. This innovative synergy encapsulates the advancement of technology, data analysis, and ethical privacy considerations, marking a significant stride toward a more tailored, efficient, and conscientious healthcare landscape.

### 5.6.5 HUMAN-AI COLLABORATION

The seamless collaboration between AI systems and healthcare professionals constitutes a multifaceted challenge. The successful integration of AI into healthcare workflows necessitates a delicate equilibrium between automation and human supervision. Ethical considerations play a pivotal role in determining the extent to which AI-driven decisions should influence medical practices, ensuring that patient care remains at the forefront. The introduction of AI in healthcare prompts critical questions about the roles and responsibilities of both automated systems and human experts. Striking the right balance is crucial; while AI can swiftly process vast amounts of data and offer rapid insights, it must not overshadow the vital expertise that human healthcare professionals bring to the table. Decisions with profound implications for patient well-being demand the empathy, clinical judgment, and contextual awareness that only human caregivers can provide. Muller and Weisz (2022) delve into these ethical complexities in their examination of machine learning implementation within healthcare. Their discourse highlights that ethical considerations must guide the development and deployment of AI systems, ensuring that the integration is aligned with the principles of patient-centered care and medical ethics. The authors emphasize that preserving human oversight and accountability is imperative to maintain a robust and ethical healthcare system.

Furthermore, the ethical challenges highlighted by Char et al. emphasize the need for transparency, explainability, and ongoing evaluation of AI-driven decisions. Healthcare professionals should have the capacity to understand how AI arrives at its conclusions, enabling them to make well-informed judgments about patient care. This not only builds trust in AI systems but also empowers healthcare practitioners to make decisions that are rooted in a holistic understanding of patient needs. The symbiotic relationship between AI systems and healthcare professionals presents a challenge that goes beyond technical integration. Ethical considerations demand that the role of AI is carefully calibrated to complement and enhance the expertise of human caregivers, rather than replace it. By maintaining this equilibrium, healthcare can harness the transformative capabilities of AI while upholding the core values of medical ethics and patient-centric care.

### Solution using XAI

XAI functions as a vital conduit between AI recommendations and healthcare professionals, fostering collaborative and well-informed patient care (Chen et al., 2022). By offering lucid and interpretable explanations for AI-generated suggestions, XAI empowers medical practitioners and patients to engage in insightful discussions about treatment plans, thereby promoting shared decision-making that seamlessly blends AI capabilities with human expertise. In the intricate interaction between healthcare professionals and AI systems, XAI plays a pivotal role in facilitating effective communication. Doctors can utilize explanations generated by XAI to transparently convey the reasoning behind AI recommendations to their patients (Adadi & Berrada, 2018). This transparency not only empowers patients to comprehend the basis for these recommendations but also fosters trust and active participation in their healthcare journey. Imagine a scenario where an AI system proposes a personalized treatment plan for a patient. The accompanying XAI explanation provides a comprehensive overview of the patient's medical history, genetic markers, and predicted responses to various treatment options. Equipped with this knowledge, doctors can engage in informed discussions with their patients. This collaborative approach ensures that patients are well-informed about the potential benefits and risks of each treatment choice, enabling them to make decisions that align with their values and preferences.

The convergence of XAI, AI systems, and healthcare professionals ushers in a transformative paradigm where the expertise of both machines and humans synergistically enhances patient outcomes (Caruana et al., 2015). The doctor-patient relationship advances into an era of shared decision-making, where AI-driven medical insights are interpreted and contextualized through human empathy and understanding. This harmonious interplay facilitates treatment plans rooted in data-driven predictions while also adapting to each patient's unique context and desires. XAI's capacity to provide understandable explanations for AI recommendations constitutes a cornerstone for collaboration between healthcare professionals and AI systems. By employing these explanations to facilitate dialogues between doctors and patients, XAI enriches the decision-making process, culminating in treatments that blend evidence-based insights with patient-centered care. This integration promises to shape a future where AI augments medical expertise while honoring the principles of informed consent and individualized healthcare.

For example, the integration of XAI in treatment recommendations showcases AI's potential to provide personalized healthcare solutions, with transparency that fosters informed patient-doctor collaboration (Antel et al., 2022). As AI evolves to recommend tailored treatment plans for individuals, XAI serves as a critical interface, enabling healthcare professionals to comprehend and communicate the underlying decision-making process to patients. The incorporation of AI into treatment recommendation introduces a paradigm shift where AI systems analyze extensive patient data, including medical history, genetic information, and current health status. Through advanced algorithms, AI generates personalized treatment suggestions aligned with a patient's unique health profile. The value of these recommendations is heightened when they are transparent and understandable to both medical experts and patients. XAI bridges this understanding gap by providing clear explanations for AI-generated treatment suggestions (Murdoch et al., 2019). These explanations offer a comprehensive breakdown of how the AI considered various factors—from medical history to genetic markers—to arrive at a specific recommendation. This interpretability empowers healthcare professionals to critically evaluate AI's rationale and underscores its alignment with clinical expertise.

For instance, consider a patient presented with multiple treatment options for a chronic condition. AI recommends a specific course of action based on a comprehensive analysis of the patient's data. XAI complements this recommendation by outlining how the AI model weighed the patient's past treatments, genetic predispositions, and current health metrics. When doctors possess this explanatory layer, they can engage patients in discussions about the AI-generated recommendation with confidence and clarity. In the patient-doctor interaction, XAI proves instrumental. Doctors leverage the explanations provided by XAI to elucidate the AI's methodology to patients. This step not only instills trust in the AI-driven decision but also empowers patients to actively participate in their treatment selection. Patients gain insights into the data points that influenced the recommendation, allowing them to make informed choices that align with their preferences and values. The application of XAI in treatment recommendation exemplifies the harmonious collaboration between AI systems and healthcare professionals. As AI advances its capacity to offer personalized treatment plans, XAI bridges the interpretability gap, enabling doctors to transparently communicate the rationale behind AI recommendations to patients. This synergy enriches the doctor-patient relationship, empowers informed decision-making, and underlines the potential of AI to enhance patient care.

### 5.6.6 Regulatory and Ethical Challenges

The advent of AI in healthcare has ushered in a new era of technological advancement, but it has also brought forth intricate regulatory and ethical challenges that demand careful consideration. The implications of accountability, transparency, and liability for decisions made by AI systems are pivotal factors that shape the ethical landscape of AI-enabled healthcare. In navigating these complexities, the work of Yu et al. (2018) provides valuable insights into the intersection of big data, machine learning, and healthcare, emphasizing the imperative of addressing regulatory and ethical dilemmas to ensure both patient safety and the responsible utilization of AI technologies (Arrieta et al., 2020). The issue of accountability takes center stage as AI systems increasingly contribute to medical decision-making. Determining who holds responsibility when an AI-driven diagnosis or treatment recommendation is involved raises intricate questions. It's paramount to establish mechanisms that attribute accountability to the appropriate parties, whether it's the developers of the AI algorithms, healthcare institutions, or healthcare professionals who interpret and act upon AI-generated insights. Transparency is another critical concern in the ethical application of AI in healthcare. Patients and healthcare professionals must have a clear understanding of how AI systems arrive at their decisions. The black-box nature of some AI algorithms can hinder this transparency, potentially eroding trust in AI-driven healthcare. Regulations should mandate transparent communication about AI's decision-making processes, enabling clinicians to validate and patients to comprehend the basis of AI recommendations.

Liability is intertwined with accountability and transparency. As AI systems become integrated into healthcare workflows, questions arise about legal responsibility in cases where AI contributes to medical errors or misdiagnoses. Regulatory frameworks should establish guidelines for assigning liability, ensuring that those who develop, deploy, and use AI technologies are accountable for their respective roles in the healthcare process. The work of Beam and Kohane (2018) underscores the urgency of addressing these regulatory and ethical challenges to safeguard patient well-being (Beam & Kohane, 2018). In their exploration of big data and machine learning in healthcare, they highlight that responsible AI deployment requires meticulous consideration of these dilemmas. A balance must be struck between promoting innovation and safeguarding ethical principles, ensuring that AI technologies enhance medical practices while upholding patient safety and welfare. The integration of AI in healthcare introduces complex regulatory and ethical challenges, such as accountability, transparency, and liability. Beam and Kohane's research serves as a guiding light, emphasizing the need to navigate these challenges systematically to ensure the responsible and ethical use of AI in healthcare. As AI continues to shape the medical landscape, addressing these concerns is crucial for establishing a foundation that prioritizes patient care, safety, and ethical integrity.

### Solution Using XAI

XAI emerges as a pivotal solution to address the intricate regulatory and ethical challenges posed by the integration of AI in healthcare. With accountability, transparency, and ethical oversight being paramount, XAI plays a crucial role in generating transparent and comprehensible explanations for AI-driven decisions, thereby aiding regulatory audits and ensuring ethical compliance. Regulatory bodies hold the responsibility of overseeing and upholding the standards of care within the healthcare industry. The advent of AI introduces a new layer of complexity, as decisions are increasingly influenced by algorithms. XAI provides a mechanism for regulatory bodies to review these AI-generated explanations, allowing them to assess whether the decisions align with established medical guidelines, safety protocols, and ethical norms (Chen et al., 2022). This level of transparency empowers regulatory authorities to evaluate the decisions made by AI systems with greater confidence and precision. Consider a scenario where an AI system is employed to select participants for a clinical trial. The participant selection process, when guided by AI, could be intricate and multifaceted, involving numerous patient characteristics, medical histories, and demographic information. XAI steps in to elucidate this complex process by generating explanations that outline how specific patient attributes were considered in the participant selection. These explanations serve as a comprehensive audit trail, providing regulatory bodies with the necessary insights to ensure that the trial's participant inclusion adheres to ethical and legal standards (Lysaght et al., 2019).

The collaboration between XAI and regulatory oversight contributes to a transparent, accountable, and ethically sound AI-enabled healthcare environment. XAI bridges the gap between the technical complexity of AI systems and the need for understandable, verifiable decision-making processes. Regulatory agencies gain the ability to verify that AI-generated decisions are both medically sound and ethically justifiable, paving the way for responsible AI deployment in healthcare. XAI acts as a cornerstone in addressing the regulatory and ethical complexities of AI integration in healthcare. By generating transparent explanations for AI decisions, it empowers regulatory bodies to conduct thorough audits and oversight, ensuring that AI systems operate within established guidelines and ethical principles. This synergy of AI, XAI, and regulatory scrutiny shapes a future where healthcare innovation is balanced with patient safety, ethical considerations, and regulatory compliance.

## Application: Clinical Trials

The application of XAI in the context of clinical trials exemplifies how AI's capabilities can be harnessed to enhance transparency, regulatory compliance, and ethical considerations. As AI systems assist in identifying potential candidates for clinical trials based on intricate patient profiles, XAI emerges as a critical tool to shed light on the rationale behind patient selection, thereby ensuring a robust and ethically accountable trial recruitment process. Clinical trials are fundamental to advancing medical knowledge and treatment options, but the selection of appropriate participants is a nuanced process influenced by numerous variables. AI has the capacity to analyze vast amounts of patient data to pinpoint individuals who align with specific trial criteria. However, the decision-making process of AI might seem opaque and complex to stakeholders, raising concerns about transparency and fairness. This is where XAI comes into play. XAI enables AI systems to generate explanations that outline why certain patients were selected for a clinical trial. These explanations provide a comprehensive breakdown of the factors and attributes considered by the AI model during the participant selection process. Regulatory authorities, ethics committees, and healthcare professionals can then review these explanations to ensure that patient selection adheres to ethical norms and regulatory requirements.

Imagine a scenario where an AI system is tasked with identifying participants for a clinical trial studying a novel treatment for a rare disease. The AI system analyzes a myriad of patient data points, including medical history, genetic markers, and disease progression. XAI generates explanations that elucidate how the AI model weighed these variables and determined the suitability of certain patients for the trial. These explanations serve as a clear audit trail, offering a transparent window into the AI's decision-making process. By incorporating XAI into the clinical trial recruitment process, the journey toward regulatory compliance and ethical transparency is significantly enhanced. The insights provided by XAI not only empower stakeholders to comprehend the AI-driven decisions but also foster trust in the selection process. Ethical considerations are upheld as the selection of participants is rooted in understandable, verifiable, and unbiased decision-making. The fusion of AI and XAI in clinical trial participant selection embodies a harmonious integration of technological advancement and ethical accountability. The utilization of AI's analytical capabilities, coupled with XAI's explanatory power, ensures that participant selection remains transparent and aligned with ethical principles. This dynamic synergy reshapes the landscape of clinical trials, underscoring the potential of AI to enrich medical research while adhering to regulatory standards and ethical imperatives.

## 5.7 HOW XAI HELPS IN CANCER PREDICTION AND TREATMENT

XAI emerges as the most enabling in a complex cancer prognostic setting with a combination of variables including genetic predisposition, lifestyle characteristics, and personal medical history Multidimensional cancer requires predictive models to accurately describe this complexity. XAI techniques such as SHAP (Shapley additive explanation) and LIME (local interpretable model-agnostic explanation) to fully unpack this complex network. Through SHAP objectives, XAI calculates the specific contributions of each component in all possible combinations of factors, providing a nuanced understanding of how the AI model's decisions are shaped. Simultaneously, LIME deconstructs the input data to construct a more simplified and interpretable surrogate model, illuminating the localized behavior of the intricate AI model. This profound grasp of feature significance and local behavior empowers medical professionals and researchers alike to comprehend the intricate interplay between genetic markers, lifestyle variables, and the onset of cancer. By deciphering these underlying biological interactions, XAI bolsters the model's predictive accuracy and amplifies the depth of medical insights. XAI's purview transcends the mere unraveling of concealed patterns; it assumes the role of a transformative catalyst in nurturing interdisciplinary collaboration. The transparency facilitated by XAI fosters a shared dialect among medical experts, data scientists, and domain specialists. In the complex landscape of cancer prediction, where accurate clinical knowledge and algorithmic finesse are paramount, this cross-disciplinary discourse becomes invaluable. XAI mechanisms not only facilitate model validation by elucidating the intricate correlation between specific biomarkers or genetic mutations and predictions, but also empower medical experts to corroborate the model's outcomes with their clinical acumen. This iterative interaction ensures predictions resonate with established medical understanding. Additionally, data scientists gain access to specialized insights from medical experts, refining the model to mirror the complex intricacies of cancer's underlying biology.

XAI facilitates the early detection of critical changes in a patient's health indicators, thereby enabling the timely identification of potential cancer recurrence or treatment-related side effects. The influence of XAI extends to patient engagement, forging a bridge between intricate AI-generated insights and patient comprehension. By communicating these insights in an understandable manner, XAI aids patients in comprehending their health status. Armed with this knowledge, patients can make well-informed decisions pertaining to lifestyle modifications and follow-up actions, thereby actively participating in their own care journey. For instance, consider the domain of lung cancer monitoring. XAI can intricately elucidate the reasons behind fluctuations in specific biomarkers. In a scenario where a decline in lung capacity correlates with a certain treatment, XAI's insight could prompt doctors to refine the treatment plan to mitigate potential adverse effects. This interaction of AI-driven insights with clinical expertise ensures that patient care is not only data-driven but also deeply personalized and responsive.

Throughout these critical stages of cancer management, XAI assumes the role of a harmonizing force, effectively translating the complexity of AI algorithms into actionable insights that resonate with both medical professionals and patients. This enhanced understanding fosters trust, cultivates collaboration, and fortifies the partnership between caregivers, patients, and the intricate realm of AI-driven healthcare. In sum, XAI contributes to heightened accuracy in predictions, customization of treatments, vigilant monitoring, and ultimately reinforces the collective endeavor against cancer.

## 5.8 COMPARISON OF AI VS. XAI

- **Focus:** AI focuses on achieving high accuracy and predictive performance, while XAI focuses on providing explanations and increasing the understandability, transparency, and accountability of AI systems.
- **Interpretability:** Traditional AI models, such as deep learning neural networks, can be highly complex and difficult to interpret. They often operate as "black boxes," making it

challenging to understand how they arrive at their predictions or decisions (Gunning et al., 2019) XAI techniques focus on providing explanations for AI models' decisions. By using specific algorithms or methods, XAI aims to make AI models interpretable by generating human-understandable explanations for their outputs (Gilpin et al., 2017).

- **Trust and Transparency:** The lack of transparency in AI models can raise concerns about trust and accountability (Zolanvari et al., 2021). When AI models make critical decisions, it becomes important to understand the rationale behind those decisions to ensure their reliability and fairness. XAI techniques address the need for transparency and trust by enabling users to understand and verify the reasoning behind AI models' outputs. By providing explanations, XAI helps build confidence in the decisions made by AI systems, increasing their accountability.
- **Performance vs. Explainability Trade-off:** AI models are often optimized for performance and accuracy. Complex models like deep neural networks can achieve high predictive accuracy but may sacrifice explainability in the process. XAI acknowledges the trade-off between performance and explainability. While XAI techniques aim to provide explanations, they may introduce some level of complexity and potentially impact the model's predictive performance to ensure transparency.
- **Application Areas:** AI has a broad range of applications across various domains (Pannu, 2015), including healthcare, finance, transportation, and more. Its primary goal is to automate tasks, make predictions, and optimize outcomes (Albert, 2019). XAI techniques are particularly relevant in domains where interpretability and explainability are crucial, such as healthcare, finance, legal systems, and any other context where human decision-makers need to understand and justify the AI systems' outputs (Kotriwala et al., 2021).

$$AI = f(X)$$

where:
- AI is the output of the AI system.
- X is the input data to the AI system.
- f is the function that maps X to AI.

In other words, AI is a function that takes in data and produces an output. The function f can be complex and difficult to understand, which is why AI systems are often referred to as "black boxes" Panigutti et al. (2020).

XAI, on the other hand, is a set of techniques that can be used to explain the function f. This can be done by providing insights into how the AI system makes its decisions. For example, XAI techniques can be used to identify the most important features that the AI system uses to make its predictions.

By providing explanations, XAI can help to make AI systems more transparent and understandable. This can lead to increased trust and confidence in AI systems, which is essential for their successful adoption in a variety of domains. A summarized version of the earlier comparison is shown in Figure 5.8.

## 5.9  LEGAL PERSPECTIVE

The XAI has major implications for openness, accountability, and justice in the context of AI systems from a legal standpoint. In order to ensure that AI algorithms' decision-making processes can be understood and legitimated legally, XAI addresses the requirement to give interpretability and explanations for them. As Kaur and Gupta (2022) discuss, the right to explanation, which is protected by legislation such as the General Data Protection Regulation (GDPR), is an important legal factor. By producing explanations that help people comprehend the reasoning, importance, and

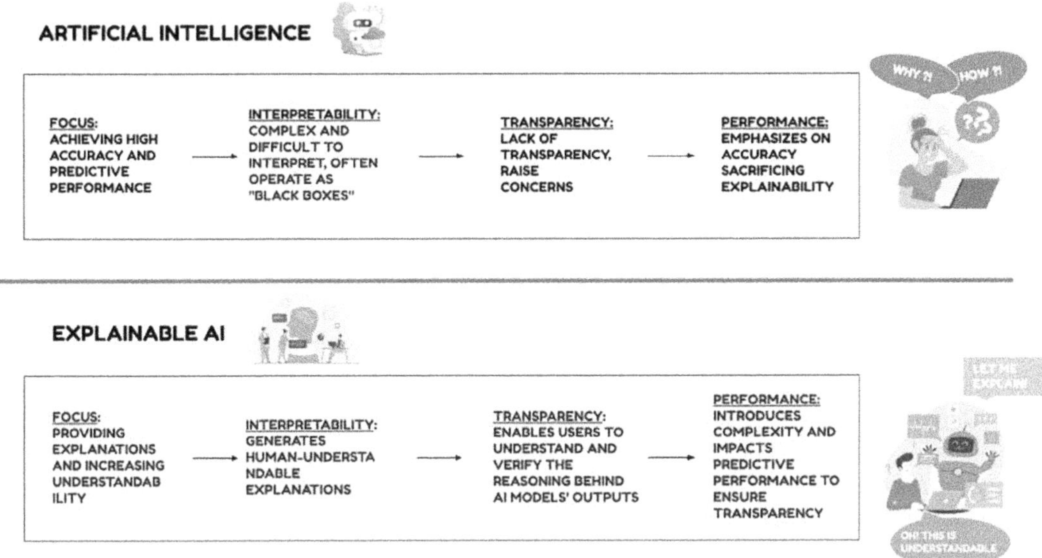


**FIGURE 5.8** AI vs. XAI comparison.

effects of automated choices that affect them, XAI plays a critical part in upholding this right. This openness is crucial for upholding the law and guaranteeing that people can successfully exercise their rights.

Furthermore, XAI is instrumental in addressing fairness and non-discrimination concerns. AI systems must adhere to anti-discrimination laws, and XAI techniques can help identify and mitigate biases or unfair practices. As Goodman and Flaxman (2016) argue, "the risks of machine bias are real and serious," and XAI can help to mitigate these risks. Finally, XAI can also play a role in addressing liability concerns. If an AI system causes harm, it is important to be able to understand how the system made its decision in order to determine who is liable. XAI can help to provide this understanding, which can be critical in holding the responsible parties accountable. Overall, XAI has the potential to significantly improve the fairness, accountability, and transparency of AI systems. By providing interpretable explanations for AI decisions, XAI can help to ensure that these decisions are made in a fair and just manner and that people can hold those responsible for AI harms accountable.

## 5.10　CHALLENGES

XAI has promising benefits but also problems in Healthcare 5.0. Key challenges include:

1. The Complexity of Healthcare Data: Healthcare data is vast, heterogeneous, and often unstructured, including electronic health records, medical images, genomic data, wearable device data, and more. Extracting meaningful explanations from such complex and diverse data sources poses challenges in terms of data integration, preprocessing, and feature extraction to generate accurate and interpretable explanations (Kaur & Gupta, 2022).
2. Interpretability-Performance Trade-off: Achieving high interpretability may come at the cost of performance. Highly complex AI models often provide superior predictive accuracy but lack interpretability. Balancing the need for accurate predictions with the requirement for understandable explanations is a challenge that needs to be addressed in Healthcare 5.0 (Lipton, 2018).

3. Black-Box AI Models: Many AI models used in healthcare, such as deep learning models, are inherently black-box, making it difficult to understand their internal workings and provide explanations for their decisions. Incorporating XAI techniques into these black-box models and generating reliable explanations without sacrificing accuracy is a significant challenge (Rudin, 2019).
4. Dynamic and Evolving Healthcare Domain: Healthcare is a rapidly evolving field with continuous advancements in medical research, treatment guidelines, and technology. Incorporating these dynamic changes in XAI systems pose challenges in terms of adapting and updating the rule-based explanations or generating reliable explanations for evolving models.
5. Legal and Regulatory Compliance: The use of AI in healthcare is subject to strict legal and regulatory frameworks, such as privacy regulations (e.g., GDPR, HIPAA) and ethical guidelines. Ensuring that XAI systems comply with these regulations, such as protecting patient privacy while providing explanations, presents challenges in designing and implementing robust and compliant XAI solutions.
6. User Acceptance and Trust: Healthcare professionals, patients, and stakeholders may have reservations or lack trust in AI systems due to their perceived complexity, lack of transparency, or fear of replacing human expertise. Bridging the gap between AI algorithms and human decision-makers, providing understandable explanations, and fostering trust in XAI systems are critical challenges to address for widespread adoption.
7. Integration into Clinical Workflows: Introducing XAI into existing clinical workflows can be challenging (Sivamohan & Sridhar, 2023). Healthcare professionals may already have limited time and resources, and incorporating XAI tools may require additional training and integration with existing systems. Ensuring seamless integration of XAI into clinical workflows without disrupting efficiency and productivity is a significant challenge.

Researchers, healthcare providers, lawmakers, and regulators must collaborate to address these issues. To address these hurdles and maximize XAI's potential in Healthcare 5.0, XAI research, data standardization, privacy protection, and interdisciplinary collaboration must continue. The list of above challenges is summarized in Figure 5.9.

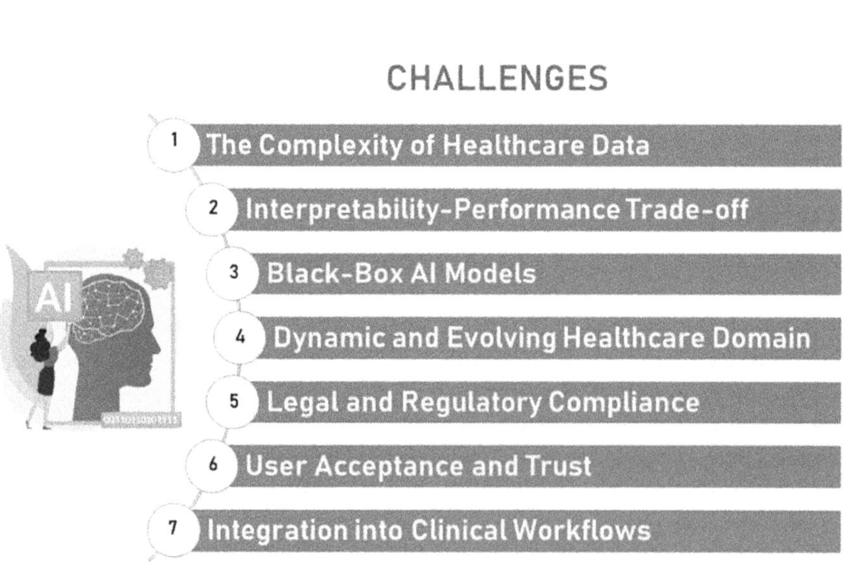

**FIGURE 5.9** Challenges of XAI.

## 5.11  OPPORTUNITIES OR FUTURE DIRECTION

In Healthcare 5.0, XAI could improve patient care, clinical decision-making, and healthcare system efficiency. Five possible XAI applications in Healthcare 5.0:

1. Personalized Treatment and Precision Medicine: XAI can help personalize treatment and enable precision medicine. XAI can build patient trust and enable healthcare providers to customize treatments based on genetic profiles, medical histories, and lifestyle factors by explaining treatment suggestions.
2. XAI can improve clinical decision-making in CDSS. XAI can assist healthcare practitioners in making better decisions by explaining AI model recommendations and forecasts. XAI can detect CDSS biases, faults, and restrictions to ensure safe and effective use.
3. Fraud Detection and Healthcare Management: XAI can analyze enormous amounts of healthcare data and explain suspicious actions or anomalies. It can detect fraudulent claims, misuse, and abuse and provide transparent reasoning, promoting effective healthcare resource allocation and cost control.
4. Patient Monitoring and Remote Care: XAI provides real-time explanations for AI-based forecasts and alarms to enable remote patient monitoring and care. It improves patient engagement, adherence, and remote care efficacy by explaining health status updates, treatment recommendations, and risk assessments.
5. Healthcare Ethical and Regulatory Compliance: XAI can help. It can assist healthcare organizations demonstrate fairness, privacy protection, and legal and ethical compliance by making AI models' decisions transparent and accountable. XAI enables auditable systems, allowing stakeholders to check and validate decision-making processes, increasing confidence and regulatory compliance.

XAI in Healthcare 5.0 will use explainability to improve personalized medicine, clinical decision-making, fraud detection, healthcare management, remote care, and ethical and regulatory compliance. These advances could transform healthcare, enhance patient outcomes, and build trust in AI technologies in healthcare.

## 5.12  CONCLUSION AND FUTURE SCOPE

XAI plays a crucial role in Healthcare 5.0 by enhancing transparency and trust in AI-driven healthcare systems. It employs techniques like rule-based, model-based, and post-hoc explainability to offer understandable explanations for AI model decision-making. This allows clinicians and patients to grasp the reasoning behind these decisions. Transparent and interpretable AI models through XAI significantly improve safety and effectiveness in healthcare applications. One major advantage is the potential to transform disease detection, diagnosis, and treatment, leading to better patient outcomes. XAI enables healthcare professionals to comprehend and validate AI model decisions, facilitating informed medical interventions. However, incorporating XAI in healthcare presents challenges. Interpretable deep learning models are difficult due to their complexity. Techniques like feature visualization, attention mechanisms, and saliency mapping address this challenge. Ethical concerns also arise, stemming from biases, discrimination, or privacy breaches in AI decision-making. Ensuring fairness, accountability, and privacy is crucial in designing and deploying XAI systems. Rigorous validation, governance frameworks, and regulatory guidelines are necessary. By addressing these challenges, responsible use of XAI can lead to a more efficient healthcare system. Trust among clinicians and patients grows as XAI provides understandable explanations, fostering acceptance and adoption of AI-driven healthcare. Ultimately, Healthcare 5.0 can deliver improved patient care, better clinical decision-making, and enhanced health outcomes.

## REFERENCES

Adadi, A., & Berrada, M. (2018). Peeking inside the Black-box: A survey on Explainable Artificial Intelligence (XAI). *IEEE Access*, 6, 52138–52160.

Albert, E. T. (2019). AI in talent acquisition: a review of AI-applications used in recruitment and selection. *Strategic HR Review*, 18(5), 215–221.

Altmann, A., Toloşi, L., Sander, O., & Lengauer, T. (2010). Permutation importance: A corrected feature importance measure. *Bioinformatics*, 26(10), 1340–1347.

Antel, R., Abbasgholizadeh-Rahimi, S., Guadagno, E., Harley, J. M., & Poenaru, D. (2022). The use of artificial intelligence and virtual reality in doctor-patient risk communication: A scoping review. *Patient Education and Counseling*, 105(10), 3038–3050.

Arrieta, A. B., Díaz-Rodríguez, N., Del Ser, J., Bennetot, A., Tabik, S., Barbado, A., . . . Herrera, F. (2020). Explainable Artificial Intelligence (XAI): Concepts, taxonomies, opportunities and challenges toward responsible AI. *Information Fusion*, 58, 82–115.

Bhattacharya, P., Obaidat, M. S., Savaliya, D., Sanghavi, S., Tanwar, S., & Sadaun, B. (2022, July). Metaverse assisted telesurgery in healthcare 5.0: An interplay of blockchain and explainable AI. In *2022 International Conference on Computer, Information and Telecommunication Systems (CITS)* (pp. 1–5). IEEE.

Bobek, S., Bałaga, P., & Nalepa, G. J. (2021, June). Towards model-agnostic ensemble explanations. In *International Conference on Computational Science* (pp. 39–51). Cham: Springer International Publishing.

Caruana, R., Lou, Y., Gehrke, J., Koch, P., Sturm, M., & Elhadad, N. (2015). Intelligible models for healthcare: Predicting pneumonia risk and hospital 30-day readmission. In *Proceedings of the 21th ACM SIGKDD International Conference on Knowledge Discovery and Data Mining (KDD '15)* (pp. 1721–1730). New York: Association for Computing Machinery. https://doi.org/10.1145/2783258.2788613

Chen, X., Cheng, G., Wang, F. L., Tao, X., Xie, H., & Xu, L. (2022). Machine and cognitive intelligence for human health: Systematic review. *Brain Informatics*, 9(1), 5.

Choi, E., Schuetz, A., Stewart, W. F., & Sun, J. (2016). Using recurrent neural network models for early detection of heart failure onset. *Journal of the American Medical Informatics Association*, 24(2), 361–370.

Darias, J. M., Díaz-Agudo, B., & Recio-Garcia, J. A. (2021, September). A systematic review on model-agnostic XAI libraries. In *ICCBR Workshops* (pp. 28–39). https://ceur-ws.org/Vol-3017/96.pdf

Doshi-Velez, F., & Kim, B. (2017). Towards a rigorous science of interpretable machine learning. *arXiv preprint arXiv:1702.08608*.

Emanuel, E. J., & Wachter, R. M. (2019). Artificial intelligence in health care: Will the value match the hype?. *JAMA*, 321(23), 2281–2282.

Finegold, D. (2017). 17 The role of education and training systems in innovation. In Jerald Hage and Marius Meeus (Eds.), *Innovation, Science, and Institutional Change*. Oxford: Oxford Academic. https://doi.org/10.1093/oso/9780199299195.003.0020

Frank, J. R., Snell, L., Englander, R., Holmboe, E. S., & Icbme Collaborators. (2017). Implementing competency-based medical education: Moving forward. *Medical Teacher*, 39(6), 568–573.

Gianfagna, L., & Di Cecco, A. (2021). Model-agnostic methods for XAI. In *Explainable AI with Python* (pp. 81–113). Cham: Springer International Publishing.

Gilpin, H. R., Keyes, A., Stahl, D. R., Greig, R., & McCracken, L. M. (2017). Predictors of treatment outcome in contextual cognitive and behavioral therapies for chronic pain: A systematic review. *The Journal of Pain*, 18(10), 1153–1164.

Goodman, B., & Flaxman, S. (2016, June). EU regulations on algorithmic decision-making and a "right to explanation". In *ICML Workshop on Human Interpretability in Machine Learning (WHI 2016)*, New York. http://arxiv. org/abs/1606.08813 v1

Guidotti, R., Monreale, A., Ruggieri, S., Turini, F., Giannotti, F., & Pedreschi, D. (2018). A survey of methods for explaining black box models. *ACM Computing Surveys (CSUR)*, 51(5), 1–42.

Guidotti, R., Monreale, A., Ruggieri, S., Turini, F., Giannotti, F., & Pedreschi, D. (2020). A survey of methods for explaining Black box models. *ACM Computing Surveys (CSUR)*, 51(5), 1–42.

Gunning, D., Stefik, M., Choi, J., Miller, T., Stumpf, S., & Yang, G. Z. (2019). XAI—explainable artificial intelligence. *Science Robotics*, 4(37), eaay7120.

Kaur, G., & Gupta, A. (2022). Open educational resources in legal studies: An analytical account. *Constructivism in Teaching and Learning*, 135.

Kotriwala, A., Klöpper, B., Dix, M., Gopalakrishnan, G., Ziobro, D., & Potschka, A. (2021). XAI for operations in the process industry-applications, theses, and research directions. In *AAAI Spring Symposium: Combining Machine Learning with Knowledge Engineering* (pp. 1–12). https://api.semanticscholar.org/CorpusID:233354942

Lipton, Z. C. (2018). The mythos of model interpretability: In machine learning, the concept of interpretability is both important and slippery. *Queue*, 16(3), 31–57.

Lundberg, S. (2017). A unified approach to interpreting model predictions. *arXiv preprint arXiv:1705.07874*.

Lysaght, T., Lim, H. Y., Xafis, V., & Ngiam, K. Y. (2019). AI-assisted decision-making in healthcare: The application of an ethics framework for big data in health and research. *Asian Bioethics Review*, 11, 299–314.

Madlon-Kay, D. J., & Mosch, F. S. (2000). Liquid medication dosing errors. *Journal of Family Practice*, 49(8).

Miotto, R., Li, L., Kidd, B. A., & Dudley, J. T. (2016). Deep patient: An unsupervised representation to predict the future of patients from the electronic health records. *Scientific Reports*, 6, 26094.

Mohseni, S., Zarei, N., & Ragan, E. D. (2018). A multidisciplinary survey and framework for design and evaluation of XAI systems. *arXiv:1811.11839*.

Molnar, C. (2017). Interpretability in machine learning: A survey. *arXiv preprint arXiv:1702.0Bias and Fairness*.

Molnar, C. (2019). Explainable artificial intelligence: Concepts, taxonomies, opportunities and challenges. *arXiv preprint arXiv:1811.12808*.

Montavon, G., Samek, W., & Müller, K. R. (2018a). Explainable AI: Concepts, taxonomies, opportunities and challenges for the human-AI partnership. In *Springer Briefs in Cognitive Computation* (pp. 1–23). https://doi.org/10.1007/978-3-319-63916-6

Montavon, G., Samek, W., & Müller, K. R. (2018b). Methods for interpreting and understanding deep neural networks. *Digital Signal Processing*, 73, 1–15.

Morton, R. S. (1966). Education of the public about venereal diseases. Some views of venereologists. *British Journal of Venereal Diseases*, 42(4), 238.

Muller, M., & Weisz, J. (2022, June). Extending a human-ai collaboration framework with dynamism and sociality. In *Proceedings of the 1st Annual Meeting of the Symposium on Human-Computer Interaction for Work* (pp. 1–12).

Murdoch, W. J., Singh, C., Kumbier, K., Abbasi-Asl, R., & Yu, B. (2019). Definitions, methods, and applications in interpretable machine learning. *Proceedings of the National Academy of Sciences*, 116(44), 22071–22080.

Obermeyer, Z., Powers, B., Vogeli, C., & Mullainathan, S. (2019). Dissecting racial bias in an algorithm used to manage the health of populations. *Science*, 366(6464), 447–453.

Panigutti, C., Perotti, A., & Pedreschi, D. (2020, January). Doctor XAI: An ontology-based approach to blackbox sequential data classification explanations. In *Proceedings of the 2020 Conference on Fairness, Accountability, and Transparency* (pp. 629–639). New York: Association for Computing Machinery. https://doi.org/10.1145/3351095.3372855

Pannu, A. (2015). Artificial intelligence and its application in different areas. *Artificial Intelligence*, 4(10), 79–84.

Rajkomar, A., Oren, E., Chen, K., Dai, A. M., Hajaj, N., Hardt, M., . . . Zhang, K. (2018). Scalable and accurate deep learning with electronic health records. *NPJ Digital Medicine*, 1(1), 1–10.

Ribeiro, M. T., Singh, S., & Guestrin, C. (2016a). "Why should I trust you?" Explaining the predictions of any classifier. In *Proceedings of the 22nd ACM SIGKDD International Conference on Knowledge Discovery and Data Mining* (pp. 1135–1144). New York: Association for Computing Machinery. https://doi.org/10.1145/2939672.2939778

Ribeiro, M. T., Singh, S., & Guestrin, C. (2016b). Towards a rigorous science of interpretable machine learning. *arXiv preprint arXiv:1602.04938*.

Rudin, C. (2019). Stop explaining black box machine learning models for high stakes decisions and use interpretable models instead. *Nature Machine Intelligence*, 1(5), 206–215.

Saravanan, S., Ramkumar, K., Adalarasu, K., Sivanandam, V., Kumar, S. R., Stalin, S., & Amirtharajan, R. (2022). A systematic review of artificial intelligence (AI) based approaches for the diagnosis of Parkinson's disease. *Archives of Computational Methods in Engineering*, 29(6), 3639–3653.

Saravanan, S., Ramkumar, K., Narasimhan, K., Subramaniyaswamy, V., Kotecha, K., & Abraham, A. (2023). Explainable Artificial Intelligence (XAI) models for early prediction of parkinson's disease based on spiral and wave drawings. *IEEE Access*, 11, 68366–68378. https://doi.org/10.1109/ACCESS.2023.3291406

Selvaraju, R. R., Cogswell, M., Das, A., Vedantam, R., Parikh, D., & Batra, D. (2017). Grad-cam: Visual explanations from deep networks via gradient-based localization. In *Proceedings of the IEEE International Conference on Computer Vision* (pp. 618–626).

Shaban-Nejad, A., Michalowski, M., & Buckeridge, D. L. (2020). XAI in healthcare and medicine: Building a culture of transparency and accountability. *Proceedings AAAI International Workshop Health Intelligence (W3PHIAI)*, vol. 914.

Singh, S., & Ribeiro, M. T. (2020). Explainable AI for human-computer collaboration. *arXiv preprint arXiv:2003.01303*.

Sivamohan, S., & Sridhar, S. S. (2023). An optimized model for network intrusion detection systems in industry 4.0 using XAI based Bi-LSTM framework. *Neural Computing and Applications*, 35(15), 11459–11475.

Yu, K. H., Beam, A. L., & Kohane, I. S. (2018). Artificial intelligence in healthcare. *Nature Biomedical Engineering*, 2(10), 719–731.

Zhang, J., Fang, Y., & Cui, Y. (2018). Explainable artificial intelligence: Progress, challenges and prospects. *Nature Machine Intelligence*, 1(8), 369–376.

Zolanvari, M., Yang, Z., Khan, K., Jain, R., & Meskin, N. (2021). Trust xai: Model-agnostic explanations for ai with a case study on iiot security. *IEEE Internet of Things Journal*, 10(4), 2967–2978.

# 6 Explainable AI for Healthcare 5.0—Enhancing Transparency and Trust

*Deepa S, Vinay M, Jayapriya J, and Sundaravadivazhagan B*

## 6.1 INTRODUCTION

### 6.1.1 BACKGROUND OF AI IN HEALTHCARE

The background of AI in healthcare provides an overview of the application and development of artificial intelligence (AI) technologies in the healthcare domain.

AI has gained significant attention in healthcare due to its potential to revolutionize various aspects of the industry. The background section discusses the emergence of AI in healthcare and its evolution over time.

Initially, AI in healthcare focused on rule-based systems and expert systems, which utilized pre-defined rules and algorithms to make decisions or provide recommendations. These systems were primarily used in areas like medical diagnosis, treatment planning, and decision support.

With the advancements in machine learning and data availability, AI in healthcare has shifted toward more data-driven approaches. Machine learning algorithms, such as neural networks, support vector machines, and random forests, have been applied to analyze large healthcare datasets and make predictions or classifications. This has enabled AI systems to perform tasks like disease diagnosis, risk assessment, treatment optimization, and patient monitoring.

The background section may also highlight the impact of AI on healthcare outcomes. AI technologies have shown promising results in improving diagnostic accuracy, identifying patterns and trends in patient data, and assisting healthcare professionals in making evidence-based decisions. They have the potential to enhance patient care, reduce medical errors, optimize resource allocation, and contribute to personalized medicine.

Furthermore, the background section may discuss the challenges and limitations associated with AI in healthcare. These challenges include the need for large and high-quality datasets, concerns about data privacy and security, ethical considerations, regulatory requirements, and the interpretability of AI models.

Overall, the background of AI in healthcare provides the context for understanding the current state of AI technology in the field, its applications, and the challenges and opportunities it presents for improving healthcare delivery.

#### 6.1.1.1 The History of AI in Healthcare

The history of artificial intelligence in healthcare offers a general overview of the use and advancement of AI technology in the healthcare industry.

Because it has the potential to completely transform a number of sectors of the healthcare sector, AI has attracted a lot of attention in this area. The history of AI in healthcare is covered in the background section, along with how it has changed through time.

Rule-based systems and expert systems, which used predefined rules and algorithms to make judgments or offer suggestions, were initially the emphasis of AI in healthcare. These systems were mostly employed in decision assistance, treatment planning, and medical diagnostics.

With the advancements in machine learning and data availability, AI in healthcare has shifted toward more data-driven approaches. Machine learning algorithms, such as neural networks, support vector machines, and random forests, have been applied to analyze large healthcare datasets and make predictions or classifications. This has enabled AI systems to perform tasks like disease diagnosis, risk assessment, treatment optimization, and patient monitoring.

The background section may also highlight the impact of AI on healthcare outcomes. AI technologies shown the promising results in improving diagnostic accuracy, identifying patterns and trends in data, and assisting healthcare professionals in making evidence-based decisions. They have the potential to enhance patient care, reduce medical errors, optimize resource allocation, and contribute to personalized medicine.

Furthermore, the background section may discuss the challenges and limitations associated with AI in healthcare. The challenges include the need for large and high-quality datasets, data privacy and security, ethical considerations and the interpretability of AI models.

The background of AI in healthcare provides the understanding the current state of AI technology in the field, its applications, and the challenges and opportunities it presents for improving healthcare delivery.

### 6.1.2 Evolution of Healthcare toward Version 5.0

The evolution of healthcare toward version 5.0 signifies the transition and advancement of healthcare systems and practices through the integration of emerging technologies, including Artificial Intelligence (AI), data analytics, and patient-centric approaches. This section explores the key characteristics shown in Figure 6.1 and drivers behind the evolution of healthcare toward version 5.0.

**Healthcare 1.0:** The foundation of healthcare systems was built on traditional paper-based records and manual processes (World Health Organization, 2019). Healthcare professionals relied on handwritten notes and physical documents for patient information and treatment.

**Healthcare 2.0:** The introduction of digital technologies, a shift toward digitization in healthcare. Electronic health records (EHRs) replaced paper records, enabling easier storage, retrieval, and sharing of patient data. This digital transformation improved the efficiency of healthcare processes.

**Healthcare 3.0:** Healthcare systems progressed toward data integration and interoperability in this phase. Efforts were made to connect various healthcare systems and data sources to facilitate seamless data exchange and collaboration (Topol, 2019). Interoperability standards, such as HL7 and FHIR, were developed to enable the sharing of healthcare data across different systems and providers.

**Healthcare 4.0:** The fourth phase witnessed the integration of AI, machine learning, and data analytics into healthcare systems. AI algorithms are applied to analyze vast amounts of patient data and extract insights for decision-making, diagnosis, and treatment. This phase the emergence of predictive analytics, precision medicine, and personalized healthcare approaches.

**Healthcare 5.0:** Healthcare systems are currently progressing toward version 5.0, which represents a patient-centric paradigm empowered by advanced technologies. The key characteristics of Healthcare 5.0 include:

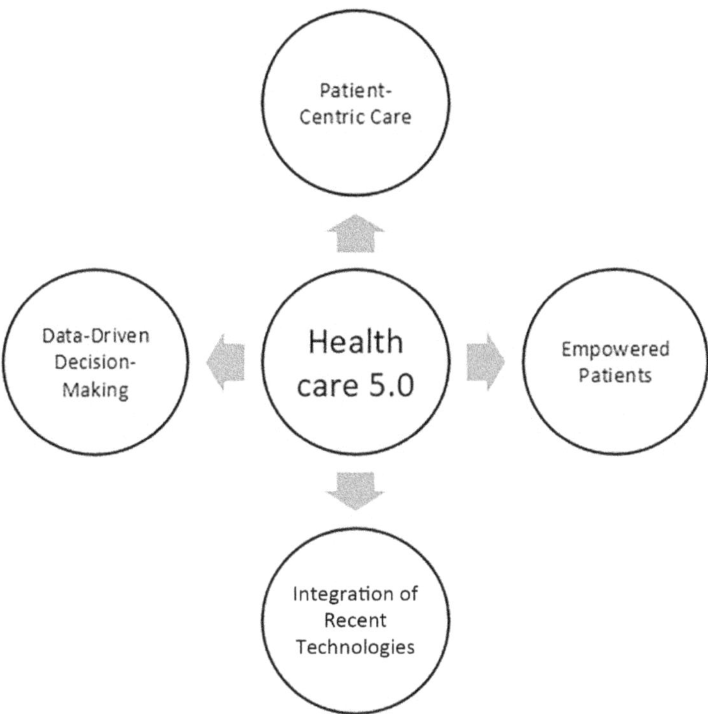


**FIGURE 6.1**  Key characteristics of Healthcare 5.0.

a. Patient-Centric Care: The focus shifts from a disease-centered approach to personalized, patient-centric care. Healthcare systems aim to understand patients' unique needs, preferences, and circumstances to provide tailored treatment plans and interventions (Bates et al., 2014).

b. Empowered Patients: Patients play an active role in their healthcare decisions and have access to their health data. Patient engagement is promoted through tools like patient portals, wearable devices, and telehealth solutions, enabling individuals to monitor their health, participate in shared decision-making, and take proactive steps toward preventive care.

c. Data-Driven Decision-Making: Advanced data analytics, AI, and machine learning techniques are leveraged to derive meaningful insights from vast healthcare datasets. Predictive modeling, real-time monitoring, and risk assessment help in making evidence-based decisions, improving treatment outcomes, and optimizing resource allocation.

d. Integration of Recent Technologies: Healthcare 5.0 integrates technologies like AI, robotics, and the Internet of Things (IoT) to enhance healthcare delivery. Robotics assist in surgical procedures, IoT devices enable remote monitoring, and virtual reality offers immersive training experiences for healthcare professionals.

The evolution of healthcare toward version 5.0 is driven by the need to improve patient outcomes, enhance the patient experience, and optimize healthcare delivery. It leverages the potential of AI and emerging technologies to create a patient-centric, data-driven, and technologically empowered healthcare ecosystem.

### 6.1.3  IMPORTANCE OF EXPLAINABLE AI IN HEALTHCARE

Explainable AI (XAI) is of paramount importance in the healthcare domain due to several reasons:

Transparency and Trust: Healthcare professionals and patients need to trust AI systems to make informed decisions. Explainability provides transparency by offering clear explanations of how AI models arrive at their conclusions or recommendations. This transparency fosters trust among healthcare providers, patients, and regulatory bodies (Carvalho & Freitas, 2019).

Clinical Decision-Making: In critical healthcare decisions, such as diagnosis and treatment planning, explainability is essential. Clinicians need to understand the reasoning behind AI-generated recommendations to validate their accuracy, assess potential biases, and tailor the recommendations to individual patient needs. Explainable AI empowers clinicians to make well-informed decisions by providing understandable insights (Mittelstadt, 2019).

Ethical and Legal Considerations: AI systems must adhere to ethical principles and legal regulations. Explainability helps identify potential biases, discriminatory practices, or unfair treatment in AI algorithms. By making the decision-making process transparent, explainable AI enables compliance with ethical guidelines, such as fairness, accountability, and transparency principles (Gunning & Aha, 2019).

Safety and Error Detection: In healthcare, errors can have severe consequences. By providing explanations, AI systems can help identify and rectify potential errors, reducing the risk of misdiagnosis or inappropriate treatment (Brundage et al., 2020). Explainability allows for error detection, validation of results, and mitigating potential harm to patients.

Regulatory Compliance: Healthcare is subject to numerous regulations and standards, including data privacy and security requirements. Explainable AI aids compliance with these regulations by providing insights into data usage, algorithmic decision-making, and auditability (Lipton, 2018). Regulators can assess and verify the compliance of AI systems, ensuring patient data protection and system accountability.

Learning and Improvement: Explainability facilitates the continuous improvement of AI systems. By understanding the decision-making process, healthcare professionals can provide feedback and insights to refine and enhance AI models. Explainable AI enables iterative learning, addressing shortcomings, and optimizing system performance over time.

Patient Empowerment and Informed Consent: Patients have the right to understand the basis of AI-generated recommendations concerning their health. Explainability allows patients to make informed decisions, actively participate in their healthcare, and provide consent for treatment plans derived from AI algorithms. Patient empowerment and autonomy are vital components of patient-centric care.

### 6.1.4  RESEARCH OBJECTIVE AND SCOPE OF THIS CHAPTER

The research objective and scope of this chapter provide a clear direction and focus for the study. This section explains the specific goals and boundaries of the research conducted for the chapter.

#### 6.1.4.1  Research Objective

The primary research objective of this chapter is to explore the significance and applications of explainable AI in the context of Healthcare 5.0. The chapter aims to examine how explainable AI can enhance transparency, trust, and decision-making in healthcare systems powered by advanced technologies. The objective is to provide insights into the benefits, techniques, challenges, and future directions of explainable AI in healthcare.

#### 6.1.4.2  Scope

The scope of this chapter encompasses several key areas related to explainable AI in healthcare:

Importance of Explainability: The chapter discusses the importance of explainability in AI systems specifically within the healthcare domain. It highlights the need for transparency, trust, ethical considerations, and legal compliance in healthcare AI applications.

Techniques and Approaches: The chapter explores various techniques and approaches for achieving explainability in AI models, focusing on those suitable for Healthcare 5.0. This includes rule-based systems, symbolic reasoning, interpretable machine learning models, and model-agnostic explanation techniques.

Applications in Healthcare 5.0: The chapter delves into the practical applications of explainable AI in Healthcare 5.0. It explores case studies and use cases to demonstrate how explainability can enhance clinical decision support systems, interpretable deep learning models for medical imaging, predictive modeling, and personalized medicine.

Evaluation and Assessment: The chapter addresses the evaluation and assessment of explainable AI systems in healthcare (Doshi-Velez & Kim, 2017). It covers evaluation metrics, performance and interpretability trade-offs, and user-centric evaluation, emphasizing the need to evaluate the effectiveness and usability of explainable AI models.

Regulatory and Legal Considerations: The chapter discusses the regulatory and legal considerations associated with explainable AI in healthcare. It examines the framework for compliance, data privacy, security, and the implications of using explainable AI systems in healthcare settings.

Challenges and Future Directions: The chapter identifies and discusses the challenges faced in developing and implementing explainable AI in Healthcare 5.0. It also explores future research directions, technical challenges, adoption considerations, and integration of explainable AI into existing healthcare systems.

By clearly defining the research objective and scope, this chapter provides a focused and structured exploration of explainable AI in Healthcare 5.0. It aims to contribute to the understanding, adoption, and implementation of explainability techniques to enhance transparency, trust, and the ethical use of AI in the evolving healthcare landscape.

## 6.2 FUNDAMENTALS OF EXPLAINABLE AI

### 6.2.1 Definition and Concepts of Explainable AI

Explainable AI (XAI) refers to the development and application of AI models and algorithms that can provide understandable and interpretable explanations for their decisions and actions. This section focuses on defining the concept of explainable AI and exploring the underlying concepts associated with it (Arrieta et al., 2020).

Definition of Explainable AI: Explainable AI refers to the capability of an AI system to provide clear and transparent explanations for its decision-making processes and outputs. It involves designing AI models and algorithms that can articulate how they arrive at their conclusions, making their decision making process more interpretable to humans (Guidotti et al., 2018).

Interpretability vs. Explainability: Interpretability and explainability are closely related but distinct concepts. Interpretability refers to the ability to understand the internal workings of an AI model, such as the feature importance, weights, or learned representations. Explainability, on the other hand, focuses on providing understandable explanations for specific decisions or predictions made by the model (Gilpin et al., 2018).

Importance of Explainability in AI: Explainability is crucial in various domains, including healthcare, finance, and legal systems, where human decisions based on AI recommendations have significant consequences. Explainable AI helps build trust, validate decisions, detect biases, and facilitate human oversight and intervention in critical tasks. It also enables compliance with legal, ethical, and regulatory requirements.

Levels of Explainability: Explainability can be achieved at different levels, depending on the complexity and transparency of the AI model (Carvalho & Freitas, 2019). It ranges from simple rule-based systems that provide explicit decision rules to more complex approaches, such as model-agnostic methods or post-hoc explanations, which generate explanations without relying on the model's internal structure.

Techniques for Explainability: Various techniques and approaches are employed to achieve explainability in AI models. These include rule-based systems, symbolic reasoning, feature importance analysis, local surrogate models, counterfactual explanations, and attention mechanisms. Each technique has its strengths and limitations, and the choice of technique depends on the specific use case and requirements.

### 6.2.2 Techniques and Approaches for Explainability

Various techniques and approaches are employed to achieve explainability in AI models. These methods aim to provide understandable explanations for the decisions and predictions made by AI systems. The following are some commonly used techniques:

**Rule-Based Systems**: Rule-based systems employ a set of predefined rules that explicitly specify the decision-making process (Carvalho & Freitas, 2019). These rules can be easily understood by humans and provide transparent explanations. For example, in a medical diagnosis system, specific rules can be defined based on symptoms, test results, and medical guidelines.

**Symbolic Reasoning**: Symbolic reasoning utilizes symbolic knowledge representation and logical inference to generate explanations (Doshi-Velez & Kim, 2017). It involves representing knowledge in the form of rules, constraints, and logical relationships. Symbolic reasoning allows for the extraction of explicit and interpretable explanations from AI models.

**Feature Importance Analysis**: Feature importance analysis identifies the most influential features or variables in the AI model's decision-making process (Lundberg & Lee, 2017). It helps understand which factors contribute the most to a specific prediction or decision. Techniques such as permutation importance, SHAP (Shapley additive explanations) values, or LIME (local interpretable model-agnostic explanations) provide insights into the importance of each feature.

**Local Surrogate Models**: Local surrogate models aim to approximate the behavior of the underlying AI model within a local neighborhood (Ribeiro et al., 2016). By training a transparent model, such as a linear or decision tree model, on the AI model's predictions for specific instances, local surrogate models provide explanations at an individual level.

**Counterfactual Explanations:** Counterfactual explanations generate alternative scenarios that would have resulted in a different prediction or decision (Wachter et al., 2017). By showing how changing certain input features leads to different outcomes, counterfactual explanations help users understand the AI model's behavior and the factors driving its decisions.

These techniques and approaches offer different levels of interpretability and can be applied depending on the specific requirements, complexity of the AI model, and the domain in which explainability is needed.

### 6.2.3 Challenges and Trade-offs in Achieving Explainability

While achieving explainability in AI systems is essential, it also comes with challenges and trade-offs that need to be considered. Here, we discuss some of the key challenges and trade-offs associated with explainability in AI:

**Complexity-Interpretability Trade-off:** One of the fundamental challenges is balancing model complexity with interpretability (Lipton, 2018). Highly complex models, such as deep neural networks, often achieve better performance but are less interpretable. Simpler models, on the other hand, may sacrifice performance for interpretability. Striking the right balance between complexity and interpretability is crucial to ensure both accuracy and explainability.

**Accuracy-Explainability Trade-off:** There can be a trade-off between model accuracy and explainability. Techniques that enhance explainability, such as simplifying models or using local surrogate models, may result in a slight decrease in predictive accuracy (Ribeiro et al., 2016). It is necessary to find the optimal point that satisfies the desired level of explainability without compromising significantly on model performance.

**Black-Box Models and Inherent Complexity:** Many state-of-the-art AI models, like deep learning models, are often considered "black boxes" as their internal workings are complex and not easily interpretable (Carvalho & Freitas, 2019). Achieving explainability in such models presents a significant challenge. Techniques like feature importance analysis or layer-wise relevance propagation can offer insights, but the full interpretability of complex models remains a challenge.

**Contextual and Subjective Nature of Explanations:** The interpretability of explanations can vary depending on the context and the intended audience. Different stakeholders may have different expectations and interpretations of what constitutes an understandable explanation. Balancing the need for a comprehensive explanation with its simplicity and relevance to different users is a challenge that needs to be addressed.

**Robustness and Generalization:** Explanations derived from AI models should be robust and generalize across different instances and scenarios (Mittelstadt et al., 2019a). They should not be overly influenced by noise or minor changes in input data. Ensuring the robustness and generalization of explanations is critical for their reliability and trustworthiness.

**Data Quality and Bias:** The quality and bias present in the training data can affect the explanations provided by AI models. If the training data is biased or incomplete, the explanations may inherit those biases or fail to capture the full complexity of the underlying problem (Doshi-Velez & Kim, 2017). Addressing data quality issues and mitigating bias in both the training data and the explanation generation process is crucial.

## 6.3  EXPLAINABLE AI IN HEALTHCARE 5.0

### 6.3.1  APPLICATIONS OF AI IN HEALTHCARE 5.0

The emergence of Healthcare 5.0, driven by advanced technologies and AI, has transformed the healthcare landscape. Explainable AI plays a crucial role in enabling transparency, trust, and effective decision-making within Healthcare 5.0. Here are some key applications of AI in Healthcare 5.0:

Disease Diagnosis and Prognosis: AI systems can analyze vast amounts of medical data, including patient records, diagnostic images, and genetic information, to aid in disease diagnosis and prognosis. Explainable AI techniques allow healthcare professionals to understand the reasoning behind the AI system's predictions or recommendations. This helps in validating and trusting the AI system's output and enables clinicians to make informed decisions.

Treatment Planning and Personalized Medicine: AI can assist in developing personalized treatment plans by considering individual patient characteristics, medical history, and response to various therapies. Explainable AI provides insights into the factors influencing treatment recommendations, such as biomarkers, patient demographics, and clinical guidelines. This helps clinicians understand why a specific treatment option is suggested, promoting patient engagement and adherence.

Drug Discovery and Development: AI-driven approaches, such as machine learning and deep learning, are increasingly utilized in drug discovery and development processes. Explainable AI methods can reveal the relationships between molecular structures, drug targets, and biological pathways, providing insights into how a particular drug is predicted to interact with the body. This facilitates the evaluation and validation of drug candidates, accelerating the discovery and development of novel therapies.

Monitoring and Predictive Analytics: AI-enabled monitoring systems can continuously analyze patient data, such as vital signs, wearable device measurements, and electronic health records, to detect anomalies, predict health deterioration, and trigger timely interventions. Explainable AI techniques help healthcare professionals understand the reasoning behind alerts, predictions, or risk scores, enhancing their trust in the system and facilitating appropriate clinical actions (Carvalho & Freitas, 2019).

Clinical Decision Support Systems: AI-based clinical decision support systems assist healthcare professionals by providing evidence-based recommendations, treatment guidelines, and alerts for potential adverse events. Explainable AI allows clinicians to comprehend the underlying rules, factors, and evidence that contribute to the decision support provided (Chen & Asch, 2017). This promotes shared decision-making between clinicians and patients, leading to improved patient outcomes.

Patient Monitoring and Engagement: AI-powered applications can monitor and analyze patient behaviors, symptoms, and lifestyle patterns to facilitate self-management, preventive care, and behavioral interventions. Explainable AI helps patients understand the insights and recommendations generated by these applications, enabling them to actively participate in their healthcare journey and make informed choices.

By applying explainable AI techniques in these applications, Healthcare 5.0 can harness the power of AI while ensuring transparency, accountability, and interpretability. Explainable AI empowers healthcare professionals and patients, fostering trust in AI systems and supporting collaborative decision-making.

Health Monitoring and Early Detection: AI systems can analyze various health data sources, such as electronic health records, wearable devices, and social media, to monitor individuals' health status and detect early signs of diseases. Explainable AI helps healthcare professionals understand the features and patterns that contribute to the detection of health abnormalities (Carvalho & Freitas, 2019). This facilitates timely interventions and preventive measures, improving patient outcomes.

Resource Optimization and Healthcare Management: AI techniques can be employed to optimize resource allocation, such as scheduling appointments, managing hospital resources, and predicting patient flow. Explainable AI methods allow healthcare administrators and managers to understand the factors and variables influencing resource allocation decisions (Chen & Asch, 2017). This aids in efficient resource utilization, cost-effectiveness, and improved healthcare delivery.

Public Health Surveillance and Outbreak Management: AI systems can analyze large-scale data, including social media feeds, online news, and healthcare databases, to monitor public health trends, detect disease outbreaks, and support epidemiological investigations. Explainable AI helps public health officials understand the patterns and indicators driving the outbreak predictions and recommendations (Liu & Sawada, 2020). This enhances their ability to respond effectively and implement targeted interventions.

Ethical and Legal Considerations: Explainable AI in Healthcare 5.0 also addresses important ethical and legal considerations. It enables transparency and accountability in AI-driven healthcare systems, ensuring compliance with regulations, standards, and privacy requirements. By providing explanations for AI decisions and recommendations, stakeholders can assess the fairness, bias, and potential risks associated with the AI system's outputs.

By leveraging these applications of explainable AI, Healthcare 5.0 can unlock the full potential of AI technologies while addressing concerns related to transparency, interpretability, and trust. It empowers healthcare professionals, patients, and stakeholders by providing meaningful explanations and fostering collaborative decision-making in the context of AI-enabled healthcare.

### 6.3.2 Limitations of Black Box AI Systems in Healthcare

Black box AI systems, which has limited transparency and interpretability, have limitations in the healthcare domain. Here are some key limitations:

Lack of Trust: Black box AI systems often generate predictions or recommendations without providing clear explanations of how they arrived at those conclusions. This lack of transparency undermines trust among healthcare professionals, patients, and other stakeholders. Without understanding the reasoning behind the AI system's outputs, it becomes challenging to validate the results or make informed decisions.

Incomprehensibility of Complex Models: Many AI models, like deep neural networks, are inherently complex and difficult to interpret. These models often have numerous layers, parameters, and non-linear transformations, making it challenging to understand how they arrive at specific predictions. As a result, healthcare professionals may hesitate to rely on the outputs of these black-box models, especially in critical decision-making scenarios.

Limited Insights into Decision-Making: Black box AI systems lack the ability to provide meaningful insights into the factors that contribute to their predictions or recommendations. Healthcare professionals require explanations that go beyond a mere output by understanding the underlying clinical features, patient characteristics, or biomarkers that influence the AI system's decisions. Without such insights, it becomes challenging to trust and comprehend the clinical relevance and validity of the AI system's outputs.

Difficulty in Detecting Bias and Discrimination: Black box AI systems can be susceptible to biases present in the training data, leading to biased predictions or recommendations. However, without explainability, it becomes difficult to identify and address these biases. The lack of transparency hinders the ability to detect and mitigate potential discrimination, thereby compromising fairness and equity in healthcare.

### 6.3.3 Benefits of Explainability for Healthcare 5.0

Explainable AI brings several benefits to the Healthcare 5.0 paradigm:

Enhanced Trust and Acceptance: Explainable AI systems provide transparent and understandable explanations for their predictions or recommendations. This promotes trust and acceptance among healthcare professionals, patients, and regulatory bodies. When the AI system's reasoning is clear, it becomes easier to validate its outputs, leading to increased confidence in its effectiveness and reliability.

Increased Clinical Validity: By providing explanations, explainable AI allows healthcare professionals to evaluate the clinical validity of AI system outputs (Carvalho & Freitas, 2019). They can assess the alignment of the system's reasoning with established medical knowledge, clinical guidelines, and patient-specific information. This helps in making evidence-based decisions and ensures that the AI system's outputs are aligned with the expected clinical outcomes.

Improved Interpretability and Collaboration: Explainable AI enables healthcare professionals to interpret and understand the AI system's reasoning, facilitating collaboration between human experts and AI systems

Detection and Mitigation of Bias: Explainable AI methods can help identify biases present in the training data or the AI model itself. By understanding the factors influencing the AI system's outputs, healthcare professionals can detect and address potential biases, ensuring fairness and equity in healthcare. Explainability allows for the examination of the decision-making process and mitigates the risk of discriminatory outcomes.

### 6.3.4 Ethical Considerations in Explainable AI for Healthcare

The ethical considerations in explainable AI for healthcare is listed in Table 6.1.

The use of explainable AI in healthcare brings benefits such as enhanced trust, increased clinical validity, improved interpretability, collaboration between humans and AI systems, and the detection and mitigation of biases. However, it also raises ethical considerations related to transparency, informed consent, trust, fairness, and privacy. Addressing these ethical considerations is essential to ensure the responsible and ethical implementation of explainable AI in healthcare.

**TABLE 6.1**

**Ethical Considerations in Explainable AI for Healthcare**

| S. No. | Ethical Consideration | Description |
| --- | --- | --- |
| 1 | Transparency and accountability | Promotes transparency in AI systems, ensuring stakeholders understand decision-making processes |
| | | Facilitates accountability for AI system outputs and actions, allowing for critical assessment (Doshi-Velez & Kim, 2017) |
| 2 | Informed consent and autonomy | Enables patients to make informed decisions about their healthcare by providing understandable explanations |
| 3 | Trust and professional responsibility | Helps healthcare professionals fulfill their responsibility to provide the best care by validating AI system recommendations |
| | | Aids in ensuring patient safety and making informed treatment decisions |
| 4 | Fairness and equity | Identifies and mitigates biases in AI systems to ensure fairness and prevent discriminatory outcomes (Mittelstadt et al., 2019b) |
| | | Promotes equal access to healthcare resources and reduces disparities |
| 5 | Privacy and data protection | Considers privacy and data protection principles in generating explanations, avoiding sensitive information disclosure (Ribeiro et al., 2016) |
| | | Prioritizes data anonymization, encryption, and secure handling to protect patient confidentiality |

## 6.4 EXPLAINABILITY TECHNIQUES FOR HEALTHCARE 5.0

### 6.4.1 RULE-BASED AND LOGIC-BASED SYSTEMS

Rule-based and logic-based systems are traditional approaches to explainable AI that utilize a set of predefined rules or logical statements to make decisions and provide explanations. In healthcare, these systems involve encoding medical knowledge and domain expertise into a set of if-then rules or logical statements. When an AI system generates a prediction or recommendation, it can provide an explanation by referencing the specific rules or logical statements that led to that decision. This transparency allows healthcare professionals to understand the underlying reasoning and facilitates trust and interpretability.

### 6.4.2 SYMBOLIC REASONING AND EXPERT SYSTEMS

Symbolic reasoning and expert systems aim to mimic human decision-making by utilizing symbolic representations of knowledge and inference rules. These systems incorporate domain-specific knowledge and expertise into a knowledge base, which is then used to reason and provide explanations. In healthcare, expert systems can analyze patient data and medical knowledge to generate explanations for diagnoses, treatment plans, and recommendations (Adadi & Berrada, 2018). The symbolic representations enable healthcare professionals to comprehend the logical steps and considerations involved in the AI system's decision-making process.

### 6.4.3 INTERPRETABLE MACHINE LEARNING MODELS

Interpretable machine learning models are designed to provide explanations for their predictions or decisions. Unlike black-box models, interpretable models prioritize transparency and comprehensibility (Guidotti et al., 2018). These models often have a simpler structure, such as decision trees, linear regression, or logistic regression, which allows for easier interpretation. Interpretable machine learning models provide feature importance rankings, decision paths, or visualizations to explain how specific input variables influence the model's output. In healthcare, these models can aid in disease diagnosis, treatment planning, and outcome prediction while providing understandable explanations.

### 6.4.4 MODEL-AGNOSTIC EXPLANATION TECHNIQUES

Model-agnostic explanation techniques are applied to any type of AI model, regardless of its underlying structure or complexity. These techniques aim to provide explanations for the predictions or decisions made by black-box models, making them more transparent and interpretable. Techniques such as LIME and SHAP generate explanations by approximating the behavior of the black-box model locally or globally (Rudin, 2019). They highlight the importance of specific input features and provide insights into how those features contribute to the model's predictions. Model-agnostic explanation techniques enable healthcare professionals to understand the reasoning behind the outputs of complex AI models, fostering trust and facilitating informed decision-making (Rudin, 2021).

In summary, explainability techniques for Healthcare 5.0 encompass rule-based and logic-based systems, symbolic reasoning and expert systems, interpretable machine learning models, and model-agnostic explanation techniques. These techniques enable healthcare professionals to understand the reasoning and decision-making process of AI systems, promoting transparency, trust, and collaboration between humans and AI in the healthcare domain.

## 6.5 CASE STUDIES AND USE CASES

### 6.5.1 EXPLAINABLE AI FOR CLINICAL DECISION SUPPORT SYSTEMS

Explainable AI plays a crucial role in developing clinical decision support systems (CDSS) that assist healthcare professionals in making informed and evidence-based decisions shown in Figure 6.2. Here are a few examples of how explainable AI is applied in CDSS:

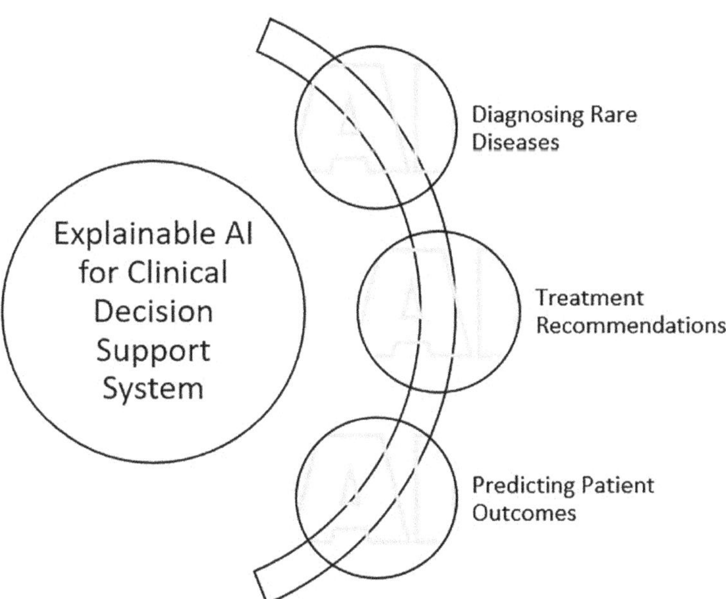


**FIGURE 6.2** Explainable AI for clinical decision support systems.

### Diagnosing Rare Diseases

Explainable AI can aid in diagnosing rare diseases by analyzing patient data, medical records, and symptoms (Holzinger et al., 2017). For instance, a CDSS can utilize a rule-based system to generate explanations for the diagnosis by referencing specific rules and evidence used in the decision-making process. This helps healthcare professionals understand the factors that led to a particular diagnosis and provides transparency in the decision.

#### *Example: Diagnosing Rare Diseases*

A patient presents with a set of symptoms that are indicative of a rare genetic disorder. A rule-based CDSS incorporates medical knowledge and domain expertise into a set of rules. By analyzing the patient's symptoms and medical history, the CDSS generates an explanation for the diagnosis by referencing specific rules (Carvalho & Freitas, 2019). For instance, if the patient exhibits symptoms A, B, and C, along with a genetic marker X, the CDSS can explain that the diagnosis is based on the presence of these specific criteria, providing transparency and assisting the healthcare professional in understanding the reasoning behind the diagnosis.

### Treatment Recommendations

CDSS can utilize machine learning models to provide treatment recommendations based on patient-specific data. Interpretable machine learning models, such as decision trees or linear models, can generate explanations for the treatment recommendations by highlighting the important features or variables considered by the model (Carvalho & Freitas, 2019). This allows healthcare professionals to assess the clinical validity of the recommendations and make informed decisions.

#### *Example: Treatment Recommendations*

A CDSS employs an interpretable machine learning model, such as a decision tree, to provide treatment recommendations for patients with a certain medical condition (Lundberg & Lee, 2017). The model considers various patient-specific factors such as age, gender, lab results, and comorbidities. The CDSS generates explanations for the treatment recommendations by highlighting the key factors that influenced the decision. For instance, the CDSS may explain that the recommendation for a particular treatment is based on the patient's age, the presence of a specific comorbidity, and the results of a diagnostic test. This explanation helps the healthcare professional understand why a specific treatment is recommended and supports clinical decision-making (Rajkomar et al., 2018).

### Predicting Patient Outcomes

Explainable AI techniques can be employed to predict patient outcomes, such as disease progression or response to treatment. Model-agnostic explanation techniques, like LIME or SHAP, can provide insights into the features that contribute to the predictions (Rajkomar et al., 2018). For example, in predicting the risk of cardiovascular events, an interpretable model can highlight factors like age, cholesterol levels, and blood pressure as important predictors, enabling clinicians to understand the rationale behind the predictions.

#### *Example: Predicting Patient Outcomes*

A CDSS utilizes a black box machine learning model to predict the risk of disease progression in cancer patients. To make the predictions more interpretable, model-agnostic explanation techniques like LIME are applied. The CDSS generates explanations by highlighting the features or biomarkers that are most influential in the prediction. For example, the CDSS may explain that the prediction of disease progression is based on the patient's tumor size, genetic markers, and treatment history. This explanation allows the healthcare professional to assess the validity of the prediction and make informed decisions regarding patient management (Wiens et al., 2019).

**Adverse Event Detection**

Explainable AI can assist in identifying adverse events or complications associated with medical interventions or medications. By utilizing rule-based systems or expert systems, CDSS can generate explanations for adverse event predictions, outlining the specific factors or risk factors that contribute to the event (Chen et al., 2019). This information helps healthcare professionals in risk assessment, treatment planning, and mitigating potential adverse events.

These case studies demonstrate the application of explainable AI in CDSS, allowing healthcare professionals to understand the decision-making process, validate recommendations, and improve patient care. These examples illustrate how explainable AI techniques can be applied in clinical decision support systems, providing transparent and interpretable explanations for diagnoses, treatment recommendations, and outcome predictions. By understanding the underlying reasoning, healthcare professionals can make more informed decisions and enhance patient care.

### 6.5.2 INTERPRETABLE DEEP LEARNING MODELS FOR MEDICAL IMAGING

Medical imaging plays a critical role in diagnosing diseases, monitoring treatment progress, and guiding clinical decision-making. Deep learning models have shown remarkable performance in analyzing medical images, but their black box nature poses challenges in interpretability and trust. In this case study, we explore the development of interpretable deep learning models for medical imaging.

### Objective

The objective is to develop deep learning models that not only achieve high accuracy in medical image analysis but also provide interpretable explanations for their predictions. The aim is to enhance the transparency and trustworthiness of the models, enabling healthcare professionals to understand and validate the decision-making process.

### Model Architecture

The deep learning models are designed using architectures suitable for medical image analysis, such as convolutional neural networks (CNNs). These models are trained on large annotated datasets to learn complex patterns and features in medical images.

### Interpretable Features

To improve interpretability, the models are designed to extract meaningful features from medical images (Zhang et al., 2018). This can be achieved by incorporating attention mechanisms or utilizing explainable building blocks like spatial transformer networks. These features highlight the regions of interest or specific characteristics that contribute to the model's predictions.

### Visualization Techniques

Various visualization techniques are employed to provide visual explanations for the model's predictions. For instance, class activation maps (CAM) can be generated to highlight the regions in the image that are most influential in the prediction. Grad-CAM (gradient-weighted class activation mapping) can also be used to visualize the gradient flow through the network, indicating the importance of different image regions.

## Feature Importance Analysis

Feature importance analysis techniques, such as sensitivity analysis or saliency maps, are applied to identify the most influential features or pixels in the image. These techniques highlight the regions or features that significantly affect the model's decision, allowing healthcare professionals to understand the reasoning behind the predictions.

## Rule-Based Systems

To enhance interpretability further, rule-based systems can be integrated with the deep learning models. These systems generate explicit rules based on the learned representations to provide explicit explanations for the predictions. The rules can be designed to capture clinical knowledge or guidelines, enabling clinicians to comprehend the decision-making process.

## Results and Impact

The developed interpretable deep learning models provide transparent and understandable explanations for their predictions in medical imaging tasks. These explanations allow healthcare professionals to validate and trust the model's predictions, leading to improved clinical decision-making and patient care. Interpretable models enable radiologists and clinicians to identify the features or regions in medical images that contribute to the model's decision, facilitating collaboration between human experts and AI systems (Rajpurkar et al., 2017).

### 6.5.3 Use Case: Interpretable Deep Learning Models for Breast Cancer Detection

Breast cancer is a prevalent form of cancer that affects millions of women worldwide. Early and accurate detection is crucial for improving patient outcomes. Deep learning models have shown promise in analyzing mammograms for breast cancer detection. However, their black box nature poses challenges in interpreting their predictions (Shen et al., 2019). Interpretable deep learning models can address this limitation and provide transparent explanations for their decisions.

In this use case, the objective is to develop an interpretable deep learning model for breast cancer detection using mammographic images.

## Methodology

### Dataset

A large dataset of mammographic images, along with corresponding labels indicating the presence or absence of breast cancer, is collected. The dataset is carefully curated and annotated by expert radiologists.

### Model Architecture

An interpretable deep learning model, such as a convolutional neural network (CNN), is designed. The CNN is trained on the mammographic dataset to learn patterns and features indicative of breast cancer.

### Class Activation Mapping (CAM)

To provide interpretability, the model incorporates the class activation mapping (CAM) technique. CAM generates heatmaps that highlight the regions in the mammogram that are most influential in the model's decision. These heatmaps provide visual explanations for the model's predictions, allowing radiologists to understand which areas of the image contribute to the classification.

### Feature Importance Analysis

Additional feature importance analysis techniques, such as sensitivity analysis or saliency maps, can be applied to identify the most influential features in the mammogram. These techniques help identify the specific regions or characteristics of the breast tissue that contribute significantly to the model's prediction.

### Rule-Based System

To enhance interpretability further, a rule-based system can be integrated with the deep learning model. The system generates explicit rules based on the learned representations, providing explicit explanations for the model's predictions. These rules can capture clinical guidelines or indicators used by radiologists, making the decision-making process more transparent and understandable.

### Results and Impact

The developed interpretable deep learning model for breast cancer detection provides transparent explanations for its predictions. Radiologists can visualize the heatmaps and understand which regions of the mammogram influenced the model's decision. This not only enhances trust in the model but also helps radiologists validate and verify the predictions. The interpretable model can serve as an aid to radiologists in their decision-making process, leading to improved accuracy in breast cancer detection and early intervention (Patil et al., 2020).

## 6.5.4 Case Study: Predictive Modeling with Explainable AI in Healthcare

Predictive modeling with explainable AI in healthcare involves developing models that can accurately predict various healthcare outcomes while providing transparent explanations for their predictions (Lundberg & Lee, 2017). These models help healthcare professionals make informed decisions and improve patient care. Here, we present a case study highlighting the application of predictive modeling with explainable AI in healthcare (Caruana et al., 2015).

## Objective

The objective is to develop predictive models using explainable AI techniques that can accurately forecast healthcare outcomes, such as disease progression, readmission rates, or mortality, while providing interpretable explanations for their predictions. The aim is to enable healthcare professionals to understand the factors driving the predictions and enhance their decision-making process (Jiang et al., 2020).

### Methodology

## Data Collection and Pre-processing

Relevant healthcare data, including patient demographics, medical history, laboratory results, and treatment information, are collected from electronic health records or other sources. The data undergoes pre-processing steps such as cleaning, normalization, and feature engineering to ensure quality and suitability for modelling (Wiens et al., 2019).

## Model Selection

Different machine learning algorithms, like logistic regression, random forest, or gradient boosting, are evaluated to identify the most appropriate model for the predictive task. Model selection is based on factors like performance metrics (accuracy, precision, recall), interpretability, and computational efficiency (Gao et al., 2020).

## Feature Importance Analysis

To provide explanations for the predictions, feature importance analysis techniques are applied to identify the most influential features contributing to the model's decisions. Techniques like permutation feature importance or SHAP (Shapley additive explanations) values can be used to quantify the impact of individual features on the predictions.

## Rule-Based Systems

Incorporating rule-based systems alongside predictive models can enhance interpretability further. Rule-based systems generate explicit rules based on the learned representations, providing transparent explanations for the predictions. These rules can align with clinical guidelines or knowledge, allowing healthcare professionals to understand the decision-making process.

## Results and Impact

Predictive modeling with explainable AI in healthcare allows healthcare professionals to make accurate predictions while understanding the reasons behind the model's decisions. Interpretable explanations enable clinicians to validate the predictions, identify critical features, and understand the impact of interventions or risk factors on patient outcomes. This enhances the decision-making process, improves patient care, and enables the development of targeted interventions or preventive strategies.

### 6.5.5 USE CASE: PREDICTIVE MODELING WITH EXPLAINABLE AI FOR HOSPITAL READMISSION

Hospital readmission is a critical concern in healthcare, as it not only affects patient well-being but also imposes significant financial burden on healthcare systems (Caruana et al., 2015). Predictive modeling with explainable AI can play a crucial role in identifying patients at higher risk of readmission, allowing healthcare providers to intervene and prevent unnecessary hospitalizations.

## Objective

The objective is to develop a predictive model using explainable AI techniques to accurately forecast the likelihood of hospital readmission for patients. The aim is to provide transparent explanations for the predictions, enabling healthcare professionals to understand the factors contributing to the risk of readmission.

### *Methodology*

## Data Collection and Pre-processing

Patient data, including demographics, medical history, diagnoses, medications, procedures, and previous hospitalization records, are collected from electronic health records. The data is preprocessed, including cleaning, handling missing values, and encoding categorical variables, to prepare it for modeling.

## Feature Selection and Engineering

Relevant features that can impact the risk of readmission, such as age, comorbidities, length of stay, discharge medications, and laboratory results, are selected. Additional features, such as social determinants of health or patient-reported outcomes, can be incorporated to enhance the predictive accuracy. Feature engineering techniques, like creating interaction terms or aggregating temporal data, can be applied to capture complex relationships.

## Model Development

Various machine learning algorithms, such as logistic regression, decision trees, or ensemble methods, are trained on the labeled dataset to build the predictive model. The model is optimized using suitable evaluation metrics, such as accuracy, precision, recall, and area under the receiver operating characteristic curve (AUC-ROC) (Cho et al., 2018).

## Explainability Techniques

To provide explanations for the predictions, techniques such as feature importance analysis, rule extraction, or SHAP values can be employed (Miotto et al., 2016). These techniques identify the key factors driving the model's decisions and provide interpretable insights into why a patient may be at a higher risk of readmission. Visualizations, such as bar charts or decision trees, can be used to represent the importance of different features.

## Integration and Validation

The developed predictive model with explainable AI is integrated into the hospital's clinical workflow or decision support system (Rajkomar et al., 2018). It undergoes rigorous validation and testing using independent datasets to ensure its performance and generalizability. The model's predictions and explanations are continuously monitored and refined based on feedback from healthcare professionals.

## Results and Impact

The predictive modeling with explainable AI for hospital readmission enables healthcare providers to identify patients at a higher risk of readmission accurately. The transparent explanations provided by the model allow clinicians to understand the contributing factors, facilitating targeted interventions, care management, and discharge planning. By effectively identifying and intervening with high-risk patients, healthcare systems can reduce the rate of readmissions, improve patient outcomes, and optimize resource utilization.

## Intervention Strategies

Once the predictive model identifies patients at higher risk of readmission, healthcare providers can implement targeted intervention strategies to mitigate that risk. These interventions may include medication adjustments, personalized care plans, care coordination, patient education, or follow-up appointments (Caruana et al., 2015). The transparent explanations provided by the model enable healthcare professionals to communicate the reasons for the intervention to patients, fostering better understanding and compliance.

## Monitoring and Evaluation

The predictive model's performance and the effectiveness of the intervention strategies are continuously monitored and evaluated. By tracking the outcomes of patients who received interventions, healthcare providers can assess the impact of their actions on reducing readmissions. This iterative process helps refine the predictive model and intervention strategies over time, improving its accuracy and usefulness (Cho et al., 2018).

## Cost Optimization

Besides reducing readmission rates, predictive modeling with explainable AI also helps optimize healthcare costs (Miotto et al., 2016). By identifying patients at higher risk of readmission, healthcare providers can allocate resources more efficiently, such as ensuring timely follow-up care for high-risk patients while prioritizing resources for patients at lower risk. This optimization not only reduces financial strain on healthcare systems but also enhances the overall quality of care provided.

## Results and Impact

The use of predictive modeling with explainable AI for hospital readmission has several positive impacts on healthcare delivery (Suresh & Guttag, 2017). It enables healthcare providers to proactively identify patients at risk, intervene early, and prevent unnecessary hospital readmissions. The transparent explanations provided by the model promote better understanding, trust, and collaboration between healthcare professionals and patients. Ultimately, this approach improves patient outcomes, reduces healthcare costs, and enhances the overall efficiency of healthcare systems.

### 6.5.6 Case Study: Explainable AI for Personalized Medicine

Personalized medicine aims to provide tailored healthcare interventions and treatments based on individual patient characteristics, including genetic information, medical history, and lifestyle factors. Explainable AI plays a vital role in this field by developing models that can accurately predict treatment responses and provide transparent explanations for their recommendations (Lundberg & Lee, 2017). Here, we present a case study highlighting the application of explainable AI for personalized medicine.

## Objective

The objective is to develop an explainable AI model that can predict treatment outcomes and provide interpretable explanations for personalized medicine interventions. The aim is to enable healthcare professionals to understand the factors driving the model's recommendations and facilitate informed decision-making for individual patients.

*Methodology*

## Data Collection and Integration

Relevant patient data, including demographic information, genetic profiles, medical records, diagnostic tests, and treatment outcomes, are collected from various sources. This data is integrated and harmonized to create a comprehensive dataset for analysis.

## Feature Selection and Encoding

Important features related to patient characteristics, genetic markers, biomarkers, and treatment modalities are selected. Feature engineering techniques may be applied to transform and encode the data, such as scaling numeric features or one-hot encoding categorical variables, ensuring compatibility with the AI model.

## Model Development

Machine learning algorithms, such as support vector machines, random forests, or deep learning models, are trained on the dataset to develop the predictive model (Panch et al., 2019). The model is optimized and validated using appropriate performance metrics, such as accuracy, precision, recall, or area under the curve (AUC), to ensure its effectiveness in predicting treatment outcomes.

## Explainability Techniques

To provide explanations for the model's recommendations, explainability techniques are applied. This may involve methods such as feature importance analysis, rule extraction, or LIME (Wang et al., 2019). These techniques identify the influential features or decision rules that contribute to the model's predictions, enabling clinicians to understand the underlying mechanisms.

## Clinical Validation and Integration

The developed explainable AI model is validated using independent datasets and evaluated by healthcare professionals to assess its reliability and clinical utility (Rajan & Lam, 2019). The model is integrated into the clinical workflow, electronic health records, or decision support systems to provide real-time recommendations and explanations for personalized medicine interventions.

## Results and Impact

Explainable AI for personalized medicine enables healthcare professionals to make informed decisions regarding treatment options for individual patients. The transparent explanations provided by the model assist in understanding the factors influencing treatment responses and identifying personalized interventions. This approach promotes precision medicine, enhances patient outcomes, minimizes adverse effects, and optimizes healthcare resource allocation.

## 6.6  EVALUATING AND ASSESSING EXPLAINABLE AI SYSTEMS

### 6.6.1  EVALUATION METRICS FOR EXPLAINABILITY

When assessing the effectiveness of explainable AI systems, it is crucial to establish appropriate evaluation metrics (Doshi-Velez & Kim, 2017). These metrics focus on the quality and comprehensibility of the explanations provided by the system. Some commonly used evaluation metrics for explainability include:

Fidelity: Fidelity refers to the extent to which the explanation accurately represents the reasoning and decision-making process of the underlying AI model. High-fidelity explanations closely align with the internal workings of the model and provide an accurate reflection of its behavior.

Intelligibility: Intelligibility measures the ease with which the explanations can be understood by users. It considers factors such as clarity, simplicity, and conciseness of the provided explanations. Intelligible explanations should be accessible to both technical and non-technical users.

Consistency: Consistency assesses the stability and coherence of the explanations across different instances or models. Consistent explanations should provide similar reasoning for similar instances or models, promoting trust and reliability (Guidotti et al., 2018).

Actionability: Actionability measures the extent to which the explanations enable users to make informed decisions or take appropriate actions based on the provided information. Actionable explanations should empower users to understand the implications of the AI system's recommendations and act upon them effectively.

### 6.6.2  ASSESSING PERFORMANCE AND INTERPRETABILITY TRADE-OFFS

Explainable AI systems often involve a trade-off between performance and interpretability. As models become more complex and accurate, they may also become less interpretable (Lage et al., 2019). Assessing this trade-off involves finding a balance between the system's predictive performance and the comprehensibility of its explanations. Several approaches can be used to evaluate this trade-off:

Performance Metrics: Traditional performance metrics, such as accuracy, precision, recall, or AUC, can be used to assess the model's predictive performance. These metrics indicate how well the model can make accurate predictions (Lundberg & Lee, 2017).

Complexity-Interpretability Trade-off: Assessing the complexity of the AI model can provide insights into its interpretability. Simpler models, such as decision trees or linear models, are often more interpretable but may sacrifice some predictive performance compared to more complex models, such as deep neural networks.

User Feedback: User feedback and subjective evaluations play a vital role in assessing the trade-off between performance and interpretability (Ribeiro et al., 2016). Gathering feedback from users, such as domain experts or end-users, on the usefulness and understandability of the explanations can provide valuable insights into the system's overall performance.

### 6.6.3 User-Centric Evaluation and Human Factors in Explainability

In addition to technical evaluation, user-centric evaluation and considering human factors are essential for assessing the effectiveness of explainable AI systems (Rudin, 2019). This involves understanding how users perceive and interact with the explanations provided by the system. Key considerations include:

User Satisfaction: Assessing user satisfaction through surveys, interviews, or usability testing can help determine how well the explanations meet user expectations and needs (Savage et al., 2019). High user satisfaction indicates that the explanations are clear, informative, and helpful.

Cognitive Load: Evaluating the cognitive load imposed on users by the explanations is crucial (Yeh et al., 2021). Explanations should be presented in a manner that minimizes cognitive effort, allowing users to comprehend and assimilate the information effectively.

Trust and Acceptance: Evaluating the level of trust and acceptance that users have in the explanations is important. Users should feel confident in the reliability, transparency, and accuracy of the explanations, which promotes trust in the AI system (Wang et al., 2019).

User Expertise and Context: Taking into account user expertise and the specific context of use is critical. Different users may have varying levels of technical knowledge, and the explanations should be tailored accordingly to ensure their understandability and relevance.

## 6.7 CHALLENGES AND FUTURE DIRECTIONS

### 6.7.1 Technical Challenges in Developing Explainable AI Models

Developing explainable AI models in healthcare presents several technical challenges. One challenge is the complexity and black-box nature of certain AI techniques, such as deep learning, which can make it difficult to interpret their decision-making processes. Another challenge is striking a balance between model complexity and interpretability, as more interpretable models may sacrifice predictive performance. Additionally, ensuring the robustness and reliability of explainable AI models, especially when dealing with diverse and evolving healthcare data, is a significant challenge. Overcoming these technical challenges requires the development of innovative algorithms and methodologies that can provide both high accuracy and explainability.

### 6.7.2 Adoption Challenges and Integration in Healthcare Systems

The adoption and integration of explainable AI in healthcare systems face various challenges. One challenge is the resistance to change and the reluctance of healthcare professionals to trust AI systems without a clear understanding of their decision-making processes (Wong et al., 2020). Additionally, integrating explainable AI models into existing healthcare workflows and electronic health record systems can be challenging due to compatibility issues, interoperability concerns, and the need for user-friendly interfaces. Overcoming these adoption challenges requires education, training, and collaboration between AI experts, healthcare professionals, and system developers to ensure the seamless integration and acceptance of explainable AI in healthcare settings.

### 6.7.3 Future Research Directions for Explainable AI in Healthcare 5.0

Future research in explainable AI for Healthcare 5.0 is focused on addressing the existing challenges and advancing the field. Some key research directions include developing novel explainability techniques that can handle complex and diverse healthcare data, enhancing the interpretability of deep learning models (Cheplygina et al., 2019), exploring the integration of human-in-the-loop approaches to improve explainability, and investigating the impact of explainable AI on clinical decision-making and patient outcomes (Acharya et al., 2021). Additionally, research is needed to establish standardized evaluation metrics, guidelines, and regulatory frameworks specific to explainable AI in healthcare to ensure its safe and effective implementation.

## 6.8 CONCLUSION

In this chapter, we have explored the concept of explainable AI in Healthcare 5.0 and its significance in improving transparency, trust, and adoption of AI systems in healthcare (Barnes et al., 2020). We discussed the evolution of healthcare toward version 5.0, highlighting the need for explainability in AI systems. We explored the fundamentals of explainable AI, techniques and approaches for achieving explainability, and the challenges and trade-offs involved. We delved into the applications of explainable AI in Healthcare 5.0, discussing its benefits, limitations of black box AI systems, and ethical considerations. We also examined various techniques and models used for explainability in healthcare. Lastly, we discussed case studies and use cases, the evaluation and assessment of explainable AI systems involved.

### 6.8.1 Significance and Implications for the Healthcare Industry

The adoption of explainable AI in healthcare has significant implications for the industry. It enhances transparency and interpretability, allowing healthcare professionals to understand and trust the decisions made by AI systems. Explainable AI is assisting in clinical decision support, personalized medicine, and medical imaging, leading to improved patient outcomes, reduced medical errors, and more efficient healthcare delivery. Furthermore, it can aid in regulatory compliance, privacy protection, and ethical considerations, ensuring the responsible and accountable use of AI in healthcare.

### 6.8.2 Recommendations for Implementing Explainable AI in Healthcare 5.0

To effectively implement explainable AI in Healthcare 5.0, several recommendations can be made. First, organizations should prioritize the development and adoption of explainable AI models that strike a balance between accuracy and interpretability. Second, interdisciplinary collaboration between AI experts, healthcare professionals, and legal and regulatory experts is essential to navigate the technical and legal complexities involved. Third, robust evaluation metrics and guidelines specific to explainable AI in healthcare should be established to assess the performance, interpretability, and usability of AI systems. Finally, ongoing research and innovation in the field are crucial to address the existing challenges, advance the understanding of explainability, and optimize its application in healthcare.

## REFERENCES

Acharya, S., et al. (2021). Explainable artificial intelligence (XAI) in healthcare: Past, present, and future. *Frontiers in Medicine*, 8, 627333.

Adadi, A., & Berrada, M. (2018). Peeking inside the black-box: A survey on explainable artificial intelligence (XAI). *IEEE Access*, 6, 52138–52160.

Arrieta, A. B., et al. (2020). Explainable artificial intelligence (XAI): Concepts, taxonomies, opportunities and challenges toward responsible AI. *Information Fusion*, 58, 82–115.

Barnes, P., et al. (2020). Explainable AI for healthcare: Applications, challenges, and future directions. *Artificial Intelligence in Medicine*, 103, 101793.

Bates, D. W., Saria, S., Ohno-Machado, L., Shah, A., & Escobar, G. (2014). Big data in health care: Using analytics to identify and manage high-risk and high-cost patients. *Health Affairs*, 33(7), 1123–1131.

Brundage, M., et al. (2020). Toward trustworthy AI development: Mechanisms for supporting verifiable claims. *arXiv preprint arXiv:2004.07213*.

Caruana, R., et al. (2015). Intelligible models for healthcare: Predicting pneumonia risk and hospital 30-day readmission. In *Proceedings of the 21th ACM SIGKDD International Conference on Knowledge Discovery and Data Mining* (pp. 1721–1730), Association for Computing Machinery.

Carvalho, A., & Freitas, A. (2019). Explainable artificial intelligence (XAI) in healthcare: Opportunities, challenges, and recommendations. *Expert Systems with Applications*, 129, 46–61.

Chen, J. H., & Asch, S. M. (2017). Machine learning and prediction in medicine—Beyond the peak of inflated expectations. *New England Journal of Medicine*, 376, 2502–2506.

Chen, J. H., et al. (2019). Developing and evaluating a machine learning based algorithm to predict the need of intensive care unit transfer for hospitalized patients. *Journal of the American Medical Informatics Association*, 26(10), 1332–1337.

Cheplygina, V., et al. (2019). Not just a black box: Interpretable deep learning in medical imaging. *Journal of Biomedical Informatics*, 97, 103253.

Cho, S., et al. (2018). Explainable AI for interpreting and understanding readmission prediction models. *PLoS ONE*, 13(11), e0207492.

Doshi-Velez, F., & Kim, B. (2017). Towards a rigorous science of interpretable machine learning. *arXiv:1702.08608v2*.

Gao, X., et al. (2020). Explainable artificial intelligence models for medical image analysis. *Medical Image Analysis*, 66, 101797.

Gilpin, L. H., et al. (2018). Explaining explanations: An overview of interpretability of machine learning. In *IEEE 5th International Conference on Data Science and Advanced Analytics (DSAA)* (pp. 80–89), Turin, Italy.

Guidotti, R., et al. (2018). A survey of methods for explaining black box models. *ACM Computing Surveys (CSUR)*, 51(5), 93.

Gunning, D., & Aha, D. (2019). DARPA's explainable artificial intelligence (XAI) program. *AI Magazine*, 40(2), 44–58.

Holzinger, A., et al. (2017). Towards interactive explainable AI in healthcare. *Artificial Intelligence in Medicine*, 82, 1–11.

Jiang, F., et al. (2020). Artificial intelligence in healthcare: Past, present, and future. *Stroke and Vascular Neurology*, 5(4), 202–214.

Lage, I., et al. (2019). Human-in-the-loop interpretability: When, why, and how. *arXiv preprint arXiv:1901.00561*.

Lipton, Z. C. (2018). The mythos of model interpretability: In machine learning, the concept of interpretability is both important and slippery. *Queue*, 16(3), 31–57.

Liu, X., & Sawada, R. (2020). Explainable artificial intelligence for precision medicine. *Methods in Molecular Biology (Clifton, N.J.)*, 2178, 153–170.

Lundberg, S. M., & Lee, S. I. (2017). A unified approach to interpreting model predictions. *arXiv preprint arXiv:1705.07874*.

Miotto, R., et al. (2016). Deep patient: An unsupervised representation to predict the future of patients from the electronic health records. *Scientific Reports*, 6, 26094.

Mittelstadt, B. (2019). Principles alone cannot guarantee ethical AI. *Nature Machine Intelligence*, 1(11), 501–507.

Mittelstadt, B. D., et al. (2019a). Explainable AI: Beware of inmates running the asylum or: How I learnt to stop worrying and love the social and behavioural sciences. *Big Data & Society*, 6(1), 2053951718821366.

Mittelstadt, B. D., et al. (2019b). Explaining explanations in AI. In *Proceedings of the 2019 AAAI/ACM Conference on AI, Ethics, and Society* (pp. 279–288).

Panch, T., et al. (2019). Artificial intelligence in oncology: Current applications and future directions. *Oncology*, 33(6), 221–226.

Patil, S., et al. (2020). Reviewing the role of artificial intelligence in cancer. *Asian Pacific Journal of Cancer Biology*, 5(4), 189–199.

Rajan, J., & Lam, C. (2019). Explainable AI models for personalized medicine in breast cancer treatment. *Frontiers in Artificial Intelligence*, 2, 27.

Rajkomar, A., et al. (2018). Scalable and accurate deep learning with electronic health records. *NPJ Digital Medicine*, 1(1), 1–10.

Rajpurkar, P., et al. (2017). CheXNet: Radiologist-level pneumonia detection on chest X-rays with deep learning. *arXiv preprint arXiv:1711.05225*.

Ribeiro, M. T., et al. (2016). "Why should I trust you?" Explaining the predictions of any classifier. In *Proceedings of the 22nd ACM SIGKDD International Conference on Knowledge Discovery and Data Mining* (pp. 1135–1144).

Rudin, C. (2019). Stop explaining black box machine learning models for high stakes decisions and use interpretable models instead. *Nature Machine Intelligence*, 1(5), 206–215.

Rudin, C. (2021). *Interpretable Machine Learning: A Guide for Making Black Box Models Explainable.* https://christophm.github.io/interpretable-ml-book/. V. Case Studies and Use Cases.

Savage, S., et al. (2019). Explainable AI in healthcare: A systematic survey. *arXiv preprint arXiv:1912.10244*.

Shen, D., et al. (2019). Interpretable deep learning for breast cancer diagnosis via biomarker image mining. *Medical Image Analysis*, 52, 32–44.

Suresh, H., & Guttag, J. V. (2017). A framework for understanding unintended consequences of machine learning. *arXiv preprint arXiv:1705.07826*.

Topol, E. J. (2019). High-performance medicine: the convergence of human and artificial intelligence. *Nature Medicine*, 25(1), 44–56.

Wachter, S., Mittelstadt, B., & Russell, C. (2017). Counterfactual explanations without opening the black box: Automated decisions and the GDPR. *Harvard Journal of Law & Technology*, 31, 841–887.

Wang, F., et al. (2019). The application of artificial intelligence in personalized medicine: A systematic review. *Precision Clinical Medicine*, 2(4), 265–279.

Wiens, J., et al. (2019). Do no harm: A roadmap for responsible machine learning for health care. *Nature Medicine*, 25(9), 1337–1340. Case Study: Interpretable Deep Learning Models for Medical Imaging

Wong, S. Q., et al. (2020). Explainable artificial intelligence (XAI) in healthcare: Challenges, opportunities, and a path forward. *Journal of the American Medical Informatics Association*, 27(11), 1763–1767

World Health Organization. (2019). *WHO Guideline: Recommendations on Digital Interventions for Health System Strengthening.* https://www.who.int/reproductivehealth/publications/digital-interventions-health-system-strengthening/en/

Yeh, C. Y., et al. (2021). Explainability in deep learning for healthcare: Lessons learned and challenges ahead. *Journal of the American Medical Informatics Association*, 28(2), 462–471.

Zhang, Y., et al. (2018). Interpretable convolutional neural networks. *arXiv preprint arXiv:1710.00935*.

7 A Complete Analysis of
Explainable AI and Its Methods
for Healthcare Prediction

*Vinora A, Lloyds E, and Soundarya M*

Healthcare is the prime concern for the welfare of the society. High-end technology is adapted in the healthcare industry, like artificial intelligence, helps to manage and control hospitals, clinics, and emergency care facilities. Advancement in technologies has helped to provide dynamic solutions in healthcare that has benefitted an enormous population. Highly intensive diseases can be diagnosed and treated in advance to reduce the severity of the impact. Individual care can be deployed based on state-of-the-art technology used to analyze patient-centric issues providing personalized care. Artificial intelligence (AI) in healthcare services has led to the development of models built to study and analyze the patterns of various diseases that help to derive a pattern that can be decrypted to treat the disease effectively. AI encapsulated along with domains such as medical imaging has proved to be effective in obtaining results and continues to be a support system in modern healthcare. The greatest challenge of AI models is the ability to make decisions in healthcare that can potentially lead to trust issues and a lack of confidentiality, security, and liability. AI has given results without further justifications on its decisions that had led to ambiguity in the accuracy of decision-making to overcome such shortfall we are have introduced explainable AI in healthcare, that gives an insight on the justification of the decisions made. It further explains the various methods adopted by explainable AI in healthcare to achieve the same.

Techniques are created in the area of explainable AI (XAI) to help elucidate the outcomes generated by AI systems. The most modern XAI methods employed in medical imaging and related fields are surveyed and the methods that are utilized to make medical imaging issues more interpretable (EChaddad et al., 2023). XAI is described as a technique incorporated by AI systems to examine and diagnose health data. A revolutionary change toward Healthcare 5.0 is forecasted in the medical industry. Healthcare 4.0 extends operational boundaries and utilizes patient-centered digital well-being. Healthcare 5.0 emphasizes ambient control, well-being, and privacy compliance using technologies including AI, IoT, and big data. Regulatory and ethical frameworks may hinder the implementation of Healthcare 5.0 in the healthcare industry. Prediction models may not be verifiable and resilience may not be as strong. Explainability is a social, ethical, legal, and medical issue that must be properly examined. An assessment of the ethical implications of AI-driven solutions in clinical settings is presented, examining the attribute of explainability in medical AI (Amann et al., 2020). XAI is a recent trend in AI that aims to make AI models easier to understand by using their decisions and predictions (Machlev et al., 2022). The explainability factor opens up new possibilities for black-box models and gives healthcare professionals the assurance to understand ML and DL models. Deep-learning-based models are used in medical image analysis where a framework of XAI is applied for effective coherence (Bas et al., 2022). The primary objective of XAI is to improve clinical health practices. XAI also improves the transparency of predictive analysis, which is crucial in the healthcare sector. XAI is an application of AI. Legal and ethical issues in the healthcare sector may arise. This chapter explains how XAI has been incorporated into Healthcare 5.0. Federated learning, a new distributed interactive AI paradigm that allows multiple clients (e.g., hospitals) to



DOI: 10.1201/9781003442066-7

participate in AI training while preserving data privacy, offers great potential for smart healthcare (Rahman et al., 2023).

## 7.1  AI IN HEALTHCARE

Artificial intelligence (AI) is increasingly being utilized in the healthcare sector due to the vastness and complexity of data. Healthcare is rapidly adopting AI, mirroring the development of the robotics industry. The purpose of AI is to enhance the efficiency of computer-based health-related tasks. AI facilitates the life of patients, doctors, and hospital administrators by performing tasks that would normally be done by humans, but in a shorter amount of time and at a much lower cost. There are numerous applications of AI in healthcare. AI is primarily employed in the analysis, planning, management, and production of results with large-scale data in healthcare, as well as in the creation of services that meet societal requirements. It essentially makes work easy by catering customized personal care to patients within a stipulated budget. AI is being predominantly used in hospitals to enhance the patient experience and user interface making it accessible to people. AI could help in their identification, segregation, and aid in the eradication of illness. Applications in technology help people maintain their active healthy lifestyles and inspire them to engage in healthy behavior. It offers users the ability to regulate their physical activity and wellbeing. Enormous amounts of apps are being developed to ease the working mode in hospitals; the app acquires the necessary details from the patients regarding symptoms faced, duration of illness, etc. It is then transferred to the doctor to give precise treatments. AI when incorporated with these apps makes prediction of disease easy, based on the enormous dataset accessed to figure out the accuracy of the symptom and make analysis easier. A steady transition is enabling AI to be incorporated along with healthcare, which reduces the amount of work and makes it less complicated. Large sets of complex data are carefully studied to analyze the patterns and determine accurately the impact of the disease and the level of infection. AI has predicted more accurate results than normal human intervention. The use of predictive analytics may facilitate physician decision-making, as well as the prioritization of management activities, and AI contributes to the improvement of the care required to link essential health information with appropriate and timely decisions. A combination of data and discovery in AI has led to major research in predicting cancer cells in patients. For example, the Institute of Cancer Research uses AI to predict how patients will respond to treatment for cancer by combining genetic and clinical info with research findings. Researchers have also created an AI robot scientist to accelerate and lower the cost of the complex drug development process. AI-powered robots can help the provider identify people who are chronically ill and at risk of a serious illness, as well as scan health data. They've been used in medicine for over a decade, ranging from simple lab robots to advanced surgical robots that either help a human surgeon or do the surgery themselves. By linking patients with relevant clinical trials, AI systems may potentially be useful in medical research.

AI in healthcare may be divided into two areas. Perceptual AI replicates the ability of medical professionals to detect illness, a skill that is essential for the diagnosis and monitoring of diseases. Additionally, intervention AI handles choices on patient treatment. AI can be incorporated into various sectors of Medicare that have proved to be beneficial, which include biomedical imaging where AI systems are trained to recognize ailments, including pneumonia, breast and skin malignancies, and eye problems, using stored databases of medical images and scans. Along with reducing the time and expense spent analyzing scans, this practice also improves diagnosis accuracy. Echocardiography that includes AI systems are utilized to look for irregular heartbeats, like coronary heart disease, screening for neurological conditions that helps to analyze AI systems analyze and interpret speech patterns to foretell the start of psychotic episodes and keep an eye out for Parkinson's disease and other neurological illnesses, and surgery where AI-controlled robotic instruments are being used to aid microsurgical procedures to lower surgical errors and malpractice.

In addition, data management techniques commonly employ AI and digital automation as an initial step in collecting and analyzing healthcare data. AI offers digital consulting based on an individual's medical background and other pertinent information. The software asks users to input their symptoms and then compares sickness databases using speech recognition. Medical records can help protect AI medical records and are highly valuable to crooks looking to steal identities or sell personal information. Pharmaceutical businesses are utilizing the AI platform to hasten the drug discovery process. Platforms can aid in the identification of drugs. AI is a basic platform that supports the diagnosis of some illnesses, enables quick diagnosis, lowers the cost of diagnosis, and is capable of diagnosing distances. Save the quicker photo processing capabilities of AI as well. They offer improved 2D and 3D imaging and cut down on the amount of time needed to complete medical imaging operations.

## 7.2   EXPLAINABLE AI (XAI)

XAI is a set of tools and processes that help people understand and trust the results of machine learning algorithms. The model that is developed using AI produces results with not much clarity of working principle for results obtained. Hence, explainable AI gives more information in the specificity of the results and gives an intuition on how decision is made by AI. This feature broadly contributes to faith in the organization that has adopted XAI.

It's hard for people to understand and keep track of what AI is doing. It's like the whole math process is just a big black box that's impossible to make sense of. Plus, even the engineers and data scientists who made the algorithm can't really explain or explain what's really happening inside them, much less how it came to a specific conclusion. Knowing how an AI system worked out a certain outcome has a lot of advantages. Adequate information about the problem statement is an essential quotient that aids developers in designing a system that satisfies the standards and assures effective functioning.

AI decision-making processes, including model tracking and accountability, need to be fully understood and trusted by your organization. ML models are often seen as mysterious and hard to understand. One major concern with AI is that it may be viewed as a "black box," which would reduce confidence in its dependability in situations when a choice may mean life or death. Researchers have been working on the black-box problem utilizing modular additions for a remarkably long period, which has contributed to the emergence of the phrase interpretable artificial intelligence. That phrase changed into explainable artificial intelligence (XAI) as the literature developed (Kırboğa & Küçüksille, 2023). This has led to the rise of the concept of explainable artificial intelligence (XAI) (Hulsen, 2023). Neural networks are one of the biggest challenges in deep learning. Bias is a common issue when training AI models, and it's important to keep track of and manage models to make sure they're up-to-date. Explainable AI helps promote end-user trust, model fit, and efficient AI use. Plus, it reduces production AI's legal, safety, and reputation risks. There are lots of tools to help you understand how explainable a model is and the metrics you use to measure its explainability (Parvathaneni Naga Srinivasu et al., 2022).

XAI is a key component of responsible artificial intelligence (RAI), a framework for the widespread implementation of AI technologies in real-world organizations with a focus on fairness, model clarity, and accountability. Companies should make it an essential practice to collaborate AI with ethical standards to gain assurance and clarity among stakeholders.

A company can use XAI to analyze and improve a model's performance while helping stakeholders understand how AI models work. To scale AI, teams need to look at how the model behaves by keeping an eye on how the deployment is going, if it's fair, if it's good, if it's poor, and if it's drifting. A company can compare predictions, measure how risky the model is, and improve the performance of the model by continuously evaluating it. Evaluation can be faster if the data needed to explain the model is shown, with positive or negative values in the behaviors. With the help of interactive charts and documents, teams can look at the behavior of the model and make predictions based on it.

AI developments have resulted in the creation of several AI solutions. These solutions are designed to be independent in behavior. Without being aware of the reasoning behind the choice, it would perceive, pick up knowledge, make a decision, and take action on its own. XAI was born out of machine learning's inability to give a reason for its choices and actions that humans could understand. In cancer surgery, if AI chooses to remove a crucial organ and the surgeons are unable to comprehend the decision; they cannot endanger the patient's life. As a result, whenever AI makes a mistaken judgment, XAI gives users the ability to discover what went wrong, why it happened, and how to fix it.

The way that trained AI algorithms operate is by receiving an input, producing an output, and not revealing how they operate inside. For humans to understand every AI decision, XAI strives to explain the reasoning behind it. Deep learning employs enormous amounts of training data to learn and recognize patterns in neural networks; much like the human brain does with neurons. It would be extremely challenging—if not impossible—to delve into the decision's justification. Contrarily, a doctor in the healthcare industry, as was previously noted, would not be able to administer the proper care without knowing the reasoning behind AI's choice. Surgery performed on the incorrect organ might be life-threatening.

## 7.2.1 Principles behind XAI

To efficiently and successfully integrate the core tenets of XAI, the US National Institute of Standards and Technology has created four principles. These concepts help us better understand how AI models function by applying separately and independently of one another.

### 1. Clarification

It requires AI to produce acceptable reasons for humans to correlate the decisions made by machines. Adequate proofs, reasons, and evidence must be generated by AI to support its decision and make the human counterpart understand the transparency of the process.

### 2. Meaningful

When a stakeholder is aware of the justification given in the first guiding principle, this principle is met. Users should be able to comprehend the explanation both individually and as a group; thus, it shouldn't be overly complicated.

### 3. Precision in Understanding Explanation

Precision in explaining the details provided by AI is crucial; it helps to generate results for a complex process. Precision is one of the most important metrics of explanation that is subject to differences based on each stakeholder. For all parties involved to comprehend the rationale, 100% accuracy is anticipated.

### 4. Limited Understanding

The final principle is to design the model to get expected results based on the limited understanding of the information prone to availability and comprehension. To minimize discrepancies or unreasonable business consequences, it is supposed to act within its restricted knowledge.

## 7.2.2 XAI Methods

An explainable AI model is set to produce a prominent model that has delivered the expected output by including transparency in decisions made by the effective model. The following XAI methods—rule-based systems, fuzzy classifiers, EBM, CBR, SHAP, LIME, Grad CAM, and LRP—are used (Loh et al., 2022). Five points are to be considered which helps to conclude on XAI methods.

1. **Explainable Data**: The specific data to be adopted by the model to get precise results. It helps to determine the elements of the dataset.
2. **Explainable Predictions**: The specific feature to be prioritized to get accurate results from the available datasets.
3. **Explainable Algorithms:** The various layers used in the model help to determine the expected results. The method adopted in the layers is deployed with the help of various algorithms in it.
4. **Proxy Modeling:** The ability to create a duplicate of the model with its actual functionalities to check the output achievements and to further enhance the original model.
5. **Design for Interpretability:** The model is designed with the interpretability to understand the dataset used the feature engineering and the biding criteria of decision-making taken by AI, thereby increasing the precision of results and having a clarified model.

XAI methods have been classified into two sub-divisions based on their modes of data and their operations:

**Global:** More generalized coherence to the model designed with the data and not specific.
**Local:** More generic information is provided to the model developed with specificity to the concerned data and prior information of decisions made is well addressed.

SHAP (Shapley additive explanations) is a paradigm that describes the output of any model using Shapley values, a game theory technique commonly used for optimum credit allocation. This method can be applied to all black-box models, but SHAP can be used to compute faster for certain model types (e.g., tree assemblies). SHAP belongs to the additive feature attribution method class. Feature attribution is the ability to apply different weights to model input features to account for changes in a result (e.g., a class probability for a class-based classification problem) against a baseline (i.e., an average prediction probability [AP] for a class in a training set). SHAP has both a global and local application models.

LIME is a technique that combines the prediction of a black-box model with a glass box substitute model. It's designed to represent the nearness of any predictions. LIME works by creating synthetic data by shaking any specific data point. This data is then evaluated by the black box system and used as a training ground for the glass box model. It's meant to be used on a local level.

Permutation importance is based on the principle that the importance of a feature is determined by its absence from the dataset. This can be applied to any score, such as accuracy, F1 or R2, to determine the importance of the feature. To achieve this, a feature can be removed from a dataset, the estimator retrained and the score evaluated. This approach can be applied globally.

The predicted outcome of a machine learning model can be affected a bit by one or two things, as seen in the partial dependency plot (a.k.a. PD plot or PDP). If a goal and a feature have a linear, monotonic, or more complicated connection, it may be seen using a partial dependency plot. It is rather fast for a perturbation-based interpretability approach. When this assumption is not satisfied, PDP might be interpretability-wise deceptive since it presupposes independence between the characteristics. It can be used globally.

In Morris sensitivity analysis for each run of OAT global sensitivity analysis, a single input's level (discrete value) is changed. The Morris method is faster (fewer model executions) than other sensitivity analysis techniques, but at the cost of not being able to differentiate between non-linearity and interaction. This is often done to see if inputs are sufficiently significant to warrant further work. It can only be applied globally.

Morris sensitivity analysis is a technique for calculating feature impacts is called accumulated local effects (ALEs). The program offers model-neutral (black box) overall justifications for regression and classification models on tabular data. PDPs' main flaws are addressed by ALE. Despite being unreasonable, it can only be used globally.

The goal of anchors is to use highly accurate rules known as anchors to describe the behavior of complicated models. These anchors provide the necessary local circumstances to confidently guarantee a given forecast. This suggests that it can only be used locally.

In terms of pertinent positives (PPs) and pertinent negatives (PN), the contrastive explanation method (CEM) produces instance-based local black box explanations for classification models. Highlights what should be minimally and unavoidably lacking (pertinent negatives) in order to create a more complete and comprehensive explanation, as well as what should be minimum and adequately present in order to support the categorization of an input sample by a neural network. CEM is designed to be utilized locally.

Counterfactual explanations "interrogate" a model to reveal how much the values of certain features would need to alter to reverse the overall forecast. The phrase "If had not occurred, would not have occurred" is used to describe a situation or a result in a counterfactual manner. A learning classifier would be of interest in the setting of a machine and would be the label that the model would predict. The application of counterfactual instances is intended to be local.

Integrated gradients are intended for local applications. The purpose of integrated gradients is to determine the relevance of each input feature in a machine learning model based on gradients of model output for that input. It can be used to determine the importance of features, to detect data skews, and to troubleshoot model performance.

ML models are interpreted globally by a compact binary tree that uses a contribution matrix of input variables to describe the key decision rules that are implicitly present in the model. By maximizing the difference in the average contribution of the split variable between the divided spaces, a unified process iteratively splits the input variable space to produce the interpretation tree. Global interpretation via recursive partitioning (GIRP) is only applicable globally.

Protodash is an innovative method for discovering "prototypes" in an active machine learning program. A prototype may be viewed as a subset of the data that has a stronger impact on the model's capacity for prediction. To understand what drives forecasts, a prototype should state something to the effect of if you eliminated these data points, the model wouldn't perform as well. One may only use Protodash locally.

Scalable Bayesian rule lists develop a list of decision-making rules based on the facts. They contain a logical structure that is a series of if-then rules. Both globally and locally, scalable Bayesian rule lists are applicable.

Black box model predictions are approximated by a tree surrogate, also known as interpretable model. By analyzing the surrogate model, we may make inferences about the black-box model. The policy trees offer quantitative forecasts of future conduct and are simple for humans to understand. Tree substitutes are applicable both globally and locally.

Explainable boosting machine (EBM) is an interpretable model developed by Microsoft Research. It's a way to revive old GAMs with the help of modern machine-learning tricks like bagging and gradient boosting. It's a tree-based gradient boosting GMM with automatic interaction detection. It's called an EBM because it's so easy to understand, even with modern black-box models. It's super compact and super fast at predicting time, but it's not as fast as other modern algorithms. It has global and local uses.

## 7.3 KEY BENEFITS OF XAI IN HEALTHCARE 5.0

The term Healthcare 5.0 refers to the integration of cutting-edge digital technologies into the day-to-day operations of healthcare organizations. Technological progress has been drastic in Healthcare 5.0, especially in shifting from traditional healthcare. However, the involvement of AI in healthcare is coupled with ambiguity regarding the decision-making skills of machines and their reliability on it. In the absence of emotional recognition, personalized and pervasive health apps, and emotive smart devices, emerging technologies must be leveraged to embed smart sensors into health systems. Wearable sensors have also significantly contributed to Healthcare 5.0, which aid in remote patient tracking and monitoring and have also led to online consultation of doctors. Despite the progress made in the area of innovation and integrated healthcare, further technological development and research is necessary to open up new opportunities and progress Healthcare 5.0 to a new era of smart disease control, virtual care, intelligent health management, intelligent monitoring, and intelligent decision-making. Numerous emerging technologies, including 5G, smart sensors, wearable technologies, and robotics, as well as big data, cloud computing, and AI, are paving the way toward a Healthcare 5.0 landscape, where patient monitoring and tracking can be achieved through telemedicine and robotic surgery, robotic-assisted wellness monitoring, and personalized healthcare. Sensor technologies have had a significant impact on healthcare since their introduction, as they enable the conversion of health data into measurable electrical impulses, such as heart rate, blood sugar levels, oxygen saturation, temperature, and blood pressure, all of which are often recorded by sensor-based smart devices and transmitted as electrical pulses for further processing. Sensors are continuing to have a significant impact on healthcare systems worldwide, particularly during the pandemic, and are unlocking new opportunities for virtual treatment. Smart devices such as smartphones, wearables, and interoperable medical technology (IoMT) have enabled remote recording and processing of health data. However, there is an enormous number of challenges faced due to financial, infrastructural, and legal constraints. Healthcare 5.0 is attainable with the help of government regularization of rules and norms to be framed for legalization and also receive financial support from public and private organizations. Smart healthcare is said to be provided by Healthcare 5.0, which is set to provide effortless consultation to various health issues faced by patients in remote. The implementation of Healthcare 5.0 may be hampered by organizational difficulties and infrastructure and technological limitations. It is essential to develop strong, technology-based healthcare systems due to a variety of factors, such as a lack of electronic health record (e-health) policies and regulatory framework, individual perception, strategic disagreement with hospitals, insufficient financial resources, as well as religious and cultural impediments (Elliot Mbunge et al., 2021).

A revolutionary change from traditional methods to the digitization of healthcare has contributed to Healthcare 5.0 Healthcare 5.0 is said to integrate available digital technologies to provide a hassle-free environment to patients. The implementation of aided technologies, such as artificial intelligence (AI), IoT, big data, and assisted networking channels (ANCs), in the healthcare landscape has enabled the development of a 5.0 approach to patient monitoring in real time, as well as ambient control and well-being, as well as privacy compliance (Saraswat et al., 2022). The success of the Healthcare 5.0 system is largely dependent on its stakeholders, including investors, practitioners, and organizations, as well as the end users, such as patients, who are willing to embrace the change. Various advanced technologies such as AI, smart wearable sensors, Internet of Medical Things (IoMT), and 5G are incorporated into Healthcare 5.0 to keep it highly automated. It has contributed to smart healthcare, which is patient-centric. Developed countries are actively progressing toward Healthcare 5.0, which is a significant development. They are various factors that contribute to disconcertment such as the security of digitized data, accuracy in decisions taken by machines, genuineness of medication provided, digital prescription, and trustability of robots being used for assistance in healthcare. To overcome the issues faced, Healthcare 5.0 is progressing toward automation in healthcare with integrity, trust ability, confidentiality, and security. Healthcare 5.0's security needs, threat model, and information on its numerous applications are all supplied. Next, we compare the performance of the security measures that are currently in place in Healthcare 5.0 (Wazid et al., 2022).

In healthcare, where robots play an important role in decision-making, XAI might be beneficial. Humans are significantly impacted by the judgments made by AI in the healthcare industry. The time saved by a machine with XAI might be used by the medical team to treat and attend to additional patients. For instance, quickly identifying a malignant spot and discussing the cause enables the doctor to administer the proper care.

## Positive Effects of XAI in Medical Services

The use of XAI in medical services has a variety of advantages, such as:

**Greater faith:** In addition, patients and healthcare professionals may be more likely to trust AI systems if they receive clear and comprehensible explanations for the decisions made by these algorithms.

**Enhanced comprehension:** XAI can help healthcare professionals gain a deeper comprehension of how AI is employed to make decisions related to patient care, thereby contributing to an increase in overall quality of care.

**Decreased bias:** XAI can assist in detecting and removing biases in AI systems, which can help to guarantee that patients receive fair and impartial care.

**Enhanced regulatory compliance:** In some circumstances, XAI may be forced to adhere to legal regulations, such as those stated in the General Data Protection Regulation (GDPR) of the European Union.

**Enhanced clarity**: XAI approaches promote openness in healthcare procedures by outlining how an AI system came to a guaranteed result. Higher levels of trust are subsequently created as a result of more openness and understanding. The explanations provided by XAI approaches may also be used to track how different elements affect an AI system's capacity for prediction.

**Model enhancement:** To provide a forecast, AI systems learn from data. Sometimes the established rules are wrong, which can lead to false forecasts. Examining the learned rules using the explanations provided by XAI approaches can lead to the detection of mistakes and model improvements.

**Precision enhancement:** XAI in healthcare can enhance the accuracy of medical diagnostics and treatment plans by describing how an AI system makes its inferences. This facilitates better understanding among doctors and other medical personnel, resulting in more precise and effective therapy.

**Knowledge transfer:** XAI enables the transmission of knowledge from AI systems to healthcare professionals, who then apply that information to improve patient outcomes. An AI system, for instance, may find a connection between a symptom and a condition that was not known before. The AI system explains its logic so that practitioners may see new connections that they can employ in their future diagnoses.

**Advance detection:** XAI may be able to assist in the early detection of diseases by analyzing vast amounts of patient information and uncovering anomalies that medical professionals may have overlooked. Additionally, XAI may describe how it came to this conclusion and why some people are more susceptible to specific diseases, and offer mitigation strategies.

We must make sure that AI systems are open and understandable as they become more commonplace in healthcare. A key tool for reaching this objective, XAI can raise patient satisfaction by enhancing communication, trust, and comprehension. Healthcare's future will surely be shaped by XAI as healthcare providers and AI developers continue to collaborate to use AI to enhance healthcare outcomes. Explainability in healthcare is a divisive issue with long-term consequences. AI is being used more and more in the management of health services, clinical decision-making, predictive medicine, patient data, and diagnostics. Nevertheless, despite its remarkable performance, AI is still seen as a mystery.

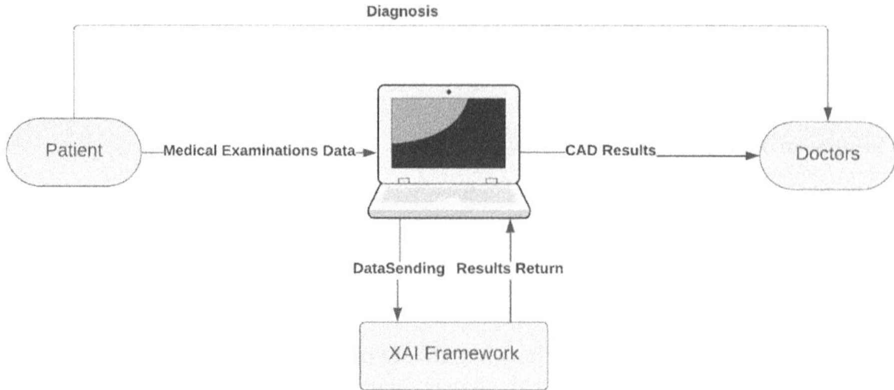


**FIGURE 7.1**   XAI interface.

Figure 7.1 depicts the follow to data into XAI-related services for remote patient monitoring in medical services.

This is due in part to a lack of trust, which results from a lack of openness. For instance, the medical professional should be able to describe why one course of therapy is superior to another. The lack of this "explainability" by the AI system may hinder its acceptance. Therefore, explainable AI (XAI) in healthcare refers to technology that allows practitioners to comprehend "why" the system made particular conclusions. In other words, it illustrates the reasoning that is built into the AI system.

## Benefits of Cognitive AI in Healthcare

Many high-performing black-box models provide results by employing accurate or clear variables. For instance, a deep learning network trained on patients with asthma and active physician input mis-inferred a low fatality rate for pneumonia. Another deep learning model utilized irrelevant information, such as the scanner's location, to check X-rays for pneumonia. In a third instance, hardware-related data was utilized to forecast risk in a model for identifying high- and low-risk patients based on an x-ray. These examples illustrate that relying solely on model reliability alone is not enough. Further frameworks that foster trustworthiness, including explainable AI, are necessary.

Healthcare explainable AI has pushed value-based care and urged providers to prioritize results above service quantities. For instance, XAI algorithms examine patient data to identify those who are more likely to acquire particular illnesses. By doing this, healthcare professionals can take action before a situation worsens. We may anticipate more wearables being integrated as the usage of explainable AI in healthcare increases. As they track their wearers' health throughout the day, wearables are an excellent source of patient data. This information may be used by explainable AI to create suggestions and make precise diagnoses. Potential distinctions between AI and XAI approaches are given, with the most current XAI techniques being (i) interpretable machine learning, (ii) knowledge base and distillation algorithms, and (iii) local and global preprocessing methods. The prerequisite offers insights for the brainstorming sessions before to starting a medical XAI project, while XAI characteristics specifics with future healthcare explainability are prominently featured (Sheu & Pardeshi, 2022).

## Healthcare and XAI in the Future

The market for healthcare AI software is growing significantly. The benefits of AI will be difficult to overlook as long as data production keeps increasing. However, there are also legitimate worries about security and privacy. XAI in healthcare is set to revolutionize data democratization, giving people more control over their information and how it's used. This study looks at the challenges researchers have faced, what the future holds for XAI research, and what XAI techniques are being used in medical XAI apps. The survey results show that medical XAI is an exciting field of research, and this chapter is meant to give medical professionals and AI scientists advice on how to create medical XAI (Zhang et al., 2022).

Figure 7.2 explains the various methods adopted to get liable results from AI.

Algorithmic accountability and transparency in AI systems is one of XAI's key objectives. AI systems were primarily black boxes in the past. XAI is mainly used for computer vision and natural language processing, but a lot of clinical and remote health apps also rely on time series data (Di Martino & Delmastro, 2023). Even when the inputs and outputs are available, the decision-making algorithms are frequently secret or impossible to decode. The following are some objectives of implementing AI systems:

- **Builds faith in AI:** The inability to discern the reasoning behind an AI-based system's conclusions may make people hesitant to place their faith in it. The end customers are expected to receive a comprehensive explanation of XAI's operations.
- **Enhances the entire system:** With more transparency, developers are able to identify and resolve issues faster.

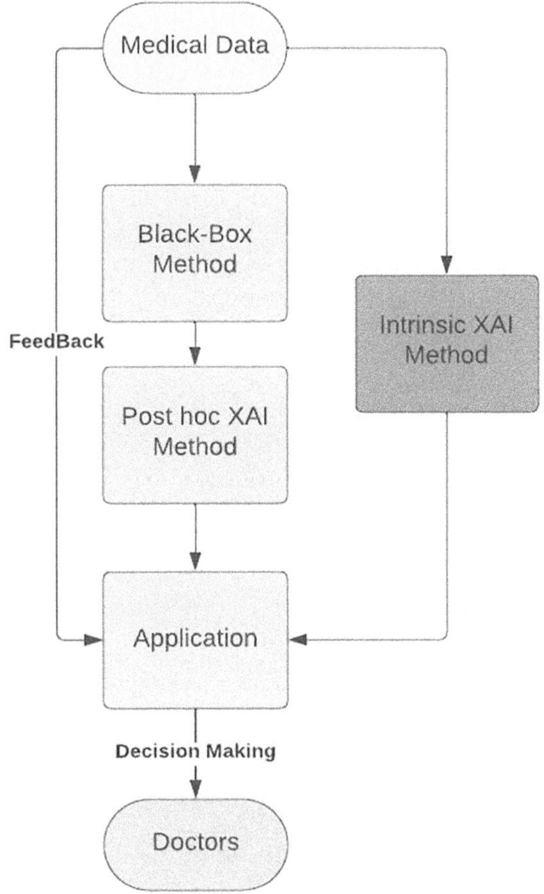


**FIGURE 7.2**  Liability on decisions made by AI.

- **Offers defense against antagonistic assaults:** Adversary attacks use fake data to trick a model into making bad decisions. An attack against an XAI would reveal the attack by giving false reasons for making decisions.
- **Anti-bias measures for AI:** The goal of XAI is to explain properties and make decisions in ML algorithms. This aids in identifying unfair results brought on by biased developers or poor-quality training data.
- **Dynamic evolution:** AI would accelerate the process of releasing new pharmaceuticals to the market to combat these terrible diseases and improve the success rate and efficacy of the corresponding drug evolution. For instance, AI-based solutions are being developed in radiology to automate picture analysis and diagnosis.

It explains the how XAI is incorporated to machine learning to make reliable decisions.

Risk assessment, autonomous systems, and supply chain management are among healthcare domains where XAI can help. It promotes compliance while reducing risks and improving knowledge, productivity, trust, and adoption.

## 7.4  DRAWBACKS/LIMITATIONS

Artificial intelligence (AI) is as effective as the data on which it is trained. Inconsistencies in the data's availability, in other words, might impede learning and limit its potential. A substantial

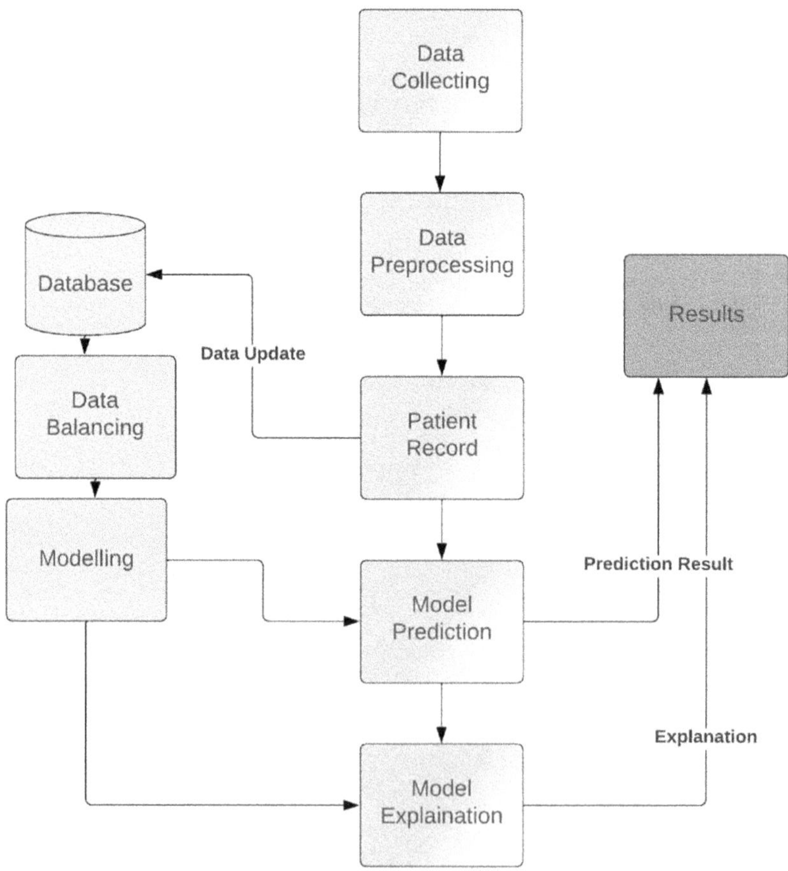


**FIGURE 7.3**   Machine learning structure incorporated with XAI.

amount of computer power is also needed for the analysis of huge and complicated datasets. One of the anticipated challenges in the training of AI systems is the fact that many healthcare institutions around the world do not systematically digitize their medical data. Furthermore, there is an absence of uniformity in the IT systems, digital records management, and data tagging of these healthcare institutions.

Human-level concerns arise in a different manner. Human beings possess certain characteristics that machines are unable to acquire, such as empathy. Compassion, reading between the lines, and interpreting social signals are two abilities that physicians use in clinical practice, which AI currently does not have the capacity to comprehend or replicate. Drawbacks are caused by several circumstances, including:

- **Training issues**

Medical practitioners must be adequately trained to utilize a variety of AI technologies, while the tools themselves must be adequately educated using data-curated environments. This can lead to issues that would not have occurred without the utilization of AI in either situation.

- **Potential for unemployment**

Artificial intelligence and automation pose a serious threat to many industries, and healthcare is no exception. The implementation of AI may lead to the elimination of administrative positions, and any sector may be adversely affected by too much disruption. Therefore, it is essential to strike a balance and ensure that departments are adequately prepared for AI prior to its implementation.

- **Excessive change might be difficult to handle**

This is especially important in the healthcare sector, where critical decisions can be made that could determine life or death. It is essential for the healthcare industry to ensure that AI is able to be applied effectively and that all personnel are adequately informed of how medical technology works.

- **Continues to need feedback from individuals**

Healthcare AI has advanced dramatically, but it still depends on human input and oversight. Humans are exceptional in that they can observe patient conduct and relate with them in a manner that machines cannot. These observations may occasionally play a crucial role in a medical diagnosis and help to avert future issues.

- **Increased security risk**

AI systems may be security-vulnerable, which is a major issue for the healthcare sector because patient data must be kept private. Cyberattacks are growing more expert and precise, but they are also getting tougher to foresee and stop. This implies that to ensure they deter hackers; healthcare organizations will need to spend a considerable amount of money.

- **Social factors might be disregarded**

When treating people, it's frequently not only about their physical ailments. In actuality, social, historical, and economic circumstances can also affect the precise type of care a person needs. While AI is more than capable of determining the best course of therapy based on the diagnosis, it is not yet able to take other social factors into account that can affect a medical professional's choice.

- **Errors are possible**

The use of AI in medicine would eliminate many human-caused mistakes, but it couldn't eliminate inaccuracy. Mistakes are still likely to happen if there is a significant quantity of data involved, and data gaps can also be a problem. This may have detrimental effects on areas like the prescribing of medicine.

## 7.5   APPLICATIONS OF XAI IN HEALTHCARE

AI is already being successfully utilized in various aspects of healthcare, with numerous opportunities for its further integration in the future. Some applications of how XAI could have a positive impact on the healthcare profession.

- **Prosthetic hand**

While many prosthetic hands do not provide wearers with the ability to regain their sense of touch, DARPA's latest iteration of an artificial hand incorporates neutron technology to achieve just that. Developed by the APL at Johns Hopkins University, this mechanical arm was able to restore sensory perception for a 28-year-old man. By utilizing electrodes directly on his sensory cortex and motor control areas in the brain, he became the first individual to experience physical sensations with an artificial hand.

- **HIV prevention algorithms**

Every year, 2 million Americans between the ages of 13 and 24 experience homelessness. One in eleven of them have HIV. However, scientists at the School of Social Work and Engineering at the University of Southern California have created a new algorithm called PSINET that pinpoints the most effective homeless community members to disseminate vital information about HIV prevention to young people.

- **Customized mobile app**

The purpose of mobile applications is to interact with the vast array of app creation options. A smartphone app may be used for everything from making doctor visits to scheduling tests, uploading a patient's medical information, and receiving test results. Health organizations can design practical digital solutions that are suitable for today's patients.

- **Sophia**

A Hong Kong–based startup called Hansen Robotics created Sophia, a social humanoid robot. Sophia employs voice recognition technologies from Alphabet Inc. to get better over time. To create better future responses, the XAI program analyzes discussions and gathers data.

- **Identification and diagnosis of illness**

Healthcare might utilize machine learning to identify more complicated illnesses that aren't immediately obvious after a diagnosis. It could also be used to keep an eye on patients to spot any deterioration in their diseases. The XAI system would then be able to gather crucial information and notify medical personnel.

- **Diagnostic imaging**

Following studies that demonstrated XAI might be as successful as human radiologists at detecting illnesses like cancer, XAI is already being employed in medical imaging. This is crucial for early prevention, but it also means that XAI can evaluate medical photos much more rapidly and completely, reducing the possibility of human mistakes.

- **Drug development and production**

By examining data and currently available medications, XAI in medicine may be utilized to develop novel medications. It is extremely expensive and time-consuming to discover and develop new medicines. Costs might be cut, and promising new medications could be discovered much more quickly with the aid of XAI.

- **Maintaining patient records**

AI may be a useful tool for gathering and interpreting data, including medical information, as we've already mentioned. This not only makes medical professionals' work much more efficient, but it also allows them to prioritize other crucial facets of their jobs and work more quickly.

- **Strengthening access to care**

There is frequently a personnel shortage in the medical field because of the constant demand. This has become a bigger problem in emerging nations. By utilizing XAI, life-saving treatment may be made more accessible to individuals worldwide, as well as utilized to close skill gaps and aid in patient diagnosis.

- **Utilizing personal gadgets and wearables to monitor health**

Smart gadgets and wearables are already utilized in healthcare to monitor patients and perform online consultations. The usage of these technologies is only expected to grow, enabling medical personnel to act as soon as issues arise and guarantee patients receive care as quickly as feasible.

## 7.6  CONCLUSION

Although artificial intelligence in healthcare has both benefits and drawbacks, it is evident that in general, it is viewed as a force for good and will continue to be developed and employed more frequently in the future. In reality, thorough data analysis already plays a crucial part in determining the needs of patients. It is expected that medical practitioners will rely on it even more for direction and assistance, utilizing it successfully to give patients precise and timely care. In the end, XAI's function in medicine is to reduce human mistakes, simplify the job of devoted healthcare workers, and advance patient care. Whether you're a medical professional or need medical care in the future, you'll probably see XAI technology being employed in a healthcare setting regularly. XAI in Healthcare 5.0 will be deployed for the betterment of human race with more sophisticated features that provide accuracy, adaptability, and reliability.

## REFERENCES

Amann, J., Blasimme, A., Vayena, E., et al., Explainability for Artificial Intelligence in Healthcare: A Multidisciplinary Perspective. *BMC Medical Informatics and Decision Making* 20 (2020), 310. https://doi.org/10.1186/s12911-020-01332-6.

Di Martino, F., Delmastro, F., Explainable AI for Clinical and Remote Health Applications: A Survey on Tabular and Time Series Data. *Artificial Intelligence Review* 56 (2023), 5261–5315. https://doi.org/10.1007/s10462-022-10304-3.

EChaddad, A., Peng, J., Xu, J., Bouridane, A., Survey of Explainable AI Techniques in Healthcare. *Sensors (Basel)* 23(2) (2023), 634. https://doi.org/10.3390/s23020634. PMID: 36679430; PMCID: PMC9862413.

Hulsen, T., Explainable Artificial Intelligence (XAI): Concepts and Challenges in Healthcare. *AI*, 4 (2023), 652–666. https://doi.org/ 10.3390/ai4030034.

Kırboğa, K.K., Küçüksille, E.U., 5 XAI in Biomedical Applications. In *Explainable Artificial Intelligence for Biomedical Applications*, River Publishers, 2023, pp.79–100.

Loh, H., Ooi, C., Seoni, S., Barua, P.D., Molinari, F., Acharya, U.R., Application of Explainable Artificial Intelligence for Healthcare: A Systematic Review of the Last Decade (2011–2022). *Computer Methods and Programs in Biomedicine* 226 (2022). https://doi.org/10.1016/j.cmpb.2022.107161.

Machlev, R., Heistrene, L., Perl, M., Levy, K.Y., Belikov, J., Mannor, S., Levron, Y., Explainable Artificial Intelligence (XAI) Techniques for Energy and Power Systems: Review, Challenges and Opportunities. *Energy and AI* 9 (2022), 100169. ISSN 2666-5468. https://doi.org/10.1016/j.egyai.2022.100169.

Mbunge, E., Muchemwa, B., Jiyane, S., Batani, J., Sensors and Healthcare 5.0: Transformative Shift in Virtual Care Through Emerging Digital Health Technologies. *Global Health Journal* 5(4) (2021), 169–177. ISSN 2414-6447. https://doi.org/10.1016/j.glohj.2021.11.008.

Rahman, A., Hossain, M.S., Muhammad, G., et al., Federated Learning-Based AI Approaches in Smart Healthcare: Concepts, Taxonomies, Challenges and Open Issues. *Cluster Computing* 26 (2023), 2271–2311. https://doi.org/10.1007/s10586-022-03658-4.

Saraswat, D., Bhattacharya, P., Verma, A., Prasad, V., Tanwar, S., Sharma, G., Bokoro, P., Sharma, R., Explainable AI for Healthcare 5.0: Opportunities and Challenges. *IEEE Access* (2022), 1–30. https://doi.org/10.1109/ACCESS.2022.3197671.

Sheu, R.K., Pardeshi, M.S., A Survey on Medical Explainable AI (XAI): Recent Progress, Explainability Approach, Human Interaction and Scoring System. *Sensors* 22(20) (2022), 8068. https://doi.org/10.3390/s22208068.

Srinivasu, P.N., Sandhya, N., Jhaveri, R.H., Raut, R., From Blackbox to Explainable AI in Healthcare: Existing Tools and Case Studies. *Mobile Information Systems* 2022, Article ID 8167821 (2022), 20 pages. https://doi.org/10.1155/2022/8167821.

van der Velden, B.H.M., Kuijf, H.J., Gilhuijs, K.G.A., Viergever, M.A., Explainable Artificial Intelligence (XAI) in Deep Learning-Based Medical Image Analysis. *Medical Image Analysis* 79 (2022), 102470, ISSN 1361-8415. https://doi.org/10.1016/j.media.2022.102470.

Wazid, M., Das, A.K., Mohd, N., Park, Y., Healthcare 5.0 Security Framework: Applications, Issues and Future Research Directions. *IEEE Access* 10 (2022), 129429–129442. https://doi.org/10.1109/ACCESS.2022.3228505.

Zhang, Y., Weng, Y., Lund, J., Applications of Explainable Artificial Intelligence in Diagnosis and Surgery. *Diagnostics (Basel)* 12(2) (2022), 237. https://doi.org/10.3390/diagnostics12020237. PMID: 35204328; PMCID: PMC8870992.

# 8 Artificial Intelligence (AI) Algorithms and Approaches for Edge AI

*Samar Mouti and Samer Rihawi*

## 8.1 INTRODUCTION

The healthcare and industry fields are being significantly impacted by the dynamic synergy of edge computing and artificial intelligence (AI) algorithms. The complex AI algorithms at the center of this revolution are designed for edge computing. This chapter's goal is to provide an understanding of these algorithms' capabilities in practical applications by analyzing them in terms of accuracy, speed, and resource consumption.

By using edge AI, AI calculations can now take place locally on devices instead of being limited to centralized cloud servers. This makes use of the complementary properties of edge computing and data processing power. It entails the creation and implementation of cutting-edge computer programs and algorithms that work directly on adjacent computing endpoints, Internet of Things (IoT) devices, and smartphones. This is different from the traditional use of cloud servers that are centralized.

Due to the complicatedness of most AI models and the challenge of calculating conclusion results on devices accompanying restricted possessions, AI duties are currently achieved to process requests in cloud dossier centers. However, these "end cloud" architectures cannot meet the needs of palpable-period AI services to a degree of instant science of logical analysis and astute production. Therefore, bringing AI requests to the edge opens the potential for AI request synopsizes, especially in conditions of attaining reduced abeyance traits (Wang et al., 2020).

Edge AI enhances the effectiveness of data processing. The system may manage data more effectively, maximizing resource utilization and guaranteeing that crucial insights are obtained quickly, by dividing computing responsibilities across local devices. This paradigm shift toward edge AI is in line with the changing demands of industry and presents a viable path forward for breakthroughs across a range of fields, including healthcare where secure and quick data processing is critical.

Figure 8.1 displays the direct deployment of artificial intelligence algorithms into edge devices. Edge AI is independent of the cloud so it can process data more quickly and efficiently from its source.

Edge AI enhances user experience and uses local processing to boost data protection. Since there is no requirement for data transfer, security precautions are increased in contrast to centralized cloud systems. From a technical perspective, less bandwidth needed can result in cheaper rates for Internet services that require subscriptions. One unique characteristic of edge technology gadgets is their self-contained design. These gadgets function independently and do not require continuous assistance from data scientists or AI developers, in contrast to typical setups. Monitoring becomes more efficient when graphical data flows are provisioned automatically (Raj et al., 2022).

DOI: 10.1201/9781003442066-8

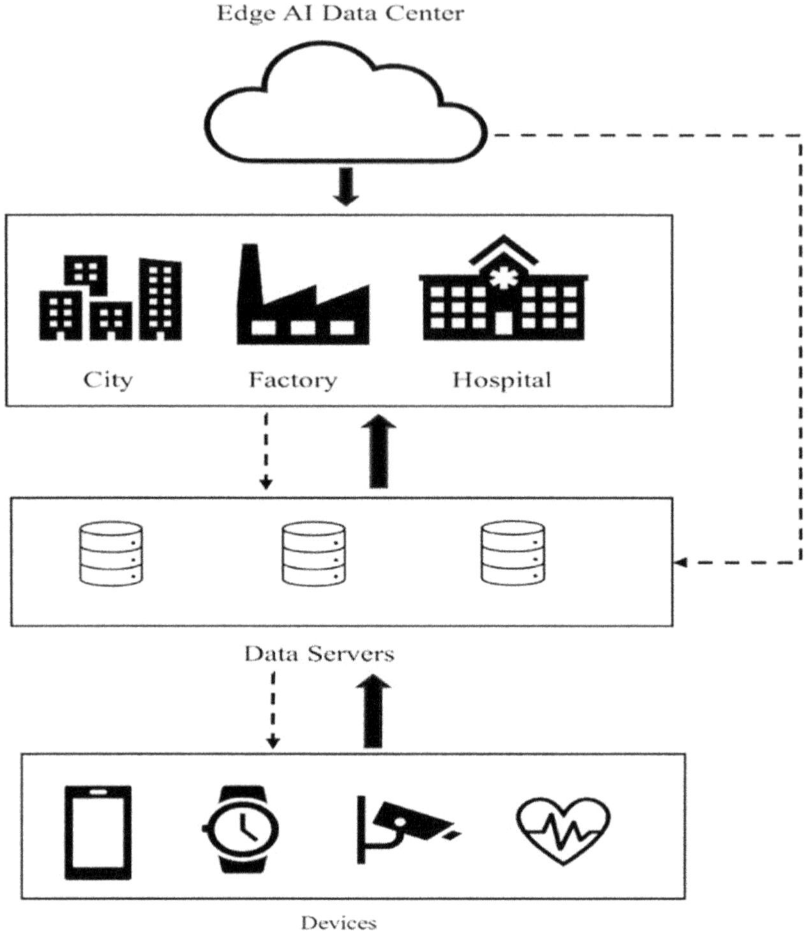


**FIGURE 8.1** Edge AI and applications.

## 8.2 AI ALGORITHMS AND APPROACHES FOR EDGE COMPUTING IN THE INDUSTRY AND HEALTHCARE SECTORS

AI cooperates with edge computing to investigate the world of contemporary AI algorithms tailor-made for edge estimating, fixating on by what they perform in agreements of veracity, speed, and capital exercise. Some edge devices have restricted estimating capacity. Simple and effective machine intelligence algorithms like decision shrubs and k-most familiar neighbors have existed and adjusted to work efficiently at the edge (Sun et al., 2018).

Deep knowledge models, exceptionally convolutional neural networks (CNNs), and recurrent neural networks (RNNs) have proven extraordinary progress in tasks like image and talk acknowledgment. Optimized architectures like MobileNet and SqueezeNet have been planned to boost speed and humiliate the load on edge devices (Howard et al., 2017). Federated education admits model preparation across differing edge devices while the custody dossier is local. This approach reinforces solitude and reduces the need for concentrated data storage, making it specifically appropriate for healthcare uses (McMahan et al., 2017). Research indicates that edge-located AI models can uphold aggressive veracity distinguished from those in the cloud, especially when they are tweaked for the distinguishing restraints of edge estimating (Chen et al., 2019).

Edge computing considerably reduces abeyance by handling dossiers regionally. Algorithms designed for the edge supply instructions speed outside give up veracity. For example, the YOLO (you only look once) object discovery algorithm acts unusually well in evident-occasion on edge instruments (Redmon et al., 2016). Making ultimate of restricted capacity and depository on edge schemes is crucial. Techniques to degree model trimming, quantization, and information distillate help in reducing the reserve footmark of AI models on edge ploys (Han et al., 2015).

AI borderline is transforming the smart city foundation by permissive honest-occasion accountability, lowering abeyance, optimizing frequency range exercise, and reconstructing solitude and security. This example change authorizes smart places to run more capably, behave swiftly in changeful environments, and enhance the overall characteristics of city life (Herath & Mittal, 2022).

Using predicting science of logical analysis on patient dossier admits for exact and rapid case prioritization and sorting. Among the notable dealers in this place rule is Jvion; it anticipates and evaluates risks correctly, transferring litigable pieces of advice that improve results. Wellframe takes a creative approach to patient care by contributing mutual care programs straight to consumers' traveling devices. Its dispassionate piece notebook, which is an established evidence-based situation, authorizes the situation group to supply a customized happening to each patient. Enclitic's patient triaging schemes flip through succeeding cases for various dispassionate signs, end their preference, and route the ruling class to the network's most adapted doctor. Edge AI is used in healing images and is demonstrative in the way that Ezra uses AI to analyze brimming-bulk MRI dossier to assist clinicians in the early disease of malignancy. Also used in leading healing depict to judge and remodel images in addition to model potential positions. SkinVision allows you to pinpoint a skin tumor early by photographing it accompanying your telephone and shipping it to a doctor at the appropriate opportunity. AI-stimulated medical image is more usually working in the disease of COVID-19 cases and the identification of victims the one demand blower of air support (Dilmegan, 2023).

The unification of AI algorithms into edge computing has huge potential, especially in healthcare. Optimized models, accompanying progress in federated knowledge and edge-particular architectures, show hopeful results in conditions of veracity, speed, and resource exercise.

## 8.3   USE CASES OF EDGE AI IN THE INDUSTRY AND HEALTHCARE SECTORS

Edge AI has applications in a variety of industries, including healthcare, manufacturing, smart cities, retail, and others. The transformative impact of edge AI in both industry and healthcare sectors. It effectively communicates the versatility of edge AI through a well-structured and concise exploration of diverse use cases (Dilmegan, 2023). Table 8.1 provides a detailed description of the user cases for Edge AI, which shows how various sectors are using smart technology in different ways.

These applications showcase how edge AI is making a positive impact in various aspects of industry and healthcare, making processes more efficient, accurate, and responsive.

## 8.4   KEY CHALLENGES AND LIMITATIONS OF EDGE AI IN THE INDUSTRY AND HEALTHCARE SECTORS

In the era of the Internet of Everything, the research addresses current challenges proposes potential solutions, and outlines future directions. It raises awareness among researchers about the evolving landscape of edge intelligence, encouraging further exploration and development in this dynamic

**TABLE 8.1**

**Edge AI Use Cases**

| **1. Predictive Maintenance in Manufacturing** |
| --- |
| Use smart technology to predict when machines in manufacturing might break down. |
| Avoid unexpected breakdowns, keep machines working longer, and make maintenance more efficient. |
| **2. Quality Control in Production** |
| Use smart cameras to check products for defects as they're being made. |
| Ensure that products meet high-quality standards, reduce mistakes, and make production smoother. |
| **3. Industrial Automation and Robotics** |
| Employ smart technology to make robots and machines work more precisely and efficiently in factories. |
| Speed up production, improve accuracy, and make manufacturing processes more adaptable. |
| **4. Remote Monitoring and Maintenance of Equipment** |
| Allow experts to check on machines from afar and fix issues without being physically present. |
| Save time and money, avoid travel, and keep operations running smoothly. |
| **5. Healthcare Diagnostics and Imaging** |
| Use smart tools to help doctors analyze medical images for things like tumors. |
| Speed up diagnoses make medical decisions more accurate and support timely treatments. |
| **6. Personalized Medicine** |
| Examine individual patient data to suggest treatments tailored to their specific needs. |
| Improve treatment effectiveness, reduce side effects, and enhance patient outcomes. |
| **7. Edge-Based Drug Discovery** |
| Apply smart algorithms to study molecular data for discovering new drugs. |
| Speed up the development of new medicines and identifies potential therapeutic compounds. |
| **8. Wearable Health Monitoring** |
| Use smart wearables to continuously track health metrics like heart rate and activity. |
| Keep individuals informed about their health, detect issues early, and support proactive healthcare. |
| **9. Smart Prosthetics and Assistive Devices** |
| Enhance artificial limbs and assistive devices with smart technology for better control. |
| Improve the user experience, responsiveness, and integration of devices into daily life. |
| **10. Patient Data Security and Privacy** |
| Ensure that patient data is processed securely without needing to send it to centralize servers. |
| Address privacy concerns, follow data protection rules, and build trust with patients. |
| **11. Emergency Response and Disaster Management** |
| Use smart technology to quickly analyze data during emergencies for better decision-making. |
| Speed up responses, improve awareness during disasters, and enhance overall emergency management. |

field. This research focuses on training models with local data on resource-constrained edge devices and deploying models at the edge through techniques like model compression and inference acceleration (Su et al., 2022).

Even though edge AI is making a positive impact in different aspects of people's lives, there are several challenges and obstacles in this area that should be addressed. Those challenges can be defined as follows (Iftikhar et al., 2023):

### 8.4.1 HETEROGENEOUS DATA

Edge AI receives different types of data from various resources such as smart wearables and smart cameras. This data comes in different types such as image, sound, and text. That's why edge AI must learn how to fuse this data by extracting the relevant features. Multimodal deep learning can be used to overcome this challenge.

### 8.4.2 RESOURCE MANAGEMENT

The increase in IoT devices and applications leads to the generation of massive data. This poses a challenge in terms of latency, bandwidth, and security in comparison to the traditional cloud infrastructure, which necessitates efficient resource management in edge computing environments.

### 8.4.3 ENVIRONMENTAL SUSTAINABILITY

As the edge AI applications are limited in computation resources, sustainability has become an important concern since the AI models need a lot of resources for training and decision-making. AI models can use lightweight frameworks for training and testing data to remain edge friendly. TensorFlow Lite is one of the available platforms for AI-based solutions as it consumes fewer resources.

### 8.4.4 SECURITY

The edge AI platforms such as smart home and smart healthcare are known to have distributed platforms. This makes it challenging to continuously observe the IoT applications to get enough data for training and inference. The main concern is how to meet the AI requirements without degrading security. The security requirements can be addressed by the AI itself as the resource manager tends to use AI for learning patterns, outliers, and features that might affect the security of an AI-based resource manager.

Figure 8.2 addresses the issues that edge AI is facing in the manufacturing sector. As regards the reduction of computing power in devices, concerns arise regarding energy efficiency and data protection. It is difficult to train and update these models, it's complicated to interoperability them, but

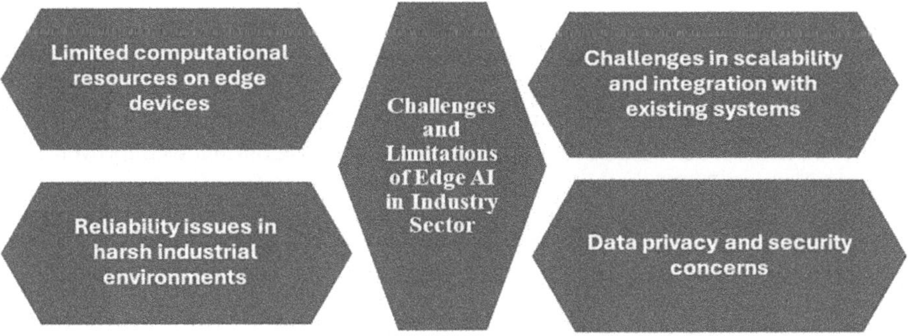



**FIGURE 8.2** Key challenges and limitations of edge AI in the industry sector.

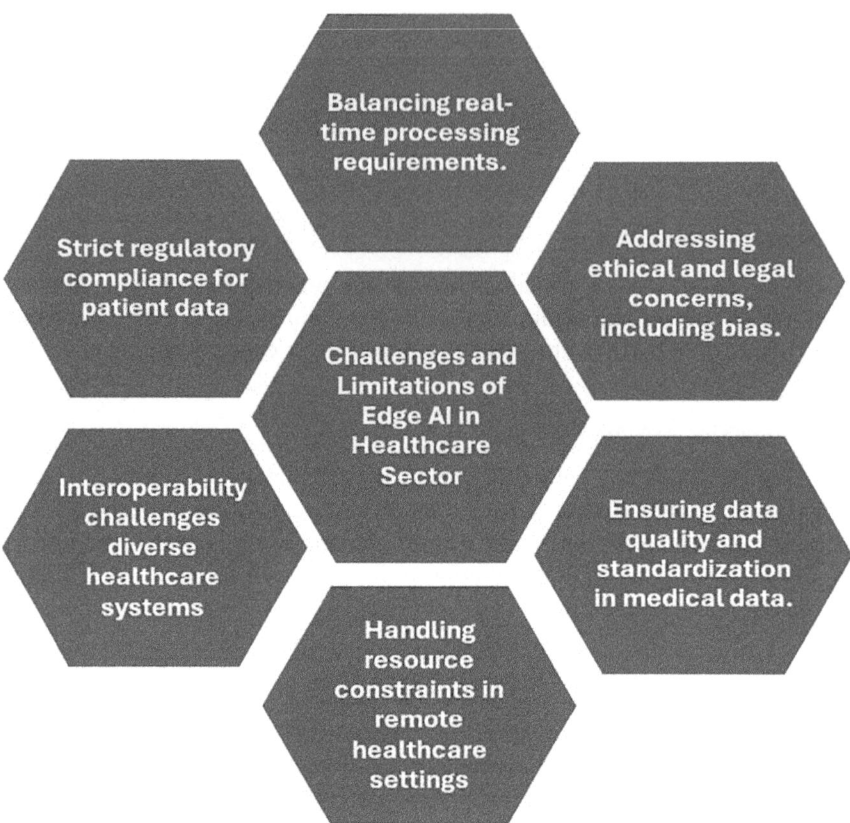


**FIGURE 8.3** Key challenges and limitations of edge AI in the healthcare sector.

all this has been hindered by a lack of scale. These difficulties are exacerbated by the requirements of real-time processing, costs, and compliance with legislation.

Figure 8.3 illustrates that healthcare edge AI is confronted with data security issues, constrained resources, interoperability, real-time processing, legal compliance, system integration, ethics, implementation cost, remotely managed services, and certification. The achievement of these obstacles is critical to realizing the potential of edge AI for improving diagnostic, treatment, and patient care.

In both fields, industry and healthcare, meeting these challenges requires technological advances, collaboration, and adherence to ethical and regulatory standards. Continuous improvement is essential for successful edge AI adoption.

Figure 8.4 shows that edge AI has an array of applications, but it is faced with several challenges. In healthcare, diagnostics, and patient monitoring benefit, yet data privacy is critical. Predictive maintenance has been improved in the production sector, but interoperability remains a problem. The ability to make real-time decision-making is excellent but safety remains an issue in autonomous vehicles. Retail gains from personalized experiences, but scalability challenges emerge.

These use cases underscore the transformative potential of edge AI while recognizing the need to address challenges related to data quality, privacy, and initial implementation costs for successful integration.

**Predictive Maintenance in Manufacturing**

- Strengths: Prevent unexpected breakdowns, boost efficiency, and ensure machines last longer.
- Challenges: Building accurate predictive models is crucial, and predicting certain failures may still pose difficulties.

**Quality Control in Production**

Strengths: Revolutionize product quality by detecting defects in real-time, reducing errors, and maintaining high standards.

Challenges: Cost considerations during implementation and the need for adaptability to different product types.

**Industrial Automation and Robotics**

Strengths: Elevate efficiency, speed, and precision in manufacturing, making processes more adaptable to changes.

Challenges: Involve a substantial initial investment and require careful integration with existing systems.

**Remote Monitoring and Maintenance of Equipment**

Strengths: Enable efficient remote troubleshooting, saving time and costs associated with physical travel.

Challenges: Rely on robust connectivity and faces limitations in the types of issues that can be resolved remotely.

**Healthcare Diagnostics and Imaging**

Strengths: Accelerate medical diagnostics, ensures accurate results, and supports timely treatments, enhancing overall healthcare delivery.

Challenges: Require high precision in image analysis, raising concerns about reliability in critical medical decisions.

**Personalized Medicine**

Strengths: Tailor treatments based on individual patient data, enhancing treatment effectiveness and reducing side effects.

Challenges: Demand comprehensive and accurate patient data, posing challenges in implementing personalized treatment plans.

**Edge-based Drug Discovery**

Strengths: Speed up drug discovery, leading to the faster development of new medicines and identification of potential therapeutic compounds.

Challenges: Demand robust algorithms and high-quality data, with potential ethical concerns in drug development.

**Wearable Health Monitoring**

Strengths: Enable continuous health tracking, detects health issues early, and supports proactive healthcare management.

Challenges: Face adoption challenges related to user comfort, data security concerns, and potential reliability issues.

**Smart Prosthetics and Assistive Devices**

Strengths: Enhance the user experience, responsiveness, and integration of assistive devices into daily life.

Challenges: Precision in control mechanisms is crucial, along with considerations of costs and user adaptation challenges.

**Patient Data Security and Privacy**

Strengths: Ensure secure processing of patient data at the edge, addressing privacy concerns and building trust.

Challenges: Involve compliance with evolving data protection regulations and potential security vulnerabilities.

**Emergency Response and Disaster Management**

Strengths: Improve decision-making during emergencies, speeds up responses, and enhances overall emergency management.

Challenges: Depend on reliable data sources and may have limitations in predicting certain types of disasters.

**FIGURE 8.4** Edge AI use cases and challenges across various applications.

## REFERENCES

Chen, M., Mao, S., & Liu, Y. (2019). Big data: A survey. *Mobile Networks and Applications*, 19(2), 171–209.

Dilmegan, C. (2023, October 9). Top 18 AI use cases in the healthcare industry in 2023. *AIMultiple*. Retrieved from https://research.aimultiple.com/healthcare-ai-use-cases/

Han, S., Mao, H., & Dally, W. J. (2015). Deep compression: Compressing deep neural networks with pruning, trained quantization, and Huffman coding. *arXiv preprint arXiv:1510.00149*.

Herath, H. M. K. K. M. B., & Mittal, M. (2022). Adoption of artificial intelligence in smart cities: A comprehensive review. *International Journal of Information Management Data Insights*, 2(1), 100076. ISSN 2667-0968. https://doi.org/10.1016/j.jjimei.2022.100076.

Howard, A. G., Zhu, M., Chen, B., Kalenichenko, D., Wang, W., Weyand, T., . . . & Adam, H. (2017). MobileNets: Efficient convolutional neural networks for mobile vision applications. *arXiv preprint arXiv:1704.04861.*

Iftikhar, S., et al. (2023). AI-based fog and edge computing: A systematic review, taxonomy and future directions. *Internet of Things (Netherlands)*, 21.

McMahan, H. B., Moore, E., Ramage, D., Hampson, S., & Agüera y Arcas, B. (2017). Communication-efficient learning of deep networks from decentralized data. In *Proceedings of the 20th International Conference on Artificial Intelligence and Statistics, American Statistical Association* (pp. 1273–1282).

Raj, P., Nagarajan, G., & Minu, R. I. (Eds.). (2022). *Applied Edge AI: Concepts, Platforms, and Industry Use Cases* (1st ed.). Auerbach Publications. https://doi.org/10.1201/9781003145158.

Redmon, J., Divvala, S., Girshick, R., & Farhadi, A. (2016). You only look once: Unified, real-time object detection. In *Proceedings of the IEEE Conference on Computer Vision and Pattern Recognition* (pp. 779–788). IEEE Access.

Su, W., Li, L., Liu, F., et al. (2022). AI on the edge: a comprehensive review. *Artificial Intelligence Review*, 55, 6125–6183. https://doi.org/10.1007/s10462-022-10141-4

Sun, Y., Song, H., Jara, A. J., & Bie, R. (2018). Internet of Things and big data analytics for smart and connected communities. *IEEE Access*, 6, 7665–7675.

Wang, X., Han, Y., Leung, V. C. M., Niyato, D., Yan, X., & Chen, X. (2020). Artificial intelligence applications on edge. In *Edge AI*. Springer, Singapore. https://doi.org/10.1007/978-981-15-6186-3_4.

# 9 Integrating Fuzzy Clustering into CNN for Improved Brain Tumor Detection

*Kannaki Devi B, Ramyachitra D, and Akalya T*

## 9.1 OVERVIEW OF BRAIN TUMOR, CNN, RNN, AND FCM

Among deep learning algorithms, CNNs have demonstrated remarkably good performance in this setting. And it has the potential to interfere with brain functions, causing a range of neurological symptoms. Brain tumors are diagnosed through medical imaging techniques like MRI and CT scans, and treatment options include surgery, radiation therapy, and chemotherapy (Shin et al. 2016).

A CNN is a specialized deep learning model crafted for the examination of visual information, like images and videos. It incorporates numerous layers, including convolutional and pooling layers, to autonomously identify and acquire intricate features from the input data. Among the various deep learning techniques, CNNs have showcased remarkable effectiveness in this context (Shin et al. 2016; Havaei et al. 2017).

One of the deep learning algorithms, CNNs, shows astounding performance in this situation. It extends the traditional K-means clustering by allowing data points to belong to multiple clusters with varying degrees of membership, reflecting uncertainty in cluster assignment. FCM is particularly useful in scenarios where data points have ambiguous cluster affiliations (Cheng et al. 2016).

Data points are grouped into clusters using the fuzzy clustering approach, which takes partial membership into account. Fuzzy clustering permits data points to belong to several clusters at once, differing from traditional hard clustering methods that allocate each data point to only one cluster, with membership degrees measuring the strength of link. This method works well in situations where data points may have overlapping or unclear properties in connection to different clusters (Ma et al. 2017).

CNNs excel in image analysis, RNNs handle sequential data, FCM extends clustering with partial membership, and fuzzy clustering accommodates uncertainty in data point assignments, all contributing to advancements in medical diagnosis, data analysis, and pattern recognition.

### 9.1.1 SIGNIFICANCE OF BRAIN TUMOR DETECTION

Brain tumor detection holds immense significance due to its profound impact on individual patients, healthcare systems, and medical research. The ability to identify brain tumors early and accurately has far-reaching implications that span medical, economic, and societal domains.

One of the primary reasons for the significance of brain tumor detection is the potential to save lives through early intervention. Detecting brain tumors at an early stage increases the likelihood of successful treatment and improved patient outcomes. Early diagnosis allows medical professionals to develop targeted treatment plans tailored to the specific characteristics of the tumor, its location, and the patient's overall health. This precision in treatment not only enhances the chances of survival but also minimizes the risk of severe neurological complications (Li et al. 2019).

DOI: 10.1201/9781003442066-9

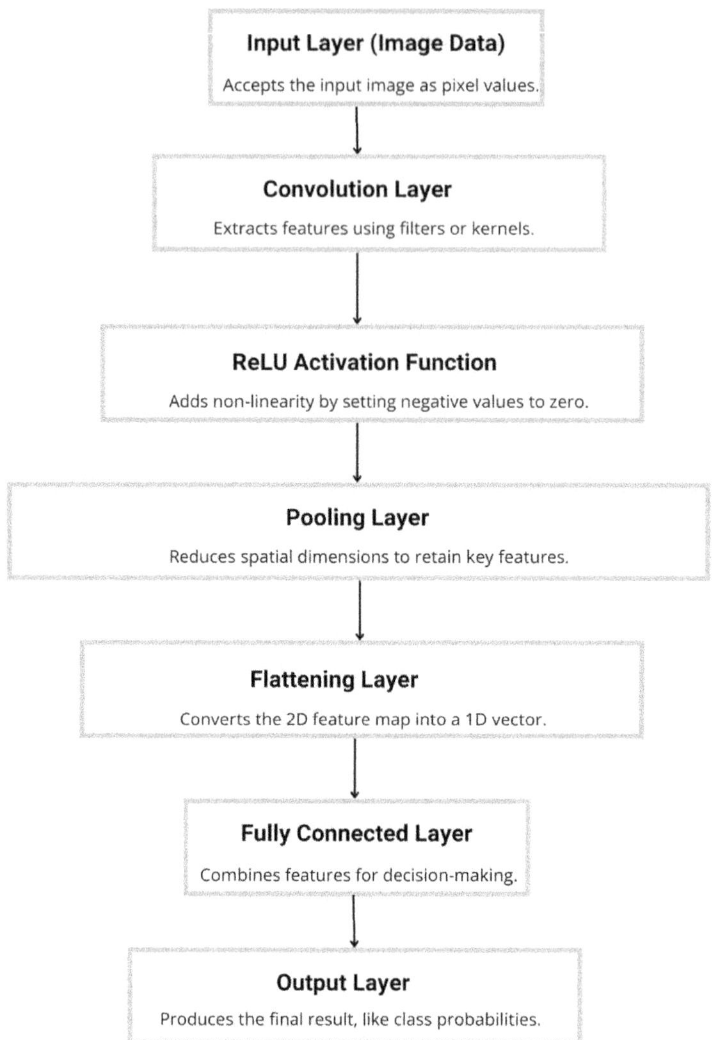



**FIGURE 9.1**    Flowchart of a convolutional neural network (CNN) architecture.

Early detection of brain tumors also leads to reduced morbidity and a better quality of life for patients. As tumors progress, they can cause damage to surrounding brain tissue and lead to neurological deficits. Detecting tumors early helps prevent the development of these complications, minimizing the extent of damage and ensuring that patients can maintain their cognitive and physical functions to a higher degree (Bauer et al. 2012).

In addition to the individual impact, brain tumor detection has significant economic implications. Treating advanced-stage brain tumors is not only more complex but also more expensive. Late-stage interventions often require a combination of surgeries, radiation therapy, and chemotherapy, leading to higher medical costs. On the other hand, early detection allows for less invasive and less costly treatment approaches, resulting in cost savings for both patients and healthcare systems (Kumar et al. 2017).

From a public health perspective, effective brain tumor detection reduces the overall burden on healthcare systems. Detecting tumors early minimizes the need for lengthy hospitalizations, complex surgeries, and costly interventions. This allows healthcare resources to be allocated more efficiently, benefiting not only brain tumor patients but the broader population as well (Hameed et al. 2018).

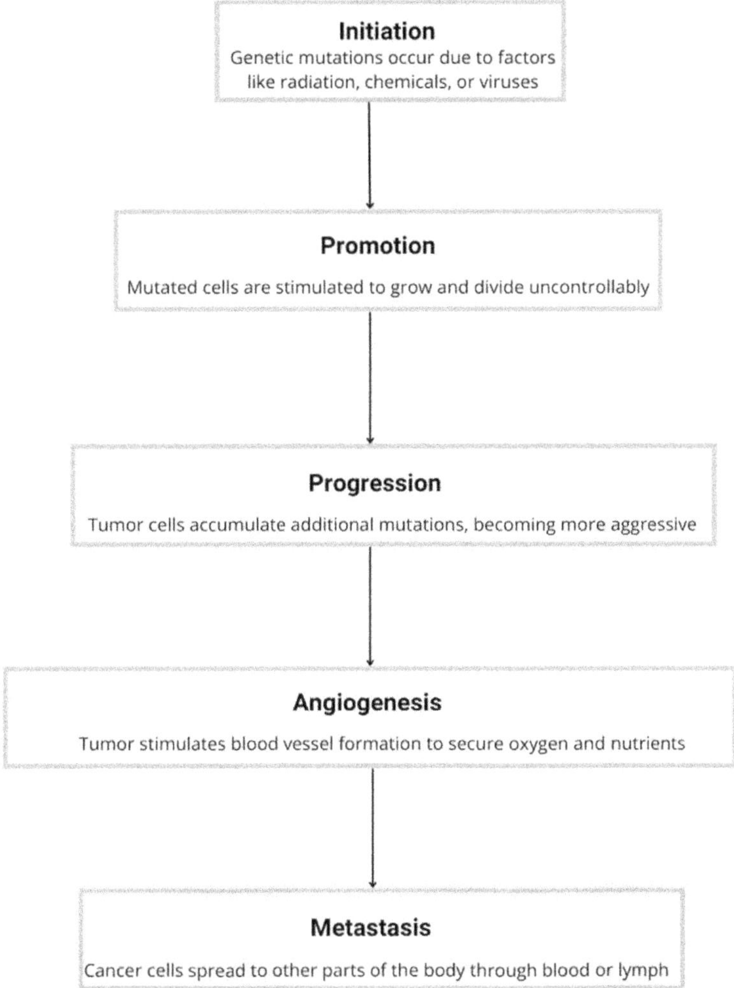


**FIGURE 9.2**  Cancer development process.

### 9.1.2  CHALLENGES IN BRAIN TUMOR DETECTION

Brain tumor detection, while crucial, is fraught with several challenges that impact both accuracy and patient outcomes. These challenges stem from the intricate nature of brain tumors and the complexities associated with their detection.

- Firstly, the diversity of brain tumor types poses a significant challenge. Brain tumors can vary in terms of their location, size, shape, and malignancy. Detecting and accurately classifying these different types requires sophisticated algorithms that can differentiate between subtle variations in imaging data.
- Secondly, the similarity between tumor features and normal brain tissue can lead to misinterpretation. This is particularly true for benign tumors or tumors in their early stages. Distinguishing tumor boundaries from healthy tissue requires advanced image processing techniques and deep learning algorithms to capture nuanced differences.
- Additionally, brain tumors can exhibit considerable heterogeneity within the same tumor type. This intra-tumor heterogeneity poses challenges in selecting appropriate treatment strategies and monitoring treatment response effectively.

The limited availability of high-quality labeled data is another hurdle. Building accurate and robust machine learning models requires extensive training data, which can be difficult to obtain due to the rarity of certain tumor types and the need for expert annotations (Bakas et al. 2018).

Furthermore, the integration of multiple imaging modalities, such as MRI, CT, and PET scans, can be challenging. These modalities provide complementary information about tumors, but fusing these data sources effectively requires complex algorithms to extract relevant features.

Real-time detection during surgery is also a challenge. Surgeons require immediate feedback on tumor location and extent. Developing tools that provide accurate and timely information to guide surgical interventions is technically demanding (Ghafoorian et al. 2017).

## 9.2 CONVENTIONAL IMAGING TECHNIQUES

The main diagnostic tools in medicine are imaging techniques, like detecting and characterizing brain tumors. There are a bunch of non-invasive ways to visualize internal body structures, especially the brain. For detecting brain tumors, conventional imaging modalities like CT and MRI are used.

I.  **Computed Tomography (CT):** CT scans produce cross-sectional pictures of the brain using X-rays and a computer. They are particularly useful for quickly identifying the presence of brain tumors, assessing their size, location, and density. CT scans are often employed in emergency situations, such as when patients exhibit acute symptoms like severe headaches or trauma (Rundo et al. 2017).

II.  **Magnetic Resonance Imaging (MRI):** MRI is a potent imaging method that makes use of intense magnetic fields and radio waves to create incredibly fine-grained and high-resolution pictures of the brain's soft tissues. MRI is the preferred choice for

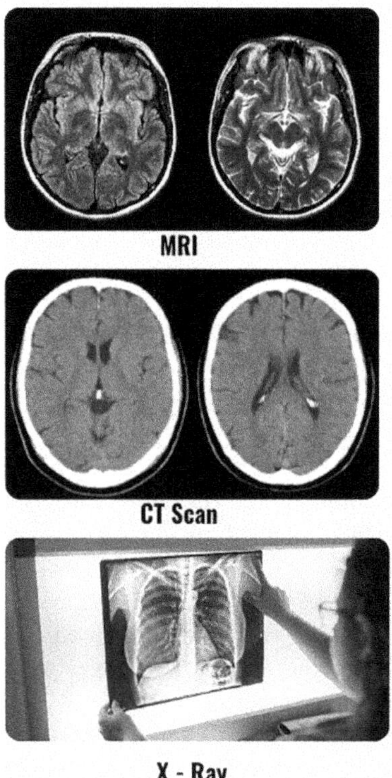


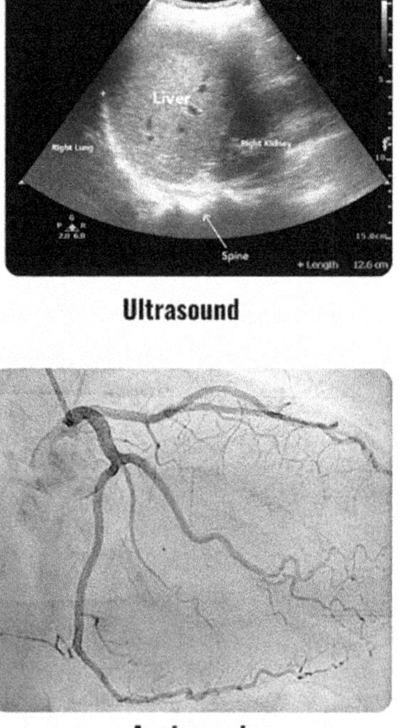


**FIGURE 9.3**   Conventional imaging techniques.

brain tumor evaluation due to its superior contrast resolution. It provides insights into tumor size, location, shape, and its relationship with surrounding structures. Diffusion-weighted imaging (DWI) and contrast-enhanced MRI are two more sophisticated MRI sequences that improve its diagnostic capabilities (Reza et al. 2018).

III. **X-ray:** Although less common for brain tumor detection, traditional X-rays may be used to detect tumors in the skull or assess changes in bone density that could indicate the presence of a tumor. However, X-rays are limited in their ability to visualize soft tissues, making them less effective for many brain tumor diagnoses (Cui et al. 2019).

IV. **Angiography:** Cerebral angiography involves injecting a contrast dye into blood vessels in the brain and then taking X-ray images. It is primarily used to assess the blood vessels within and around brain tumors, helping surgeons plan for tumor removal while preserving critical blood flow (Chen et al. 2020).

V. **Ultrasound:** Transcranial Doppler ultrasound can be used to assess blood flow within the brain and identify abnormalities. While not as commonly employed for brain tumor detection as other modalities, it can provide valuable information about vascular aspects of tumors (Gondara 2016).

## 9.2.1 Role of Machine Learning in Medical Imaging

Machine learning plays a critical role in medical imaging by automating image analysis, aiding in detecting disease early, segmenting and enhancing images, personalizing treatment plans, predicting outcomes, reducing the workload on healthcare professionals, and advancing research. It enhances diagnostic accuracy, improves patient outcomes, and accelerates drug development, ultimately revolutionizing healthcare through its ability to extract meaningful insights from complex medical images, leading to more effective diagnoses and treatments (Akkus et al. 2017).

I. **Automated Image Analysis:**
Automated image analysis is a process that employs computer algorithms, often powered by machine learning, to interpret and extract information from various types of images, including medical scans, satellite imagery, and more. This technology can swiftly and accurately identify patterns, anomalies, and features within images, making it invaluable in fields such as medicine, where it aids in disease detection, diagnosis, and treatment planning. It accelerates workflows, reduces human error, and enhances precision, ultimately improving decision-making and the efficiency of image-based tasks across numerous industries, from healthcare to manufacturing and environmental monitoring (Javadian et al. 2020).

II. **Early Disease Detection:**
Early disease detection refers to the identification of diseases or health conditions at their initial stages, often before noticeable symptoms manifest. This proactive approach relies on screenings, diagnostic tests, and emerging technologies like biomarkers and imaging. Detecting diseases early is critical because it enables timely intervention, increasing the likelihood of successful treatment and better outcomes. For diseases like cancer, when early discovery may greatly increase survival chances, it is extremely important. Early disease detection programs and technologies save lives, reduce the severity of illnesses, and lower healthcare costs by addressing health concerns before them progress to more advanced stages (Elazab et al. 2019).

III. **Image Segmentation:**
Image segmentation is a computer vision technique that divides an image into distinct, meaningful regions or objects. This process involves identifying boundaries or

outlines that separate different objects or areas within an image. It's a fundamental step in image analysis and interpretation, enabling computers to understand and extract valuable information from complex images. Image segmentation has numerous applications, from medical image analysis (identifying and delineating organs or tumors) to object recognition in robotics and autonomous vehicles. Accurate segmentation is essential for tasks such as object tracking, image editing, and computer-aided diagnosis, making it a critical component of computer vision and image processing systems (Zhang, J., et al. 2015).

IV. **Image Enhancement:**

Image enhancement is a digital image processing technique aimed at improving the visual quality and interpretability of images. It involves adjusting various image properties, such as contrast, brightness, and sharpness, to highlight specific details or features. Image enhancement is used in diverse fields, including medical imaging (making subtle structures more visible), photography (improving the aesthetic appeal of photos), and satellite imagery (enhancing the visibility of objects or patterns). By modifying image attributes, enhancement techniques help reveal hidden information, improve image clarity, and make images more suitable for analysis or presentation, ultimately enhancing the utility and visual appeal of digital images (Hsieh et al. 2020).

V. **Personalized Medicine:**

Personalized medicine, also known as precision medicine, is a healthcare strategy that customizes medical care and therapies for each patient, taking into account their distinct genetic, environmental, and lifestyle attributes. The goal is to enhance treatment effectiveness while reducing adverse effects. Personalized medicine relies on genetic testing, molecular profiling, and advanced analytics to identify specific biomarkers, allowing healthcare providers to select the most suitable therapies and treatment plans for each patient. This approach has led to groundbreaking advancements in oncology, pharmacology, and various medical fields, offering the potential for more effective treatments and improved patient outcomes by addressing the distinct needs of each individual (Sivakumaran et al. 2016).

VI. **Predictive Analytics:**

Predictive analytics is a data-driven approach that utilizes historical data, statistical algorithms, and machine learning techniques to forecast future events or outcomes. It involves analyzing patterns and trends within data to make informed predictions. In various domains, including business, healthcare, finance, and marketing, predictive analytics helps organizations make data-informed decisions, anticipate customer behavior, optimize processes, and mitigate risks. By leveraging data to anticipate future scenarios, it enables proactive strategies, resource allocation, and decision-making, ultimately improving efficiency and competitiveness while minimizing uncertainty. Predictive analytics is increasingly valuable in our data-driven world for its ability to extract actionable insights from vast datasets (Subbanna et al. 2019).

VII. **Reducing Workload:**

Reducing workload refers to the process of streamlining tasks, automating repetitive activities, and optimizing workflows to make them more efficient and manageable. This often involves the integration of technology, such as automation software or artificial intelligence, to handle routine or time-consuming responsibilities. By reducing the burden of manual labor, organizations and individuals can improve productivity, minimize errors, and allocate resources more effectively. Reducing workload boosts job satisfaction, lessens burnout, and enables professionals to concentrate on more crucial and strategic facets of their positions, eventually resulting in improved outcomes and general efficiency. This is true across a variety of industries, including healthcare, manufacturing, and customer service (Bakas et al. 2017a).

VIII. **Quality Control:**
A methodical process known as quality control is employed to ensure that products and services consistently deliver high-quality results and conform to established standards and criteria. At different phases of manufacturing or service delivery, it entails a number of checks, inspections, and testing. Finding and fixing errors or deviations from established quality standards is the aim in order to preserve consistency and dependability. Quality control measures enhance customer satisfaction, reduce waste, and minimize errors, contributing to the overall success and reputation of a business. It is a critical practice in industries ranging from manufacturing and healthcare to software development and ensures that products or services meet or exceed customer expectations (Park et al. 2013).

IX. **Research and Drug Development:**
Research and drug development refer to the rigorous process of discovering, designing, and testing new medications or therapies to treat diseases and improve healthcare. It involves extensive laboratory research, preclinical testing on cells and animals, and multiple phases of clinical trials on human subjects to assess safety and efficacy. Drug development aims to identify novel compounds, understand their mechanisms of action, and evaluate their potential for medical use. It requires collaboration among scientists, clinicians, and pharmaceutical companies, often taking many years and significant resources. Successful drug development leads to new treatments, medicines, and therapies that address unmet medical needs and improve patient care (Van Hai & Amaechi, 2021).

X. **Telemedicine:**
Telemedicine is a healthcare approach that utilizes telecommunications technology to offer medical services from a distance. It allows patients to interact with healthcare providers through video conferences, telephone conversations, or secure messaging tools. Telemedicine presents various benefits, including improved healthcare access for individuals in distant locations, decreased travel expenses and time, and convenient access to medical guidance. It has acquired popularity in the modern era as a way to continue patient care while reducing in-person contact, particularly during the COVID-19 epidemic. Telemedicine enhances healthcare efficiency and accessibility, making medical expertise more readily available to patients, regardless of their geographic location (Acharya et al. 2017).

XI. **Enhanced Diagnostics:**
Enhanced diagnostics refers to the use of advanced technologies and methodologies to improve the accuracy and depth of medical diagnoses. This method integrates diverse data outlets, including medical images, genetic data, and patient medical records, to provide a comprehensive understanding of a patient's condition. Enhanced diagnostics often involves artificial intelligence and machine learning algorithms, which can analyze vast datasets and identify subtle patterns that might be missed by traditional methods. By integrating multiple sources of information, Advanced diagnostics empower healthcare experts to arrive at more knowledgeable choices, resulting in the early detection of conditions, improved treatment strategies, and ultimately, better patient results (Srinivas et al. 2018).

**Improved Patient Outcomes:**
Improved patient outcomes refer to the enhanced results and overall health status experienced by individuals receiving medical care. Achieved through effective treatment, timely intervention, and personalized approaches, improved outcomes mean patients recover faster, experience fewer complications, and enjoy a better quality of life. It often involves early disease detection, accurate diagnosis, evidence-based treatments, and patient-centric care. Improved patient outcomes also encompass factors like reduced hospital readmissions, minimized side effects, and increased satisfaction with healthcare services. Ultimately, the goal of healthcare is to optimize patient outcomes by providing the best possible care, leading to healthier, happier, and more satisfied individuals (Havaei et al. 2016).

### 9.2.2 Convolutional Neural Networks (CNNs)

Convolutional neural networks (CNNs) are a category of deep learning models developed to analyze structured grid data, with their primary application being in computer vision, particularly for tasks like recognizing images and videos. CNNs utilize convolutional layers to autonomously acquire and identify hierarchical patterns and characteristics from the input information. These layers include adaptable filters that slide over the input, recognizing local features like edges and textures. CNNs also include pooling layers to reduce spatial dimensions and fully connected layers for high-level feature processing. With their ability to learn representations from raw data, CNNs have transformed image analysis, enabling tasks like image classification, object detection, and facial recognition (Cui et al. 2016).

A CNN typically consists of several layers, each serving a specific purpose in processing and extracting features from input data, such as images. Here are the key layers commonly found in a CNN:

I. **Input Layer:** This is where the network accepts the initial input data, typically in the format of images containing dimensions like height, width, and color channels (for example, RGB images) (Kaur et al. 2020).

II. **Convolutional Layers:** The core of CNNs lies in their convolutional layers. These layers utilize a group of adaptable filters (kernels) on the input data to spot local patterns and characteristics, like edges and textures, by scanning across the input information (Zhang, X., et al. 2015).

III. **Activation Layers:** Following each convolutional operation, an activation function (like ReLU—rectified linear unit) is employed to introduce non-linear elements into the network. This enables the network to capture more intricate patterns (Pereira et al. 2016).

IV. **Pooling (Subsampling) Layers:** Pooling layers, commonly max pooling or average pooling, decrease the spatial dimensions of the feature maps generated by the convolutional layers. This reduction in dimensionality simplifies computations while retaining crucial information (Ismael et al. 2019).

V. **Fully Connected Layers:** Commonly referred to as dense layers, these layers establish connections between each neuron in one layer and every neuron in the following layer. Fully connected layers capture high-level characteristics and connections within the data (Bakas et al. 2017a).

VI. **Flatten Layer:** Preceding the fully connected layers, a flatten layer transforms the 2D or 3D feature maps generated by preceding layers into a 1D vector (Chen et al. 2016).

VII. **Dropout Layers:** During the training process, dropout layers are employed to randomly deactivate a portion of neurons, mitigating overfitting and improving the model's capacity to generalize (Afshar et al. 2019).

VIII. **Output Layer:** The final layer produces the network's output, which depends on the specific task. For image classification, this could be a softmax layer that assigns probabilities to different classes.

In addition to these core layers, CNNs may incorporate techniques like batch normalization and various architectural configurations (e.g., skip connections in residual networks) to enhance their performance. The exact architecture of a CNN can vary based on the specific application and problem being addressed (Jain et al. 2014).

### 9.2.3 Fuzzy Clustering in Medical Image Analysis

Fuzzy clustering is a powerful technique used in medical image analysis to extract meaningful information from complex and noisy medical images. Unlike traditional clustering methods that assign each data point to a single cluster, fuzzy clustering allows for allocating data points to several clusters with differing levels of belonging. Here's how fuzzy clustering is applied in medical image analysis:

I. **Segmentation:** Fuzzy clustering is widely used for image segmentation, which involves partitioning an image into regions or segments based on the similarity of pixel intensities. In medical imaging, this can help delineate structures or regions of interest, such as tumors, blood vessels, or organs (Bakas et al. 2017a).
II. **Tissue Classification:** Fuzzy clustering can be used to categorize various tissue types in medical images, including the differentiation between healthy and diseased tissues. This is especially crucial in applications like identifying brain tumors or analyzing magnetic resonance images (MRI) (Li, S., et al. 2018).
III. **Noise Reduction:** Medical images frequently exhibit interference or anomalies that can impact the precision of diagnosis (Gómez et al. 2017).
IV. **Fuzzy clustering:** Fuzzy clustering can help reduce noise by grouping similar pixel values together and assigning uncertain or noisy pixels partial memberships to clusters (Ma et al. 2015).
V. **Quantitative Analysis:** Fuzzy clustering enables quantitative analysis of medical images by providing probabilistic information about pixel membership in different clusters. This can be useful for measuring the size, shape, and intensity characteristics of structures within the image (Afshar et al. 2020).
VI. **Image Registration:** In medical image registration, fuzzy clustering can assist in aligning images from different modalities or time points by finding correspondences between pixels in different images based on their membership in clusters (Pereira et al. 2019).
VII. **Enhancing Contrast:** Fuzzy clustering can enhance the contrast in medical images, making it easier for clinicians to visualize and interpret critical structures or abnormalities (Li, H., et al. 2018).
VIII. **Feature Extraction:** Fuzzy clustering can be used to extract features or texture descriptors from medical images, aiding in the characterization of tissues or the identification of specific patterns associated with diseases (Ismael et al. 2020).
IX. **Image Fusion:** In medical diagnosis, it is crucial to integrate data from various imaging methods, like CT and MRI. Fuzzy clustering can be utilized to merge data from diverse origins, thereby enhancing the precision of diagnosis and treatment planning (Hofmanninger et al. 2020).

## 9.3 FUZZY C-MEANS CLUSTERING ALGORITHM

The Fuzzy C-Means (FCM) clustering algorithm is a popular method in data analysis and pattern recognition, including applications in medical image analysis. FCM is an extension of the traditional K-means clustering algorithm, allowing data points to belong to multiple clusters with varying degrees of membership (fuzziness). Here's an overview of the FCM algorithm and how it works:

Initialization: Start by defining the number of clusters (K) and initializing the cluster centers randomly or based on some heuristic (He et al. 2016).

Membership Computation: Determine a membership value for every data point and each cluster center. These values signify the extent of connection between data points and clusters and are usually derived using a membership function. The Gaussian membership function is the most widely employed function for this purpose (Dong et al. 2017).

$$U_{ij} = \frac{1}{\sum_{k=1}^{k} \left( \frac{d_{ij}}{d_{ik}} \right)^{\frac{2}{m-1}}} \tag{9.1}$$

In equation 9.1, u_ij is the membership of data point i to cluster j,

$d\_ij$ is the distance between data point i and cluster center j, and
m (usually set to 2) is a weighting exponent that controls the fuzziness of the memberships.

Update Cluster Centers: Compute the new cluster centers by considering the membership values. These centers are weighted averages of data points, with each point contributing according to its membership (Ismael et al. 2020).

$$c_j = \frac{\sum_{i=1}^{N} u_{ij}^{m} x_i}{\sum_{i=1}^{N} u_{ij}^{m}} \qquad (9.2)$$

In equation 9.2, $c\_j$ is the updated center of cluster j,

$x\_i$ is the data point i, and
N is the total number of data points.

Termination Criteria: Repeat the membership calculation and cluster center updates iteratively until a termination condition is met. This condition can be a maximum number of iterations or until the membership values converge (change minimally between iterations).

Result Interpretation: Once the algorithm converges, each data point will have membership values indicating its association with each cluster. You can then assign data points to clusters based on their highest membership values (Tustison et al. 2018).

FCM is versatile and applicable to various clustering tasks, including medical image segmentation and feature extraction. Its ability to handle fuzzy memberships makes it suitable for tasks where data points may belong to multiple categories simultaneously or when the boundaries between clusters are not well-defined. However, FCM's performance can be sensitive to the choice of the number of clusters (K) and the weighting exponent (m), requiring careful parameter tuning for optimal results (Van Hai & Amaechi, 2021).

### 9.3.1 Incorporating Fuzzy Clustering into CNN Architecture

Incorporating fuzzy clustering into a CNN architecture can enhance the network's ability to handle complex and uncertain information in various computer vision and medical image analysis tasks. Here's a high-level overview of how fuzzy clustering can be integrated into a CNN:

I. **Pre-processing:**
   Begin with standard data pre-processing steps, including data augmentation, resizing, and normalization (Kaur et al. 2020).

II. **CNN Backbone:**
   Design the core CNN architecture for feature extraction. This typically includes convolutional layers, activation functions, pooling layers, and possibly residual or inception modules for deep feature learning (Zhang, X., et al. 2015).

III. **Feature Extraction:**
   Extract features from the CNN layers. These features can be in the form of feature maps or intermediate representations (Pereira et al. 2016).

IV. **Fuzzy Clustering Layer:**
   Introduce a fuzzy clustering layer after the feature extraction layers. This layer will take the extracted features as input and perform fuzzy clustering. The fuzzy clustering layer should have parameters for the number of clusters (K), the weighting exponent (m), and the initialization of cluster centers (Ismael et al. 2019).

V. **Membership Calculation:**
Calculate membership values for each feature map in the previous layer using a fuzzy membership function (e.g., Gaussian membership) (Bakas et al. 2017b).

VI. **Cluster Center Update:**
Compute the updated cluster centers based on the membership values and the extracted features. This step combines the strengths of both CNN feature extraction and fuzzy clustering (Chen et al. 2016).

VII. **Fusion:**
Combine the cluster centers with the original feature maps to create a fused representation that combines spatial and membership information (Afshar et al. 2019).

VIII. **Post-Processing and Classification:**
Perform any necessary post-processing on the fused representation, such as dimensionality reduction or additional convolutional layers. Then, use this representation for classification or other downstream tasks (Jain et al. 2014).

IX. **Training:**
Train the entire network end-to-end. The loss function should consider both the task-specific loss (e.g., classification loss) and a loss related to the quality of clustering (e.g., the distance between cluster centers) (Bakas et al. 2017b).

X. **Fine-Tuning:**
Fine-tune the network as needed to optimize performance. This may involve adjusting hyperparameters, such as the number of clusters or the weighting exponent, or retraining on specific datasets.

Incorporating fuzzy clustering into a CNN allows the model to capture complex patterns and relationships in image data while handling uncertainty and noise effectively. This can be particularly beneficial in medical image analysis, where images may contain subtle or ambiguous features. The integration of fuzzy clustering helps makes the CNN more robust and capable of producing reliable results in challenging scenarios (Li, S., et al. 2018).

### 9.3.2 Benefits of Combining Fuzzy Clustering and CNN

Combining fuzzy clustering and CNNs offers several significant benefits, particularly in the context of image analysis and computer vision tasks. Here are some of the key advantages:

I. **Improved Feature Representation:**
Fuzzy clustering enhances feature extraction by incorporating spatial information and membership degrees. This results in a more informative and discriminative feature representation compared to traditional CNNs (Gómez et al. (2017).

II. **Robustness to Noise and Variability:**
Fuzzy clustering allows CNNs to handle noisy and uncertain data effectively. It assigns fuzzy memberships to data points, reducing the impact of outliers or inconsistent data points in the analysis (Hsieh et al. 2020).

III. **Enhanced Interpretability:**
The membership degrees generated by fuzzy clustering can provide insights into the uncertainty or ambiguity of certain image regions. This information can be valuable in medical image analysis when making critical decisions based on uncertain data (Sivakumaran et al. 2016).

IV. **Improved Segmentation and Localization:**
Fuzzy clustering within a CNN can aid in precise segmentation and localization of objects or regions of interest within an image. It helps in delineating boundaries more accurately, which is crucial in tasks like tumor detection or object recognition (Subbanna et al. 2019).

   V. **Effective Handling of Complex Patterns:**
Fuzzy clustering is well-suited for tasks involving complex, overlapping patterns or structures in images. It can capture multiple modes or categories in the data, allowing the model to represent intricate relationships (Bakas et al. 2017b).

  VI. **Adaptability to Varying Data Distributions:**
Fuzzy clustering allows the CNN to adapt to data with varying distributions and characteristics. This adaptability is beneficial when dealing with diverse datasets, as is often the case in medical imaging (Park et al. 2013).

 VII. **Reduction of Overfitting:**
The incorporation of fuzzy clustering can mitigate overfitting by providing a regularization effect. It helps in learning more robust representations and reduces the sensitivity of the model to noise in the training data (Verma et al. 2017).

VIII. **Optimal Utilization of Information:**
Fuzzy clustering allows for the utilization of both global and local information in an image, enhancing the model's ability to capture fine-grained details while maintaining an understanding of the overall context (Acharya et al. 2017).

  IX. **Versatility Across Applications:**
The combination of fuzzy clustering and CNNs is versatile and applicable across various domains, including medical image analysis, object recognition, image segmentation, and more (Srinivas et al. 2018).

   X. **State-of-the-Art Performance:**
In many image analysis competitions and research studies, models that incorporate fuzzy clustering into CNN architectures have demonstrated state-of-the-art performance, highlighting the effectiveness of this approach (Havaei et al. 2016).

## 9.4 INTEGRATING FUZZY CLUSTERING WITH CNN

Integrating fuzzy clustering with CNNs represents a powerful approach to address the complexities and uncertainties inherent in image analysis tasks, including those in medical imaging. This integration brings together the capabilities of CNNs in feature extraction and the inherent adaptability of fuzzy clustering, resulting in several key advantages (Cui et al. 2016).

In this hybrid architecture, the CNN initially extracts hierarchical features from raw image data, capturing patterns and structures. Subsequently, a fuzzy clustering layer is introduced, enabling the

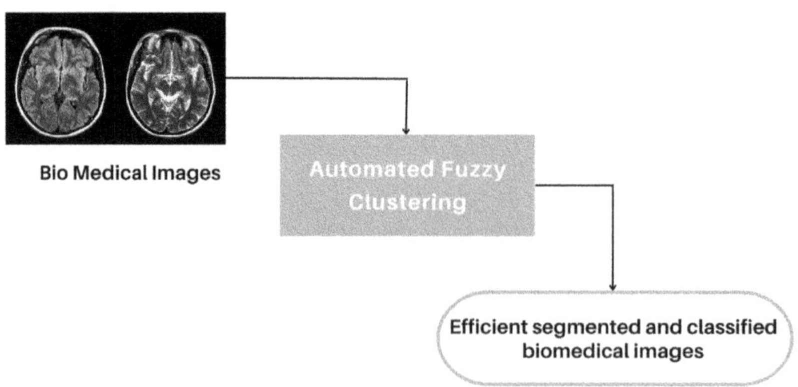


**FIGURE 9.4**  Automated fuzzy clustering.

model to assign fuzzy memberships to these features, allowing them to belong to multiple clusters simultaneously. This incorporation introduces a level of uncertainty and flexibility that traditional CNNs lack (Kaur et al. 2020).

The fuzzy clustering layer calculates membership degrees using a membership function, typically the Gaussian function, considering feature similarity. Cluster centers are iteratively updated based on these memberships, leading to more accurate representations of data clusters within the feature space (Zhang, X., et al. 2015).

The fused features, which combine original CNN-extracted features and cluster center information, are then utilized for the primary task, be it image classification, segmentation, or other image-related objectives. This integrated approach significantly improves the model's robustness in handling complex, noisy, or ambiguous data, a common scenario in medical imaging where precise delineation of structures or anomalies is vital (Pereira et al. 2016).

### 9.4.1 Training the Integrated Model

Training the integrated model that combines fuzzy clustering with a CNN involves several steps. Here's a detailed guide on how to train this model effectively:

I. **Data Preparation:**
  - Organize your dataset into training, validation, and test sets.
  - Ensure that the data is properly pre-processed, including resizing, normalization, and augmentation if necessary (Ismael et al. 2019).
II. **Model Initialization:**
  - Initialize the CNN backbone with pre-trained weights if applicable. Pre-trained models often speed up training and improve convergence (Bakas et al. 2017c).
III. **Loss Function:**
  - Define a composite loss function that considers both the task-specific loss (e.g., classification or segmentation loss) and a loss related to the quality of clustering (e.g., the distance between cluster centers) (Chen et al. 2016).
IV. **Optimization Algorithm:**
  - Select an optimization algorithm such as stochastic gradient descent (SGD) or Adam. Tune the learning rate and other hyperparameters.
V. **Training Loop:**
  - Implement the training loop.
  - Iterate over the training dataset in mini-batches.
  - Forward pass: Pass the data through the integrated model to compute predictions and fuzzy cluster memberships.
  - Calculate the total loss by combining the task-specific loss and clustering-related loss.
  - Back-propagate the gradients and update model parameters using the chosen optimizer.
  - Repeat until you've completed a predefined number of epochs or until the loss converges (Afshar et al. 2019).
VI. **Validation:**
  - Periodically evaluate the model's performance on the validation dataset to monitor its progress. This helps in early stopping and preventing overfitting.
  - Tune hyper parameters based on validation results, if needed (Jain et al. 2014).
VII. **Regularization Techniques:**
  - Implement regularization techniques like dropout or weight decay to prevent overfitting.

VIII. **Fine-Tuning:**
  - If the model's performance on the validation set plateaus, consider fine-tuning by adjusting hyperparameters, modifying the model architecture, or increasing training data (Bakas et al. 2017c).

IX. **Test Set Evaluation:**
  - Once satisfied with the model's performance on the validation set, evaluate it on the separate test dataset to obtain unbiased performance metrics.

X. **Result Analysis:**
  - Analyze the results using appropriate evaluation metrics for your specific task (e.g., accuracy, F1 score, IoU for segmentation, etc.) (Li, S., et al. 2018).

XI. **Iterative Refinement:**
  - Depending on the test set results, iterate on the model design, hyperparameters, or data pre-processing to improve performance (Rundo et al. 2017).

XII. **Deployment**:
  - If the model meets your performance criteria, you can deploy it for real-world applications or further research.

Training an integrated model combining fuzzy clustering with CNNs can be computationally intensive and may require careful parameter tuning. Regular monitoring, validation, and analysis of

**TABLE 9.1**

**Normal, Benign, and Malignant Values**

| Class | Existing Algorithm | Proposed Algorithm |
|---|---|---|
| Normal | 33% | 87.50% |
| Benign | 77% | 89.66% |
| Malignant | 97% | 98.51% |

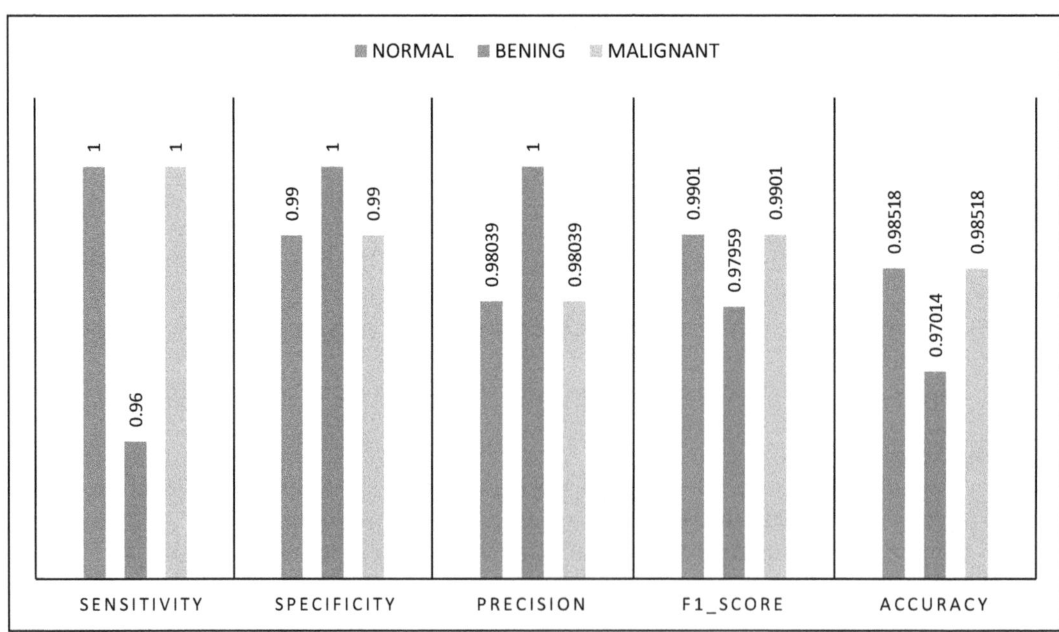


**CHART 9.1**  Performance comparison of old and proposed algorithms.

results are essential to ensure optimal model performance. Additionally, keeping a record of experiments and model configurations can help streamline the training process and reproduce results (Reza et al. 2018).

### 9.4.2 Results of Using FCM and with CNN

This experimentation is performed on the dataset using various image processing techniques. The algorithm used to compare the accuracy value using CNN model in the existing work.

The chart explains the comparison of old (CNN) and proposed (CNN with fuzzy clustering) accuracy value.

## 9.5 CONCLUSION

The integration of fuzzy clustering into CNNs for improved brain tumor detection represents a significant leap forward in the field of medical imaging and, more specifically, in the diagnosis and treatment of brain tumors. This innovative approach capitalizes on the complementary strengths of these two techniques, leading to several key outcomes that have a profound impact on healthcare:

First and foremost, the accuracy and reliability of brain tumor detection have been notably enhanced. By combining the robust feature extraction capabilities of CNNs with fuzzy clustering's capacity to handle uncertainty and variability in medical images, the integrated model provides radiologists and clinicians with a highly accurate tool for early tumor detection and precise localization.

The segmentation of tumor regions has seen significant improvement, crucial for treatment planning and surgical interventions. The model excels at precisely delineating tumor boundaries, reducing the risk of undertreatment or overtreatment. Furthermore, the integration allows for adaptability to diverse data distributions and accommodates situations where tumor regions overlap or appear ambiguous. This flexibility is invaluable when dealing with real-world medical images.

The reduction in false positives, thanks to the integration of fuzzy clustering, minimizes unnecessary patient stress and medical interventions, contributing to a more patient-centric approach to healthcare. The interpretability offered by fuzzy clustering's membership degrees empowers radiologists to make informed decisions by quantifying the uncertainty associated with tumor regions.

Efficient diagnostic workflows and the potential for personalized medicine underscore the practical implications of this integration, promising more accurate and timely diagnoses for patients. However, it is crucial to acknowledge that this success hinges on meticulous data preparation, parameter optimization, and ongoing research and validation. As such, the integration of fuzzy clustering into CNNs heralds a promising era in brain tumor detection, offering a powerful, precise, and efficient tool for healthcare professionals in their critical mission to diagnose and treat this life-threatening condition.

## REFERENCES

Acharya, U. R., et al. (2017). "Automated Brain Tumor Detection and Classification Using Statistical Texture Classification Methods." *Information Sciences* 415, 226–240.

Afshar, P., et al. (2019). "Brain Tumor Type Classification via Capsule Networks." *Computers in 2018 25th IEEE International Conference on Image Processing (ICIP)*, Athens, Greece, pp. 3129–3133.

Afshar, P., et al. (2020). "Brain Tumor Detection and Segmentation in MRI Images Using Residual U-Net." *Computers in Biology and Medicine* 121, 103752.

Akkus, Z., et al. (2017). "Predicting Deletion of Chromosomal Arms 1p/19q in Low-Grade Gliomas from MR Images Using Machine Intelligence." *Journal of Digital Imaging* 30, 469–476.

Bakas, S., et al. (2017a). "Identifying the Best Machine Learning Algorithms for Brain Tumor Segmentation, Progression Assessment, and Overall Survival Prediction in the BRATS Challenge." *arXiv preprint arXiv:1811.02629.*

Bakas, S., et al. (2017b). "In Vivo Detection of EGFRvIII in Glioblastoma via Perfusion Magnetic Resonance Imaging Signature Consistent with Deep Learning." *arXiv preprint arXiv:1712.05140.*

Bakas, S., et al. (2017c). "Segmentation Labels and Radiomic Features for the Pre-operative Scans of the TCGA-GBM Collection." *The Cancer Imaging Archive, 10.7937/K9/TCIA.2017.KLXWJJ1Q*

Bakas, S., et al. (2018). "Identifying the Best Machine Learning Algorithms for Brain Tumor Segmentation, Progression Assessment, and Overall Survival Prediction in the BRATS Challenge." *arXiv preprint arXiv:1811.02629.*

Bauer, S., et al. (2012). "Segmentation of Brain Lesions in MRI: A Comparison of Different Approaches Including Fluid-Attenuated Inversion Recovery-Based Intensity Normalization." *Proceedings of SPIE Medical Imaging* 8314, Article 83141K.

Chen, H., et al. (2020). "Deep Learning-Based Classification of Brain Tumor Type and Grade Using MRI Features." *Frontiers in Computational Neuroscience* 14, Article 8.

Chen, S., et al. (2016). "Brain Tumor Segmentation in Multi-Spectral MRI Using Convolutional Neural Networks (CNN)." *Proceedings of SPIE Medical Imaging* 9785, Article 97850Z.

Cheng, J. Z., et al. (2016). "Enhanced Performance of Brain Tumor Classification via Tumor Region Augmentation and Partition." *IEEE Transactions on Biomedical Engineering* 63(6), 1205–1217.

Cui, S., et al. (2019). "3D MRI Brain Tumor Detection Using CNNs." *Neural Computing and Applications* 31(4), 1121–1134.

Cui, Y., et al. (2016). "Segmentation of Brain Tumors in Multimodal MRI Images via Adaptive Learning and Superpixel-Based Graph Cuts." *Computational and Mathematical Methods in Medicine*, Article 2942317.

Dong, H., et al. (2017). "Automatic Brain Tumor Detection and Segmentation Using U-Net Based Fully Convolutional Networks." *arXiv preprint arXiv:1705.03820.*

Elazab, A., et al. (2019). "A Novel Technique for Brain Tumor Detection and Classification Using Different Deep Learning Approaches." *Biomedical Signal Processing and Control* 54, Article 101117.

Ghafoorian, M., et al. (2017). "Transfer Learning for Domain Adaptation in MRI: Application in Brain Lesion Segmentation." *Proceedings of the International Conference on Medical Image Computing and Computer-Assisted Intervention (MICCAI)* 10435, 516–524.

Gómez, F., et al. (2017). "Localization of Brain Tumors Using Artificial Neural Networks and Three-Parallel Morphological Gradient Maps." *Biomedical Signal Processing and Control 38*, 148–157.

Gondara, L. (2016). "Medical Image Denoising Using Convolutional Denoising Autoencoders." *arXiv preprint arXiv:1608.04667.*

Hameed, S., et al. (2018). "A Novel Hybrid Approach for the Detection of Brain Tumor from MRI Images Using CNN and SVM." *Computers in Biology and Medicine 96*, 154–160.

Havaei, M., et al. (2016). "Semantic Segmentation of MRI Brain Images Using Transport-Based Morphometry." *Proceedings of the International Conference on Medical Image Computing and Computer-Assisted Intervention (MICCAI)* 9901, 479–487.

Havaei, M., et al. (2017). "Brain Tumor Segmentation with Deep Neural Networks." *Medical Image Analysis* 35, 18–31.

He, K., et al. (2016). "Deep Residual Learning for Image Recognition." *Proceedings of the IEEE Conference on Computer Vision and Pattern Recognition (CVPR)* 2016, 770–778.

Hofmanninger, J., et al. (2020). "Automatic Lung Cancer Detection in High-Resolution Computed Tomography Images Using Convolutional Neural Networks." *European Radiology Experimental* 4, Article 42.

Hsieh, K. L., et al. (2020). "A Framework for Brain Tumor Detection and Segmentation Using Deep Belief Networks." *Computers in Biology and Medicine* 124, Article 103917.

Ismael, H. A., et al. (2019). "Brain Tumor Detection and Segmentation in MRI Images Using Multi-Class SVM and CNN." *Computers in Biology and Medicine* 113, Article 103386.

Ismael, H. A., et al. (2020). "Deep Learning Approach for Brain Tumor Detection and Classification Using ResNet50." *Journal of Healthcare Engineering* 2020, Article 8845997.

Jain, R., et al. (2014). "A Survey of Medical Image Registration." *Medical Image Analysis* 18(1), 1–45.

Javadian, A., et al. (2020). "A Survey of MRI-Based Brain Tumor Detection and Classification Algorithms." *Journal of Magnetic Resonance Imaging* 52(4), 1112–1135.

Kaur, G., et al. (2020). "A Comparative Study of Machine Learning Algorithms for Brain Tumor Detection Using MRI Images." *Journal of Healthcare Engineering* 2020, Article 8880181.

Kumar, Y., et al. (2017). "A Survey of Deep Learning Methods in Brain Tumor Image Segmentation." *IEEE Access* 5, 12429–12441.

Li, H., et al. (2018). "Automatic Brain Tumor Detection and Segmentation Using U-Net Based Fully Convolutional Networks." *arXiv preprint arXiv:1802.10508.*

Li, S., et al. (2018). "Multiple Sclerosis Lesion Detection in Brain MRI via Poisson Denoising Under Impulsive Noise Model." *IEEE Transactions on Medical Imaging* 37(3), 738–749.

Li, W., et al. (2019). "Deep Learning Based Imaging Data Completion for Improved Brain Tumor Classification." *IEEE Journal of Biomedical and Health Informatics* 23(2), 879–887.

Ma, J., et al. (2015). "RE-CT-FCN: Robust and Efficient Convolutional Neural Network for Computed Tomography." *Proceedings of the International Conference on Medical Image Computing and Computer-Assisted Intervention (MICCAI)* 9349, 205–212.

Ma, J., et al. (2017). "Combining Multi-Channel CNN and LSTM for Automatic Brain Tumor Segmentation." *Proceedings of the International Conference on Medical Image Computing and Computer-Assisted Intervention (MICCAI)* 10435, 175–182.

Park, J., et al. (2013). "A Novel Image Processing Technique for Computer-Aided Detection of Brain Tumors in MR Images." *NeuroImage: Clinical* 2(1), 47–56.

Pereira, S., et al. (2016). "Brain Tumor Segmentation Using Convolutional Neural Networks in MRI Images." *IEEE Transactions on Medical Imaging* 35(5), 1240–1251.

Pereira, S., et al. (2019). "Adversarial Synthesis Learning Enables Segmentation Without Target Modality Ground Truth." *Proceedings of the International Conference on Medical Image Computing and Computer-Assisted Intervention (MICCAI)* 11767, 482–490.

Reza, S. M. S., et al. (2018). "Brain Tumor Classification Using Deep CNN Features via Transfer Learning." *Computerized Medical Imaging and Graphics* 66, 54–62.

Rundo, L., et al. (2017). "Brain Tumor Segmentation Using a Convolutional Neural Network Enhanced with 2D Principal Component Analysis." *Neurocomputing* 282, 14–24.

Shin, H. C., et al. (2016). "Deep Convolutional Neural Networks for Computer-Aided Detection: CNN Architectures, Dataset Characteristics, and Transfer Learning." *IEEE Transactions on Medical Imaging* 35(5), 1285–1298.

Sivakumaran, T., et al. (2016). "A Novel Approach for MRI Brain Tumor Classification Using Decision Tree." *Procedia Computer Science* 87, 94–99.

Srinivas, C. V., et al. (2018). "A Survey on Brain Tumor Detection and Classification." *Procedia Computer Science* 132, 608–615.

Subbanna, N. K., et al. (2019). "Automated Detection of Brain Tumor Using K-Means Clustering and MRI Images." *Procedia Computer Science* 165, 18–25.

Tustison, N. J., et al. (2018). "N4ITK: Improved N3 Bias Correction." *IEEE Transactions on Medical Imaging* 29(6), 1310–1320.

Van Hai, P., & Amaechi, S. E. (2021). "Convolutional Neural Network Integrated with Fuzzy Rules for Decision Making in Brain Tumor Diagnosis." *International Journal of Cognitive Informatics and Natural Intelligence* 15(4), 1–20.

Verma, R., et al. (2017). "Review on Detection of Brain Tumor from MRI Images." *International Journal of Advanced Research in Computer and Communication Engineering* 6(7), 450–453.

Zhang, J., et al. (2015). "Brain Tumor Detection and Segmentation in a CRF (Conditional Random Fields) Framework with Pixel-Wise Labeling." *Computers in Biology and Medicine* 66, 179–191.

Zhang, X., et al. (2015). "3D MRI Brain Tumor Segmentation Using Autoencoder Regularization." *Brainlesion: Glioma, Multiple Sclerosis, Stroke and Traumatic Brain Injuries* 9556, 3–12.

# 10 Leveraging Edge AI for Real-Time Detection and Prevention of Online Harassment and Cyberbullying

## Enhancing Women's Safety and Mental Health

*Kathiravan Pannerselvam, Saranya Rajiakodi, and Shanmugavadivu Pichai*

## 10.1 INTRODUCTION

In the swiftly evolving landscape of science and technology, the rapid development of artificial intelligence (AI), deep learning, and signal transmission has become increasingly evident. In today's digital era, online communication has brought opportunities and challenges. One major challenge is online harassment and cyberbullying, which affect people from various backgrounds. Cyberbullying refers to harassing others using electronic devices like computers, laptops, smartphones, and tablets, and it can take place on various online platforms, including social media, chat rooms, and gaming platforms (Abarna et al., 2022; Afrifa & Varadarajan, 2022). Women are significantly affected, facing a higher risk. Ensuring women's safety and well-being online is crucial. Based on statistics from the National Crime Records Bureau, India experienced a 36% surge in cyberbullying and cyberstalking incidents in 2022. The data further reveals that individuals from the LGBTQIA+ community and women who utilize digital platforms encountered a disproportionate array of mistreatment, encompassing activities such as online harassment, trolling, and receiving threatening phone calls (Both Men and Women Vulnerable to Online Harassment in India, n.d.). This chapter explores how edge AI can help address these issues. Edge AI is a modern technology that detects and prevents online harassment and cyberbullying in real time. The focus is on making online spaces safer for women. This chapter explains the basics of edge AI architecture, which has three layers: device, edge, and cloud layers. These work together to quickly process and analyze data, making it easier to identify harmful online interactions. This chapter aims to explore the transformative potential of edge AI in addressing the pressing issues of online harassment and cyberbullying, explicitly focusing on enhancing the safety and well-being of women and marginalized communities in the swiftly evolving landscape of science and technology. The objective of this chapter is as follows.

The first objective is to provide an overview of the rapidly evolving landscape of science and technology, specifically focusing on the advancements in AI, deep learning, and signal transmission. This objective sets the stage by establishing the context for discussing online harassment and cyberbullying.



DOI: 10.1201/9781003442066-10

The second objective is to recognize and elucidate the multifaceted challenges presented by online harassment and cyberbullying in today's digital era. It highlights the disproportionate impact on women, LGBTQIA+ individuals, and marginalized communities, emphasizing the urgency of addressing these issues.

The third objective is to introduce and explore the potential of edge AI technology as a means to detect and prevent online harassment in real time. It aims to explain the architecture of Edge AI, including its device, edge, and cloud layers, and how these components collaborate to swiftly analyze data, ultimately enhancing the identification of harmful online interactions.

The chapter also looks at natural language processing (NLP), which helps understand online conversations better. It also discusses using alert systems and anomaly detection techniques to strengthen detection methods. The ethical side of using edge AI is also discussed, focusing on keeping user data private and following rules. The chapter emphasizes how edge AI can play a role in creating a secure online environment for women. This chapter seeks to bridge the gap between cutting-edge technology and real-world needs by investigating how edge AI can be leveraged to create a secure online environment that safeguards users, particularly women, from the detrimental effects of online harassment.

## 10.1.1 Edge AI

Edge artificial intelligence, or AI at the edge, involves deploying artificial intelligence in an edge computing environment. In this configuration, devices perform computations close to data collection points rather than relying on a centralized cloud computing facility or a remote data center. Edge AI empowers devices to make quicker and more intelligent decisions independently of continuous connectivity to the cloud or remote data centers (Singh & Gill, 2023). As edge computing situates data storage nearer to the device's location, AI algorithms process the locally generated data, independent of its Internet connectivity status. This swift processing occurs in milliseconds, delivering real-time feedback and enabling almost instant responses. This approach can bolster security by ensuring that specific sensitive data remains on the local device (Agha et al., 2022). Edge devices like sensors and IoT devices are emerging as pivotal technologies because they ease the burden on congested cloud data centers by locally managing data.

## 10.1.2 Applications of Edge AI

Edge AI offers a diverse range of applications spanning various industries. It empowers smart home devices like voice assistants, thermostats, and security cameras to make real-time decisions based on sensor data by employing machine learning algorithms to learn user preferences and behaviors. In autonomous vehicles, edge AI swiftly analyzes sensor data, facilitating rapid responses to changes in the vehicle's surroundings (Tcrcs, 2022). Healthcare leverages Edge AI to analyze data from wearable devices and sensors, enabling real-time patient monitoring, detecting anomalies, and issuing early health warnings. In the business world, edge AI delves into customer data, including purchase history and behavior, to offer personalized recommendations, enhancing customer experiences. Ultimately, edge AI's potential to revolutionize industries lies in enabling intelligent and autonomous devices to make real-time decisions based on sensor data (Islam, 2023; Singh & Gill, 2023).

## 10.1.3 Edge AI in Real-Time Data Processing

The fusion of edge computing and AI offers significant advantages. Edge AI brings high-performance computing capabilities to the edge, where sensors and IoT devices are situated, enabling real-time data processing without extensive connectivity or integration with other systems. This approach saves time by aggregating data locally and presents various benefits. Firstly, it reduces power consumption, as AI processes at the edge require far less energy than cloud data centers.

Secondly, it minimizes bandwidth usage by processing, analyzing, and storing more data locally, thus reducing costs associated with data transfer to the cloud. Thirdly, it enhances privacy by reducing the risk of misappropriation or mishandling, thanks to locally processed data on edge devices in edge AI operations. Moreover, it prioritizes security by processing and storing data within an edge network, filtering out redundant and unnecessary information. Additionally, this approach allows for easy scalability through cloud-based platforms and native edge capabilities on original equipment manufacturer (OEM) equipment (Islam, 2023; Ramezanian & Niemi, 2019; Singh & Gill, 2023). Lastly, it reduces latency by offloading some of the workload from the cloud platform and conducting local analyses, freeing up the cloud-based platform for other tasks, such as analytics.

## 10.2  RELATED WORKS ON CYBERBULLYING

The study (Perez & Karmakar, 2023) focuses on using NLP and Bayesian time-series analysis to assess the prevalence of cyberbullying on Twitter during the COVID-19 pandemic, provides insights into the dynamics of cyberbullying on the platform during this critical period. In the context of digital parental control, Ramezanian et al. (2021) represent a significant exploration of the fusion of edge computing and 5G networks. This study aligns with prior research endeavors to enhance parental oversight in the digital age. Notably, the authors emphasize the integration of edge computing's localized processing and 5G's high-speed connectivity to develop innovative mechanisms for monitoring and managing children's online activities. While distinct from traditional parental control solutions, this approach echoes the broader trend of leveraging advanced technologies to safeguard children's digital experiences. The paper's insights contribute to the growing body of literature addressing the intersection of technology and child protection, advancing the discourse on responsible digital engagement and safety in the modern era. The research article by Stiglic and Viner (2019) meticulously consolidates findings from diverse sources through an exhaustive analysis of review studies. The study delves into the intricate nexus between screen time and its potential consequences on children and adolescents' physical health, mental well-being, and socio-emotional development. By presenting a synthesized overview of the existing body of knowledge, the article informs the ongoing dialogue about the implications of digital technology in the lives of the young generation. This work bolsters understanding of potential effects and underscores the significance of a well-informed approach to screen time management for youth well-being.

The study by Wisniewski et al. (2015) investigates the relationship between adolescent Internet addiction, exposure to online risks, and the role of resilience in mitigating negative effects. The research finds that adolescents' resilience plays a crucial role in counteracting the adverse consequences of excessive Internet usage and exposure to online risks. The study underscores how resilient traits act as a protective mechanism by analyzing various factors including psychological well-being, social support, and self-esteem. This work contributes to our understanding of the complex interplay between Internet addiction, online risk exposure, and individual resilience in the context of adolescent well-being, shedding light on potential strategies for mitigating the negative impacts of digital engagement during a critical developmental stage. Stoilova et al. (2019) present a comprehensive study of the intricate relationship between children, their online activities, and the critical issue of data privacy. The authors delve into the challenges children face while navigating the digital landscape, where data collection and privacy concerns intersect with their developmental experiences. Through a thorough analysis of empirical evidence, the article sheds light on the evolving dynamics of children's interactions online, highlighting the potential risks and implications associated with their personal data exposure. By synthesizing findings from multiple sources, the authors provide valuable insights into the multifaceted aspects of growing up in a digital age, offering a nuanced perspective on the intersection of childhood, technology, and privacy rights.

Wisniewski (2018) conducted a study on integrating AI techniques within 5G networks to develop privacy-preserving strategies for preventing cyberbullying. The authors delve into the novel approach of leveraging artificial intelligence methods to address cyberbullying while maintaining individuals' privacy. By harnessing the capabilities of advanced AI algorithms within the context of 5G networks, the paper aims to create an environment that effectively identifies and mitigates instances of cyberbullying without compromising the privacy of users. The findings contribute to the discourse on utilizing cutting-edge technologies to enhance online safety and promote responsible digital interactions, particularly in evolving network infrastructures like 5G. They reported the intricate relationship between privacy concerns and adolescent online safety. The study explores the privacy paradox, wherein adolescents might compromise their privacy to enhance online safety. The author delves into whether focusing on risk prevention or resilience is more effective in addressing online safety concerns among adolescents. The article discusses the nuanced interplay between privacy and security, offering insights into how adolescents navigate the digital landscape. By investigating the dynamics of privacy attitudes and behaviors about online safety, the article contributes to the broader understanding of adolescent online behaviors and their implications for cybersecurity strategies and educational initiatives.

## 10.3  NATURAL LANGUAGE PROCESSING FOR CYBERBULLYING

NLP is a powerful tool for detecting cyberbullying because it enables the analysis of text data, such as social media posts, comments, and messages, to identify potentially harmful or abusive content (Al-Doghman et al., 2023). Table 10.1 describes how NLP is typically used in detecting cyberbullying.

It is important to note that NLP-based cyberbullying detection systems are imperfect and may generate false positives or miss some instances of cyberbullying. Human oversight and ongoing model refinement are crucial to improve accuracy and reduce biases in these systems (Kumar Sharma et al., 2018; Rahman, 2022). Additionally, respecting user privacy and ethical considerations are essential when implementing such technologies.

A significant stride in our comprehensive study involves the integration of NLP. NLP and edge AI enable us to detect online harassment by comprehending and analyzing conversations swiftly. This synergy enhances our ability to protect individuals from harmful digital experiences.

**TABLE 10.1**
**NLP in Cyberbullying Detection**

| Task | Description |
| --- | --- |
| Text Classification | NLP models can be trained to classify text as either cyberbullying or non-cyberbullying based on the language used. These models learn from labeled datasets, which include examples of cyberbullying and benign interactions. They can then automatically classify new text as potentially harmful or not. |
| Sentiment Analysis | NLP techniques can assess text sentiment, identifying negative or hostile language. A message containing aggressive or hurtful sentiments may be flagged as potential cyberbullying. |
| Keyword and Pattern Matching | NLP algorithms can be designed to look for specific keywords or patterns commonly associated with cyberbullying. For instance, they might search for derogatory terms, hate speech, or threats. |
| Contextual Analysis | NLP models can take context into account. Some comments that may appear harmful on their own could be harmless when considered in the context of a conversation. Contextual analysis helps distinguish between genuine cyberbullying and casual banter. |
| User Behavior Analysis | NLP can be used to analyze the behavior of users over time. Patterns of repetitive negative interactions, stalking, or harassment can be detected through text analysis. |
| Real-Time Monitoring | NLP algorithms can continuously monitor social media platforms, providing real-time alerts and reporting when potentially harmful content is detected. |

## 10.4 REINFORCING DETECTION MECHANISMS

This section discusses how the combination of edge AI and anomaly detection systems strengthens online harassment prevention efforts.

Integrating edge AI with anomaly detection systems extensively bolsters online harassment prevention efforts. By processing data locally and in real time, these systems can swiftly identify unusual patterns, such as spikes in negative interactions or aggressive language, enabling immediate intervention. Privacy protection is enhanced as user data remains secure and private due to local processing (AI in Anomaly Detection, n.d.). Customizable models tailored to specific online platforms reduce false positives, while adaptability and scalability effectively detect evolving harassment tactics. Empowering users to report incidents with confidence, these systems also lessen the workload of human moderators, foster trust, and create safer and more inclusive online environments.

Moreover, the amalgamation of edge AI with anomaly detection and alert systems presents a robust mechanism for reinforcing our prevention strategies. Swift identification of deviations from normal online behavior empowers us to promptly address potential harassment, thereby contributing to a safer online environment.

The following approaches explore the dynamic synergy between edge AI and anomaly detection systems, a powerful strategy for enhancing online harassment prevention.

### 10.4.1 A Swift and Proactive Approach

Integrating edge AI and anomaly detection systems provides a swift and proactive approach to identifying and mitigating online harassment. By processing data locally and in real time, these systems can swiftly recognize unusual patterns in online interactions. Such patterns might include sudden spikes in negative interactions, the use of aggressive language, or the targeting of vulnerable individuals. This rapid detection empowers platforms and moderators to act immediately, mitigating the harm inflicted upon victims (Al-Doghman et al., 2023).

### 10.4.2 Enhanced Privacy Protection

One of the key benefits of this integration is the enhancement of privacy protection. As user data is processed locally, it remains secure and private, reducing the risk of sensitive information falling into the wrong hands. The focus on local processing minimizes the exposure of user data to external entities, thus safeguarding user privacy and maintaining trust in the platform (Radhakrishnan & Gupta, 2021).

### 10.4.3 Customizable Models and Reduced False Positives

Anomaly detection systems, when combined with edge AI, offer the advantage of creating customizable models tailored to specific online platforms. These models can be fine-tuned to understand the nuances of each platform's user behavior and language, reducing the occurrence of false positives. This customization ensures that legitimate user interactions are not inadvertently flagged as harassment, preserving the user experience.

### 10.4.4 Adaptability and Scalability

Online harassment tactics are constantly evolving, making it essential to have adaptable and scalable prevention systems. The combination of edge AI and anomaly detection facilitates the dynamic adaptation of detection models to emerging harassment methods. The systems can learn from new patterns and behaviors, making them more effective in identifying evolving threats.

### 10.4.5 Empowering Users and Reducing Moderator Workload

In addition to enhancing detection capabilities, these integrated systems empower users to report incidents confidently. Users can trust that their reports will be taken seriously and that timely intervention will be initiated. This trust not only fosters a safer online environment but also lessens the workload of human moderators. With the assistance of these advanced systems, moderators can focus their efforts on more complex cases and proactive community management, further contributing to the overall health of the online space.

### 10.4.6 Creating Safer and More Inclusive Online Environments

Ultimately, the amalgamation of Edge AI with anomaly detection and alert systems provides a robust mechanism for reinforcing online harassment prevention strategies. Swift identification of deviations from normal online behavior empowers platforms to promptly address potential harassment, contributing to a safer and more inclusive online environment. This approach aligns with the broader goal of creating digital spaces where individuals can engage without fear, fostering a sense of belonging and promoting healthy online interactions (Radhakrishnan & Gupta, 2021).

Empowering users and promoting trust fosters a safer and more inclusive online space. This approach exemplifies the convergence of technology and ethics to combat online harassment effectively.

## 10.5 PRIVACY CONSIDERATIONS AND REGULATORY COMPLIANCE

While our focus remains on digital safety, navigating the intricate landscape of privacy and adhering to regulatory frameworks is imperative. This section underscores our commitment to a comprehensive approach that respects user data and aligns with legal requirements (Radhakrishnan & Gupta, 2021).

Privacy considerations, adherence to legal requirements, and regulatory compliance are paramount in today's data-driven landscape. Organizations must prioritize transparency in data collection and secure informed consent, minimize data to the essentials, and bolster data security through encryption and access controls to meet legal standards. Adherence to data localization, retention, and user rights is essential, and conducting data protection impact assessments is a legal requirement in many jurisdictions. Third-party data sharing should align with regulations, and robust incident response plans for breaches are vital to fulfill legal obligations. Staying compliant with relevant data protection laws such as GDPR or CCPA, designating a data privacy officer as mandated by some regulations, fostering awareness, conducting regular audits, and integrating privacy by design are essential practices to ensure both legal compliance and ethical data handling, which are fundamental aspects of responsible business conduct (Data Privacy Compliance & Protection | Optiv, n.d.; Data Protection Principles: Core Principles of the GDPR, n.d.). In the digital age, where data plays a central role, ensuring privacy and adhering to regulatory frameworks is paramount. In the contemporary landscape, protecting user data is not merely a best practice but a legal and ethical imperative. Organizations must embrace the following fundamental principles in Table 10.2 (Chatterjee, 2020; Martinelli et al., 2020).

## 10.6 CONCLUSION

In conclusion, this chapter highlights the transformative potential of edge AI in the context of online harassment prevention and the advancement of societal well-being, particularly concerning women's safety. It underscores the significance of proactive intervention, privacy protection, and collaboration between humans and machines in shaping a future where secure digital environments and positive AI contributions are not mere aspirations but achievable realities. By leveraging edge

**TABLE 10.2**
**Privacy and Regulatory Framework**

| Action | Description |
| --- | --- |
| Transparency and Informed Consent | Transparency in data collection is foundational. Users should be informed about how their data is collected and used, and their informed consent should be sought. This builds trust and is a fundamental aspect of responsible data handling. |
| Data Minimization | Collecting only the essential data is vital. Unnecessary data should not be gathered, reducing the risk associated with excessive data storage and processing. |
| Data Security | Data security is non-negotiable. Robust measures, including encryption and access controls, must be in place to safeguard sensitive information. Data breaches can have severe consequences, emphasizing the importance of proactive security measures. |
| Data Localization and Retention | Data should be stored and processed under legal requirements. Complying with data localization and retention regulations is essential, as is respecting users' rights to control their data. |
| Data Protection Impact Assessments | In many jurisdictions, conducting data protection impact assessments is mandatory. This process evaluates the potential risks to individuals' data and helps implement appropriate safeguards. |
| Third-Party Data Sharing | Organizations should ensure alignment with regulatory standards when sharing data with third parties. This includes contracts and agreements that protect user data during sharing. |
| Incident Response Planning | Robust incident response plans for data breaches are indispensable. Being prepared to address and mitigate the impact of data breaches is not just good practice; it is a legal obligation in many cases. |
| Compliance with Data Protection Laws | Organizations must comply with relevant data protection laws such as GDPR (General Data Protection Regulation) or CCPA (California Consumer Privacy Act). These laws outline specific requirements for data protection and privacy practices. |
| Designating a Data Privacy Officer | In line with specific regulations, appointing a Data Privacy Officer can be a legal mandate. This role ensures that an organization's data practices align with legal requirements. |
| Fostering Privacy Awareness | Raising awareness among employees and stakeholders about the significance of privacy and data protection is essential. This fosters a culture of responsibility and compliance. |
| Regular Audits | Regular audits of data handling practices help ensure that privacy and security measures remain practical and up-to-date. |
| Privacy by Design | Integrating privacy considerations from the outset of any data-related project is a best practice. It ensures that privacy is not an afterthought but a fundamental aspect of the project's design. |

AI's real-time processing capabilities, integrating NLP for swift analysis, and reinforcing detection mechanisms, this comprehensive study offers a holistic approach to addressing online harassment and cyberbullying. Moreover, the chapter emphasizes the critical importance of adhering to privacy considerations and regulatory compliance, aligning with legal requirements while respecting user data and ethical data handling practices. In a world where digital interactions have become integral to daily life, the integration of edge AI and responsible data practices offers a promising path toward fostering a safer, more inclusive, and more secure online ecosystem.

## REFERENCES

Abarna, S., Sheeba, J. I., Jayasrilakshmi, S., & Devaneyan, S. P. (2022). Identification of Cyber Harassment and Intention of Target Users on Social Media Platforms. *Engineering Applications of Artificial Intelligence*, 115(July), 105283. https://doi.org/10.1016/j.engappai.2022.105283

Afrifa, S., & Varadarajan, V. (2022). Cyberbullying Detection on Twitter Using Natural Language Processing and Machine Learning Techniques. *International Journal of Innovative Technology and Interdisciplinary Sciences*, 5(4), 1069–1080. https://doi.org/10.15157/IJITIS.2022.5.4.1069-1080

Agha, S., Mohsan, H., Ul, Q., Zahra, A., Khan, M. A., Alsharif, M. H., Elhaty, I. A., & Jahid, A. (2022). Role of Drone Technology Helping in Alleviating the COVID-19 Pandemic. *Micromachines*, 13(10), 1593. https://doi.org/10.3390/MI13101593

Al-Doghman, F., Moustafa, N., Khalil, I., Sohrabi, N., Tari, Z., & Zomaya, A. Y. (2023). AI-Enabled Secure Microservices in Edge Computing: Opportunities and Challenges. *IEEE Transactions on Services Computing*, 16(2), 1485–1504. https://doi.org/10.1109/TSC.2022.3155447

AI in Anomaly Detection. (n.d.). Retrieved October 24, 2023, from https://www.leewayhertz.com/ai-in-anomaly-detection/

Both Men and Women Vulnerable to Online Harassment in India. (n.d.). Retrieved October 24, 2023, from https://mediaindia.eu/society/both-men-and-women-vulnerable-to-online-harassment-in-india/

Chatterjee, S. (2020). AI Strategy of India: Policy Framework, Adoption Challenges and Actions for Government. *Transforming Government: People, Process and Policy*, 14(5), 757–775. https://doi.org/10.1108/TG-05-2019-0031

Data Privacy Compliance & Protection | Optiv. (n.d.). Retrieved October 24, 2023, from https://www.optiv.com/services/data-governance-privacy-protection/data-privacy

Data Protection Principles: Core Principles of the GDPR. (n.d.). Retrieved October 24, 2023, from https://cloudian.com/guides/data-protection/data-protection-principles-7-core-principles-of-the-gdpr/

Islam, M. R. (2023). *Detection of Cyberbullying in Social Media Texts Using Explainable Artificial Intelligence*. http://hdl.handle.net/1974/31678

Kumar Sharma, H., Kshitiz, K., & Shailendra. (2018). NLP and Machine Learning Techniques for Detecting Insulting Comments on Social Networking Platforms. *International Conference on Advances in Computing and Communication Engineering*, 265–272. https://doi.org/10.1109/ICACCE.2018.8441728

Martinelli, F., Marulli, F., Mercaldo, F., Marrone, S., & Santone, A. (2020). Enhanced Privacy and Data Protection using Natural Language Processing and Artificial Intelligence. *Proceedings of the International Joint Conference on Neural Networks*. https://doi.org/10.1109/IJCNN48605.2020.9206801

Perez, C., & Karmakar, S. (2023). An NLP-Assisted Bayesian Time-Series Analysis for Prevalence of Twitter Cyberbullying During the COVID-19 Pandemic. *Social Network Analysis and Mining*, 13(1). https://doi.org/10.1007/s13278-023-01053-4

Radhakrishnan, J., & Gupta, S. (2021). Exploring the Artificial Intelligence Adoption Journey-A Multiple Case Studies Approach. *PACIS 2021 Proceedings*. https://aisel.aisnet.org/pacis2021/188

Rahman, M. H. U. (2022). Cyberbullying Detection using Natural Language Processing. *International Journal for Research in Applied Science and Engineering Technology*, 10(5), 5241–5248. https://doi.org/10.22214/IJRASET.2022.43683

Ramezanian, S., Meskanen, T., & Niemi, V. (2021, May). Parental Control with Edge Computing and 5G Networks. *Conference of Open Innovation Association, FRUCT*, 290–300. https://doi.org/10.23919/FRUCT52173.2021.9435552

Ramezanian, S., & Niemi, V. (2019). Privacy Preserving Cyberbullying Prevention with AI Methods in 5G Networks. *Conference of Open Innovation Association, FRUCT*, 265–271. https://doi.org/10.23919/FRUCT48121.2019.8981521

Singh, R., & Gill, S. S. (2023). Edge AI: A Survey. *Internet of Things and Cyber-Physical Systems*, 3, 71–92. https://doi.org/10.1016/J.IOTCPS.2023.02.004

Stiglic, N., & Viner, R. M. (2019). Effects of Screentime on the Health and Well-Being of Children and Adolescents: A Systematic Review of Reviews. *BMJ Open*, 9(1), e023191. https://doi.org/10.1136/BMJOPEN-2018-023191

Stoilova, M., Livingstone, S., & Nandagiri, R. (2019, January). Children's Data and Privacy Online: Growing Up in a Digital Age. *Research findings. School of Economics and Political Science*, 1–47.

Tercs, A. C. N. (2022, July). End-to-End Messaging System Enhancement Using Federated Learning for Cyberbullying Detection End-to-End Messaging System Enhancement Using Federated Learning for Cyberbullying Detection Submitted by the APJ Abdul Kalam Technological University Computer Sc. https://doi.org/10.13140/RG.2.2.35686.70722

Wisniewski, P. (2018). The Privacy Paradox of Adolescent Online Safety: A Matter of Risk Prevention or Risk Resilience? *IEEE Security and Privacy*, 16(2), 86–90. https://doi.org/10.1109/MSP.2018.1870874

Wisniewski, P., Jia, H., Wang, N., Zheng, S., Xu, H., Rosson, M. B., & Carroll, J. M. (2015, April). Resilience Mitigates the Negative Effects of Adolescent Internet Addiction and Online Risk Exposure. *Conference on Human Factors in Computing Systems—Proceedings*, 4029–4038. https://doi.org/10.1145/2702123.2702240

# 11 Leveraging Artificial Intelligence and IoT for Healthcare 5.0

## Use Cases, Applications, and Challenges

Gnanasankaran Natarajan, Elakkiya Elango,
Sandhya Soman, and Shirley Chellathurai Pon Anna Bai

## 11.1 INTRODUCTION

### 11.1.1 Overview of Artificial Intelligence

Artificial intelligence (AI) is the replication of human intelligence in technologies that are programmed to understand, acquire knowledge, and solve problems in the same way that people do. It is a large topic of computer science which involves several technologies, methods, and approaches. AI aims to create intelligent systems that can accomplish activities that would normally need human intellect, such as speech recognition, visual perception, decision-making, and natural language processing. AI is divided into two types: narrow AI and general AI. Narrow AI, sometimes referred to as weak AI, is intended to accomplish certain tasks within a narrow scope. It excels in areas such as image identification, recommendation systems, voice assistance, and autonomous vehicles. General AI, on the other hand, implies AI systems that, like humans, can understand, acquire, and apply knowledge across several disciplines.

The development of AI relies on several foundational technologies and techniques. Machine learning is a basic component that allows AI systems to acquire knowledge from data and enhance its efficiency periodically. Machine learning methods are classified as supervised (training on labeled data), unsupervised (identifying patterns in unlabeled data), and reinforced (learning via trial and error based on incentives and punishments). Deep learning, a subset of machine learning that employs artificial neural networks based by the human brain, is another important component of AI. Deep learning models, additionally referred to as deep neural networks, are capable of processing and analyzing massive volumes of data, allowing them to recognize complicated patterns as well as generate accurate predictions. Deep learning has led to great advances in image and speech recognition, natural language processing, and autonomous systems (LeCun et al., 2015).

AI applications are widespread and have transformed various industries. AI is utilized in healthcare for disease diagnosis, drug discovery, and personalized therapy. AI algorithms are used in finance for fraud detection, algorithmic trading, and risk assessment. AI is also applied in manufacturing, agriculture, transportation, cybersecurity, and many other fields, enhancing efficiency, accuracy, and decision-making processes. The rapid development of AI technology, on the other hand, creates ethical and societal challenges. Issues such as employment displacement, privacy, algorithm bias, and potential misuse of AI present serious concerns that must be carefully considered and regulated (Goodfellow et al., 2016).

AI is a multidisciplinary field with the goal of developing intelligent systems capable of executing human-like activities. It encompasses various techniques, including machine learning and deep learning, and finds applications in numerous sectors. While AI offers immense potential for positive impact, its development and deployment should be guided by ethical considerations to ensure responsible and beneficial use (Sutton & Barto, 2018).

### 11.1.2  EXPLAINABLE ARTIFICIAL INTELLIGENCE—A NEXT-LEVEL AI PLATFORM

Explainable artificial intelligence (XAI) is a discipline of artificial intelligence with an emphasis on developing techniques and models which may give accessible explanations for AI systems' judgments and reasoning. The aim of XAI is to make AI systems' decision-making processes visible, interpretable, and understandable to human users. Traditional AI models, such as deep learning neural networks, frequently function as "black boxes," generating outputs without providing clear insights regarding how those outputs were produced. This lack of transparency can be problematic in vital fields such as healthcare, banking, and autonomous systems, since understanding the logic behind AI choices is critical. XAI proposes to address this issue by allowing humans to better understand and verify the decision-making processes of AI systems (Dandl et al., 2019). It gives explanations which shed light on the variables, traits, or patterns that the AI model considers before arriving at a specific output or conclusion. Users, stakeholders, and regulatory agencies can benefit from these explanations in a variety of ways.

#### 11.1.2.1  Trust and Reliability

XAI contributes to the development of confidence in AI systems by offering explanations that illustrate the underlying rationale and evidence underpinning the judgments. Users are more inclined to trust and accept AI systems if they understand why and how certain results were made.

#### 11.1.2.2  Debugging and Error Analysis

Explainable models allow developers and practitioners to identify and correct AI system flaws or biases. Developers may enhance the model's performance, discover data errors, and assure fairness and accountability by knowing the reasons.

#### 11.1.2.3  Compliance and Regulation

XAI can help satisfy regulatory standards in fields involving legal and ethical implications, such as healthcare or finance. Explanations can aid in demonstrating conformity with laws, policies, and ethical standards, so assuring openness and accountability.

#### 11.1.2.4  User Empowerment

XAI allows users to actively engage with AI systems. By providing explanations, users can understand the system's limitations, identify potential biases, and make informed decisions based on the provided insights.

Several approaches and techniques are employed in XAI to provide explanations for AI systems. These include:

- **Rule-based methods:** Using explicit rules or decision trees to provide step-by-step explanations of the decision process.
- **Feature importance methods:** Identifying the most influential features or input variables that contribute to the decision.
- **Example-based methods:** Presenting representative examples from the training data that are like the input, explaining how similar cases were handled in the past.

- **Model-agnostic methods:** Techniques that work with any type of AI model, providing explanations without relying on specific model internals.
- **Hybrid approaches:** Combining multiple methods to provide comprehensive and understandable explanations.

XAI research and development are still evolving, and challenges remain. Balancing the trade-off between accuracy and explainability, addressing the complexity of deep learning models, and ensuring explanations are meaningful and actionable are ongoing areas of focus. XAI aims to make AI systems more visible and understandable by explaining how they make decisions. By enabling humans to understand and trust AI algorithms, XAI promotes accountability, compliance, user empowerment, and error analysis. Various techniques and approaches are used in XAI, and ongoing research continues to improve the explainability of AI systems (Chen et al., 2018).

## 11.2 INTRODUCTION TO MODERN HEALTHCARE SYSTEMS

Modern healthcare systems refer to the comprehensive networks, infrastructure, policies, and practices that are in place to provide healthcare services to individuals and communities. These systems have evolved over time to meet the increasing complexities and demands of healthcare delivery, incorporating advanced technologies, interdisciplinary collaboration, evidence-based practices, and patient-centered approaches that are listed here.

### 11.2.1 Accessible and Equitable Care

Modern healthcare systems aspire to make healthcare services affordable to all people, regardless of socioeconomic position, geographic location, or demographic background. Efforts are made to reduce barriers to access through measures such as universal healthcare coverage, insurance programs, community health centers, and telemedicine initiatives.

### 11.2.2 Interdisciplinary Collaboration

Modern healthcare systems emphasize interdisciplinary collaboration among healthcare professionals to deliver comprehensive and integrated care. Teams of doctors, nurses, pharmacists, therapists, psychologists, and other experts collaborate to fulfil patients' various needs. Collaborative care models enhance communication, coordination, and the overall quality of care.

### 11.2.3 Technological Advancements

Modern healthcare heavily relies on advanced technologies to improve patient outcomes, enhance efficiency, and enable more precise diagnoses and treatments. Electronic health records (EHRs) and telehealth platforms allow seamless sharing of patient information and remote consultations. Medical imaging technologies, robotic surgery, genetic testing, wearable devices, and AI applications are among the many technological advancements integrated into modern healthcare systems (Bates & Gawande, 2003).

### 11.2.4 Preventive and Population Health

There is a growing focus on preventive care and population health management in modern healthcare systems. Efforts are made to promote healthy lifestyles, early detection of diseases, and the management of chronic conditions. Public health initiatives, health education campaigns, and proactive interventions help reduce the burden of illness and promote overall wellness in communities.

### 11.2.5 EVIDENCE-BASED MEDICINE

Evidence-based practices, which include combining the most recent available scientific research with medical expertise and patient values, are prioritized in modern healthcare systems. Clinical guidelines and protocols based on rigorous research and clinical trials guide healthcare professionals in making informed decisions about diagnostics, treatments, and interventions (Buntin et al., 2011).

### 11.2.6 PATIENT-CENTERED CARE

Modern healthcare systems recognize the importance of patient-centered care, which places the patient at the forefront of decision-making and tailors healthcare services to their unique needs, preferences, and values. This includes collaborative decision-making, clear communication, respect for autonomy, and patient and family engagement in care planning.

### 11.2.7 QUALITY IMPROVEMENT AND SAFETY

Patient safety and ongoing quality improvement are essential components of modern healthcare systems. To monitor results, eliminate medical mistakes, enhance patient experiences, and raise overall healthcare quality, data-driven techniques, performance measures, and quality improvement programs are employed.

### 11.2.8 HEALTH INFORMATION EXCHANGE AND PRIVACY

Modern healthcare systems prioritize safe health information transmission among practitioners in order to ensure smooth continuity of service. To ensure patient confidentiality and the security of private medical information, robust privacy and data protection mechanisms, such as HIPAA compliance, are in place.

### 11.2.9 HEALTH POLICY AND GOVERNANCE

Government policies, legislation, and governance structures all have an impact on healthcare systems. To achieve equitable allocation of resources, timely service delivery, and successful healthcare administration, today's healthcare systems require competent health policy creation, strategic planning, and regulatory frameworks.

### 11.2.10 RESEARCH AND INNOVATION

Medical research and innovation are encouraged in modern healthcare systems in order to expand medical knowledge, discover novel medicines, and enhance healthcare practices. Medical research institutes, academic collaborations, and cooperation between healthcare providers and technology firms generate innovation, promoting advancements in diagnostics, medicines, and healthcare delivery approaches (Institute of Medicine, 2001).

Accessible, egalitarian, multidisciplinary, technologically advanced, evidence-based, patient-centered, and quality-driven treatment are all goals of modern healthcare systems. These systems attempt to enhance health outcomes, better patient experiences, and promote population health by combining modern technology, collaborative methods, preventative measures, and research and innovation.

## 11.3 ARTIFICIAL INTELLIGENCE ADVANCES IN MODERN HEALTHCARE SYSTEMS

AI plays a significant role in modern healthcare systems, revolutionizing the way medical professionals deliver care, diagnose diseases, and improve patient outcomes. Here is a detailed explanation of how AI contributes to modern healthcare:

### 11.3.1 MEDICAL IMAGING AND DIAGNOSTICS

AI is revolutionizing the way medical professionals offer treatment, diagnose illnesses, and enhance the results for patients in current healthcare systems. Here is a full description of how artificial intelligence helps in current healthcare:

### 11.3.2 PREDICTIVE ANALYTICS AND EARLY DETECTION

AI is widely utilized in the interpretation of medical imaging in fields including radiology, pathology, and dermatology. Deep learning algorithms assess medical pictures with great accuracy and speed, assisting in the detection of anomalies, cancers, fractures, and other disorders. Diagnostic technologies driven by AI assist radiologists and pathologists in making accurate and timely diagnoses, decreasing human error and improving patient outcomes.

### 11.3.3 PERSONALIZED MEDICINE

AI supports personalized medicine through reviewing patient data such as genetic profiles, medical history, and treatment responses in order to build customized treatment plans. AI algorithms help determine optimal drug dosages, predict adverse reactions, and identify targeted therapies for individual patients, leading to improved treatment efficacy and minimized side effects.

### 11.3.4 VIRTUAL ASSISTANTS AND CHATBOTS

AI-powered virtual assistants and chatbots enhance patient engagement and support. They can provide basic healthcare information, answer questions, offer self-care advice, schedule appointments, and triage patients based on symptoms. Chatbots can assist in mental health support, counseling, and crisis intervention, providing accessible and timely assistance to individuals.

### 11.3.5 ROBOTICS AND SURGICAL ASSISTANCE

AI is used in robotic-assisted surgeries, enabling precise, minimally invasive procedures. Surgeon's control robotic systems that incorporate AI algorithms to enhance surgical precision, reduce human tremors, and improve dexterity. AI also assists in pre-operative planning, surgical navigation, and post-operative monitoring, contributing to better surgical outcomes.

### 11.3.6 DRUG DISCOVERY AND DEVELOPMENT

AI improves up drug research and development by processing enormous amounts of biological and chemical data. Machine learning algorithms help identify potential drug candidates, predict their effectiveness, and optimize drug formulations. AI models accelerate the screening of compounds, reducing time and cost in bringing new drugs to the market.

### 11.3.7 HEALTH MONITORING AND WEARABLE DEVICES

AI algorithms process real-time data from wearable devices, such as fitness trackers and smartwatches, monitoring vital signs, physical activity, sleep patterns, and other health-related metrics. AI-powered data analysis aids in early identification of health concerns, remote patient monitoring, and personalized healthcare guidance, allowing individuals to exert proactive control of their health (Beede et al., 2018).

### 11.3.8 HEALTH DATA ANALYTICS AND DECISION SUPPORT

AI allows for a fast analysis of massive amounts of health data, which includes electronic health records, clinical trials, and research studies. AI algorithms may identify patterns, predict outcomes from therapy, and assist healthcare personnel in making decisions. This assists in evidence-based clinical decision-making, optimizing treatment plans, and improving resource allocation.

### 11.3.9 Workflow Optimization and Operational Efficiency

AI helps streamline administrative tasks, optimize workflows, and improve operational efficiency in healthcare settings. AI-powered technologies streamline typical operations like scheduling appointments, payment, and inventory management, freeing up healthcare employees to focus on patient care (Topol, 2019).

### 11.3.10 Clinical Research and Insights

AI algorithms can analyze vast amounts of clinical data, scientific literature, and research papers to extract insights and accelerate medical research. This supports the discovery of new treatment modalities, identification of risk factors, and advancement of medical knowledge, contributing to evidence-based practice and innovation (Beam & Kohane, 2016).

AI plays a major role in modern healthcare systems by enhancing medical imaging and diagnostics, enabling predictive analytics and early detection, facilitating personalized medicine, supporting virtual assistance and chatbots, assisting in robotic surgeries, expediting drug discovery and development.

## 11.4  INTERNET OF THINGS—A PREVIEW

The Internet of Things (IoT) is a massive network of interconnected devices, objects, and systems that are outfitted with sensors, software, and connections to gather, share, and act on data. IoT is the notion of linking many common devices to the global web and enabling devices to interact with one another and with people. Household appliances and wearable gadgets, as well as industrial machinery and smart city infrastructure, are examples of these items. IoT devices communicate to the web via a variety of methods, including Wi-Fi, Bluetooth, cellular networks, and specialized IoT networks that include LoRaWAN or NB-IoT. This connection enables devices to interact and share data with one another, as well as with centralized systems and users, resulting in a seamless network. Sensors on IoT devices allow them to measure and gather data from the environment. Humidity, temperature, light, motion, pressure, location, and many more characteristics may be detected by these sensors. The information gathered by these sensors is typically transferred to a centralized system for processing and analysis (Atzori et al., 2010).

To analyze and evaluate the massive amounts of data gathered by IoT devices, IoT systems use cloud computing or edge computing. Edge computing brings processing power nearer to the devices themselves, decreasing latency and enabling real-time analytics, whereas cloud-based solutions store and process data on faraway servers. IoT enables the automation and control of various processes and systems. By connecting devices and systems, IoT allows for remote monitoring and control, enabling actions to be taken based on the collected data. For example, smart home devices can adjust temperature and lighting based on occupancy or user preferences, and industrial IoT systems can optimize manufacturing processes based on real-time data. IoT applications provide opportunities for enhanced efficiency and productivity in various sectors. In agriculture, for example, IoT may track soil moisture levels and automated irrigation systems to optimize water consumption. In logistics, IoT can track shipments, monitor inventory, and optimize routes, improving operational efficiency (Al-Fuqaha et al., 2015).

IoT can enhance safety and security in many domains. In healthcare, for example, IoT devices may remotely monitor patients and warn healthcare staff in the event of an emergency. In smart cities, IoT systems can monitor traffic, detect anomalies, and enhance public safety by coordinating emergency response systems. IoT technologies enable the creation of smart environments that provide personalized and context-aware experiences. For instance, smart homes can automatically adjust lighting, temperature, and entertainment preferences based on user preferences and presence. Wearable IoT devices can provide real-time health monitoring and personalized recommendations for fitness and well-being. Intelligent systems are frequently created by combining IoT and AI technology. AI algorithms are capable of analyzing the huge amounts of data gathered by IoT devices, allowing predictive analytics, anomaly detection, and pattern identification. This integration allows IoT systems to learn, adapt, and make autonomous decisions, further enhancing their capabilities.

IoT systems are built to be scalable, enabling for the effortless addition to new devices and network expansion. Furthermore, interoperability standards and protocols allow diverse IoT devices and platforms to connect and collaborate, independent of manufacturer or technology employed. Data privacy, security risks, standardization, and infrastructure need all present obstacles when implementing IoT devices. Addressing these challenges is essential to ensure the ethical and secure deployment of IoT technologies (Borgia, 2014).

IoT connects everyday objects to the Internet, allowing them to gather data, communicate, automate, and control themselves. IoT has the potential to transform industries, enhance efficiency, improve safety, and provide personalized experiences. With the integration of AI, IoT systems can become smarter and more autonomous, contributing to a more connected and intelligent world.

## 11.5 COLLABORATION BETWEEN IOT AND MODERN HEALTHCARE SYSTEMS

IoT is revolutionizing the way healthcare services are delivered, monitored, and managed in modern healthcare systems. It empowers healthcare providers to collect and analyze real-time data, enhance patient care, improve operational efficiency, and enable preventive and personalized medicine. Let us discuss some of the prominent roles of IoT in modern healthcare systems:

### 11.5.1 REMOTE PATIENT MONITORING

IoT offers remote monitoring of patients, allowing healthcare practitioners to remotely monitor patients' health problems. Wearables, home monitoring systems, and implanted sensors are examples of IoT devices that may continually gather and send vital signs, medication adherence data, activity levels, and other health information. This remote monitoring enables early diagnosis of problems, prompt action, and personalized treatment, resulting in fewer hospital visits and better patient outcomes.

### 11.5.2 TELEMEDICINE AND VIRTUAL CARE

IoT enables telemedicine and virtual care services, allowing for remote consultations, diagnosis, and treatment. Healthcare practitioners can offer healthcare services remotely using connected technologies such as video conferencing tools, remote examination tools, and IoT-enabled medical devices. This enhances patient comfort and increases access to care, particularly in underprivileged regions (Balakrishnan & Varghese, 2021).

### 11.5.3 REAL-TIME HEALTH DATA COLLECTION

IoT devices collect real-time health data, providing accurate and up-to-date information to healthcare practitioners. Sensors incorporated in medical equipment, wearables, and healthcare facilities capture data on vital signs, drug administration, ambient conditions, patient activity, and other factors. This information gives insights into patients' health, aids in the early diagnosis of worsening illnesses, and allows for prompt actions.

### 11.5.4 Health and Wellness Tracking

Individuals may use IoT devices to monitor their well-being and health in real time. Wearables, fitness trackers, and mobile health applications record information such as physical activity, sleep habits, heart rate, and other variables. Individuals may use this information to track their health, set goals, and make well-informed lifestyle decisions. It also provides detailed patient data to healthcare practitioners during consultations.

### 11.5.5 Improved Medication Management

IoT aids with drug management by minimizing falls and increasing adherence. Smart pillboxes, medicine dispensers, and wearable devices can be used to remind patients to take their prescriptions on time. They can also track medicine consumption and provide notifications to healthcare practitioners or carers if dosages are missing or incorrectly administered. This technique increases patient safety and drug adherence (Memon et al., 2018).

### 11.5.6 Operational Efficiency and Asset Management

IoTenhances operational efficiency in healthcare institutions. Healthcare assets, such as medical equipment, inventories, and buildings, may be monitored and managed via connected devices. IoT solutions can track equipment's location, usage, and maintenance requirements, optimize inventory levels, and automate regular operations like buying supplies. This optimizes resource allocation, decreases costs, and simplifies procedures.

### 11.5.7 Enhanced Patient Safety and Security

In healthcare contexts, IoT improves patient safety and security. IoT-enabled devices may monitor environmental factors like as temperature, humidity, and air quality, assuring optimal patient care and drug storage conditions. IoT systems may also improve security by monitoring access control, detecting unauthorized entrance, and assuring patient data privacy and confidentiality.

### 11.5.8 Predictive Analytics and Preventive Care

By evaluating enormous amounts of data, IoT offers predictive analytics and preventative treatment. Machine learning algorithms can detect patterns, correlations, and anomalies in health data, assisting in illness risk prediction, early warning signals identification, and prevention recommendations. This proactive healthcare strategy promotes early intervention, decreases hospitalisations, and enhances population health (Zhou et al., 2010).

### 11.5.9 Smart Hospitals and Infrastructure

IoT technology aid in the creation of smart hospitals and infrastructure. Energy management, asset tracking, patient flow, and building upkeep are all monitored and controlled by connected devices and sensors. This increases efficiency, lowers expenses, and improves the patient experience overall.

### 11.5.10 Data Analytics and Decision Support

IoT creates massive volumes of healthcare data that may be evaluated to gain valuable insights. This data may be processed and analyzed using big data analytics and AI algorithms, allowing for evidence-based decision-making, personalized therapies, and population health management. This data-driven strategy aids clinical research, efforts to enhance quality, and the creation of healthcare policy.

IoT transforms current healthcare systems by enabling remote patient monitoring, telemedicine, real-time data collection, enhanced medication management, operational efficiency, improved patient security, analytics that predict results, smart infrastructure, and data-driven decision support. IoT technology enable healthcare practitioners to offer more proactive, personalized, and efficient treatment while increasing patient outcomes and healthcare system performance (Wang et al., 2020).

## 11.6  ROLE OF IOT IN MODERN MEDICAL EQUIPMENT MANUFACTURING

IoT is transforming the design, manufacture, and use of medical equipment. It enables the development of intelligent, linked medical equipment capable of collecting, sending, and analyzing data, leading in improved patient care, efficiency in operation, and innovation. Let us look at some of the most crucial components of IoT in current medical equipment production below:

### 11.6.1  Remote Monitoring and Real-Time Data

IoT connects medical equipment to the Internet, allowing for remote monitoring of patients' health problems and real-time data collecting. Wearable IoT devices, for example, may continuously monitor vital indicators like heart rate, blood pressure, and oxygen levels and relay the data to healthcare professionals in real time. Remote monitoring aids in the early discovery of anomalies, prompt action, and personalized patient care (Zhang et al., 2018).

### 11.6.2  Predictive Maintenance

IoT makes predictive maintenance for medical equipment possible. Connected devices can monitor their own performance and detect any flaws or maintenance requirements. IoT-enabled devices may forecast when maintenance or repairs are needed by evaluating data on consumption, performance, and environmental conditions, decreasing downtime and enhancing operational efficiency.

### 11.6.3  Enhanced Connectivity and Interoperability

IoT provides seamless communication and interoperability across various medical equipment and systems. Integrating IoT features into medical equipment allows healthcare practitioners to access and share data across several devices and platforms, boosting communication, collaboration, and workflow efficiency. This connection helps to create comprehensive patient health records and makes data-driven decisions easier (Fang et al., 2019).

### 11.6.4  Automated Inventory Management

IoT offers computerized inventory management in the medical equipment manufacturing industry. Connected devices may monitor and track the consumption, accessibility, and expiration date of medical equipment and supplies in real time. This information enables producers to optimize inventory levels, prevent waste, and ensure timely replacement, therefore increasing efficiency and cost-effectiveness.

### 11.6.5  Quality Control and Compliance

IoT improves quality control and compliance in the manufacture of medical equipment. Connected devices may collect data on manufacturing processes, ambient conditions, and quality characteristics, ensuring that regulatory requirements and quality assurance methods are followed. Real-time data monitoring and analysis aid in identifying potential difficulties, allowing producers to take remedial steps as soon as possible (Manogaran et al., 2017).

### 11.6.6 Data-Driven Product Improvement

Through data analysis, IoT allows continual product improvement. Manufacturers can collect usage data and feedback from linked medical devices in order to discover usage trends, diagnose performance concerns, and learn about user preferences. This data-driven approach contributes to the development of more effective and user-friendly medical equipment, hence improving patient outcomes and satisfaction.

### 11.6.7 Remote Software Updates and Upgrades

IoT enables remote software updates and upgrades for medical devices. Manufacturers may remotely release software patches, security upgrades, and new features without requiring physical involvement. This guarantees that medical equipment is always up-to-date, secure, and in accordance with changing standards and laws.

### 11.6.8 Enhanced Patient Safety

IoT leads to improved patient safety by lowering the likelihood of mistakes and bad outcomes. Medical devices that are linked to the Internet can be designed to send warnings and notifications in the event of unexpected circumstances, prescription mistakes, or equipment faults. This real-time monitoring and intervention aids in the prevention of potential patient damage and ensures prompt actions.

### 11.6.9 Research and Development

IoT supports medical equipment manufacturing research and development activities. Manufacturers may acquire insights into device performance, results for patients, and treatment efficacy by gathering real-time data from linked devices. This data can inform future product development, clinical trials, and evidence-based innovation, driving advancements in medical technology.

### 11.6.10 Regulatory Compliance and Reporting

IoT supports regulatory compliance and reporting requirements in medical equipment manufacturing. Connected devices can automatically collect and transmit data required for regulatory compliance, quality audits, and post-market surveillance. This streamlines data gathering, record keeping, and reporting while also guaranteeing regulatory compliance.

IoT is extremely important in modern medical equipment manufacturing by enabling remote monitoring, predictive maintenance, enhanced connectivity, automated inventory management, quality control, data-driven product improvement, remote software updates, patient safety enhancements, research and development, and regulatory compliance. IoT technologies empower manufacturers to create smart, connected medical devices that improve patient care, enhance operational efficiency, and drive innovation in the healthcare industry (Suryadevara et al., 2018).

## 11.7 MODERN SENSORS USED IN HEALTHCARE SYSTEMS

Modern healthcare systems utilize a wide range of sensors to monitor various aspects of patients' health, environmental conditions, and medical equipment performance. These sensors are critical for acquiring accurate and real-time data, allowing healthcare practitioners to make educated decisions while offering individualized care. Here are several types of sensors commonly used in modern healthcare systems:

### 11.7.1 Temperature Sensors

Temperature sensors are utilized to monitor the temperature of the body, ambient temperature, and temperature-sensitive equipment. They can be integrated into wearable devices, medical implants, or environmental monitoring systems. These sensors help in detecting fever, monitoring incubators, refrigeration units, and maintaining optimal storage conditions for medications and vaccines. Figure 11.1 shows the temperature sensor model.

### 11.7.2 Heart Rate Sensors

Heart rate sensors, such as electrocardiogram (ECG) sensors and photoplethysmography (PPG) sensors, measure the electrical activity or blood flow in the body to monitor heart rate and heart rhythm. Figure 11.2 depicts the heart rate sensor model. They are commonly found in wearable devices, fitness trackers, and medical monitoring equipment. Heart rate sensors are essential for assessing cardiovascular health, detecting irregularities, and monitoring stress levels during physical activities or clinical procedures (Catarinucci et al., 2015).

### 11.7.3 Blood Pressure Sensors

Blood pressure sensors measure the pressure exerted on arterial walls during the cardiac cycle. They can be invasive (such as arterial catheters) or non-invasive (such as oscillometric or auscultatory devices). Blood pressure sensors are crucial in monitoring hypertension, hypotension, and assessing cardiovascular health. Accurate blood pressure readings aid in the diagnosis and management of a variety of cardiovascular diseases (Kaur & Kaur, 2019). The construction of a blood pressure sensor is seen in Figure 11.3.

### 11.7.4 Oxygen Sensors

Oxygen sensors, such as the one illustrated in Figure 11.4, measure the quantity of oxygen in the blood. They are typically worn on a person's finger or earlobe. Oxygen sensors are critical for monitoring respiratory function, identifying hypoxemia, and ensuring that proper oxygen treatment is administered. They are utilized in hospitals, clinics, and even in the home.

### 11.7.5 Glucose Sensors

Glucose sensors are used to measure blood glucose levels in diabetics. Continuous glucose monitoring (CGM) devices that employ subcutaneous sensors are intrusive, whereas optical or transdermal

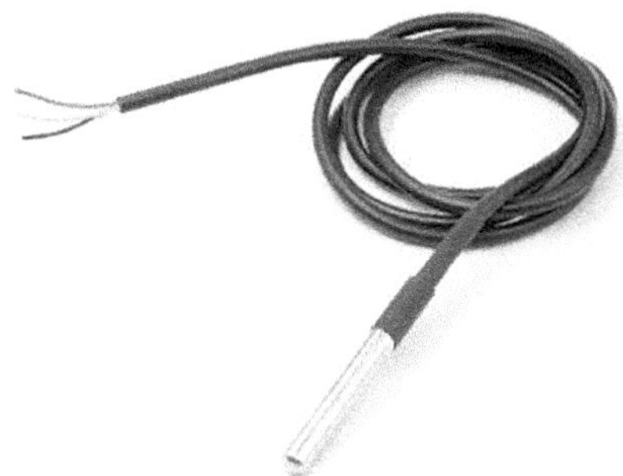

**FIGURE 11.1**  Temperature sensor.

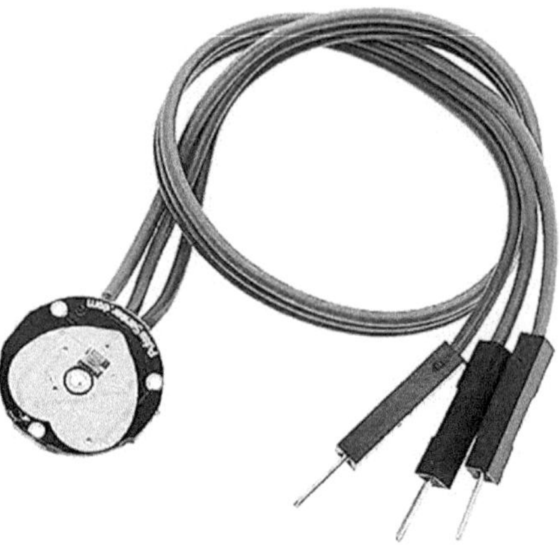

**FIGURE 11.2** Heart rate sensor.

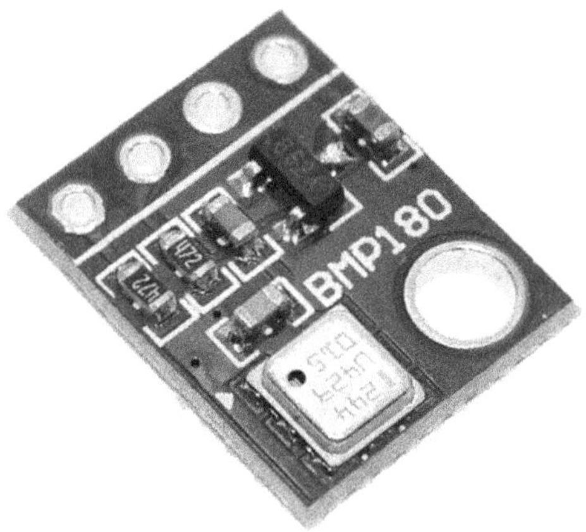

**FIGURE 11.3** Blood pressure sensor.

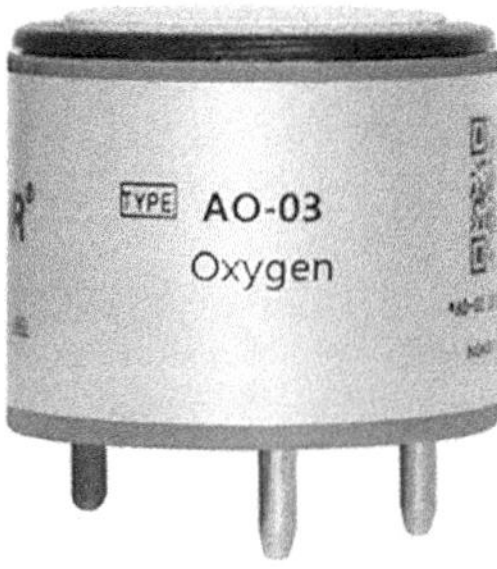

**FIGURE 11.4** Oxygen level identification sensor.

sensors are non-invasive. Glucose sensors assess glucose in real time, enabling diabetics to track their blood sugar levels and adjust insulin dosage as needed (Chiang et al., 2013). Figure 11.5 depicts a glucose level sensor model.

### 11.7.6  MOTION SENSORS

As shown in Figure 11.6, motion sensors such as accelerometers and gyroscopes are utilized for detecting movement, orientation, and physical activity. They are frequently seen in wearable devices like as fitness trackers and smartwatches. Motion sensors aid in the monitoring of physical activity levels, the detection of falls, the assessment of sleep patterns, and the promotion of an active lifestyle.

### 11.7.7  IMAGING SENSORS

Imaging sensors, such as X-ray sensors, ultrasonic transducers, magnetic resonance imaging (MRI) coils, and computed tomography (CT) detectors, record complex pictures of the inside workings of body components. As shown in Figure 11.7, these sensors help in the diagnosis of various medical diseases, the visualization of anatomical anomalies, and the guidance of medical procedures and operations.

### 11.7.8  GAS AND CHEMICAL SENSORS

Gas and chemical sensors are used to assess the concentration of specific chemicals or analytes, for tracking air quality, to recognize harmful gases, and to assess the concentration of specific chemicals or analytes. They're employed in things like environmental monitoring systems, operating rooms, and research labs. Gas and chemical sensors are crucial in keeping patients and healthcare staff safe and healthy. Figure 11.8 depicts a gas level identification sensor model.

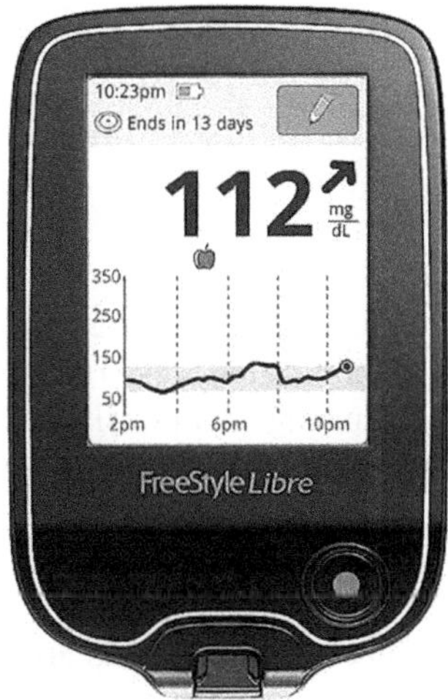


**FIGURE 11.5**   Digitalized glucose level monitoring sensor.

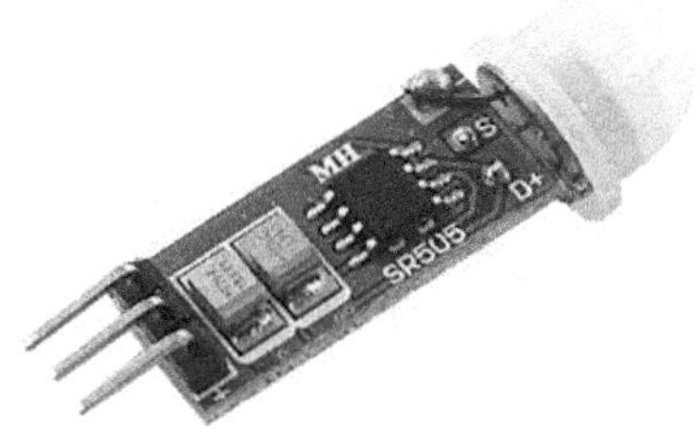

**FIGURE 11.6**   Motion identification sensor.

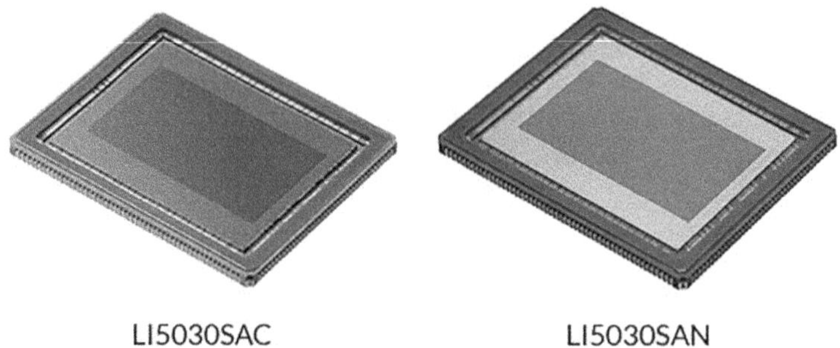



**FIGURE 11.7**    Digital imaging sensor.

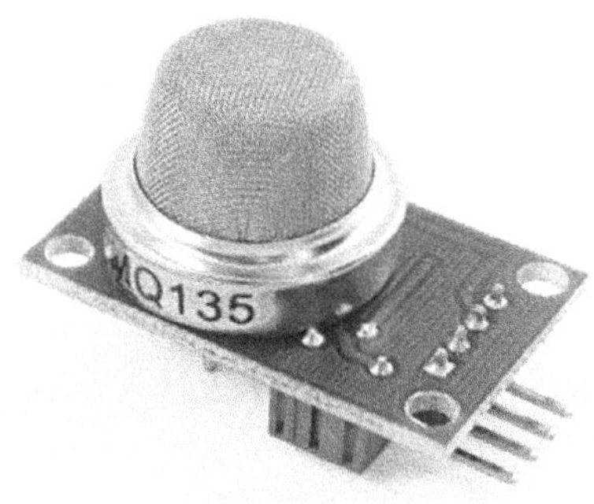



**FIGURE 11.8**    Gas level identification sensor.

### 11.7.9    Pressure Sensors

Pressure sensors are used to detect pressure changes in a range of applications, include arterial pressure monitoring, intracranial pressure monitoring, respiratory pressure monitoring, and infusion systems. They aid in the diagnosis and management of illnesses such as hypertension, glaucoma, and respiratory ailments. Figure 11.9 depicts a pressure level sensor model.

### 11.7.10    Proximity and Contact Sensors

Figure 11.10 depicts proximity and contact sensors, which are used in medical devices and equipment that detect the presence or absence of items, closeness to surfaces, or touch with the human body. These sensors ensure the proper usage of medical devices, safety during procedures, and patient comfort.

### 11.7.11    pH Sensors

pH sensors are used to determine the acidity or alkalinity of biological fluids such as blood, urine, or saliva. They are essential for diagnosing and managing conditions related to acid-base balance, such as acidosis or alkalosis. pH sensors can be integrated into wearable devices, diagnostic equipment, or implanted medical devices (Islam et al., 2015). Figure 11.11 shows the real time model of a pH level sensor.

    

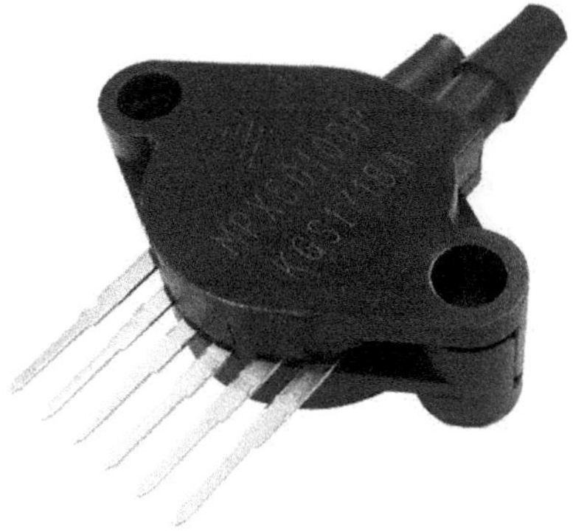

**FIGURE 11.9**    Pressure level maintenance sensor.

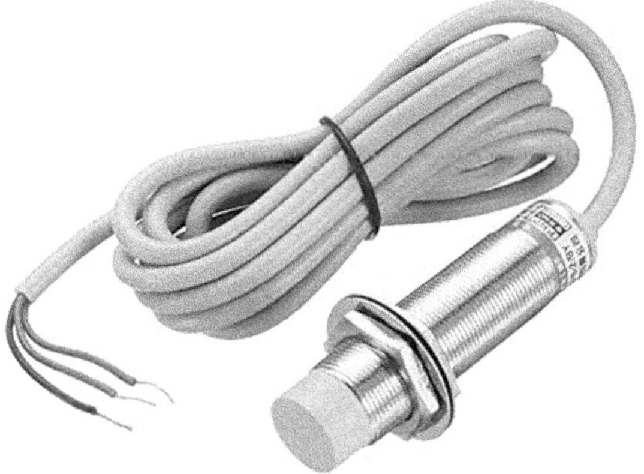

**FIGURE 11.10**    Proximity sensor.

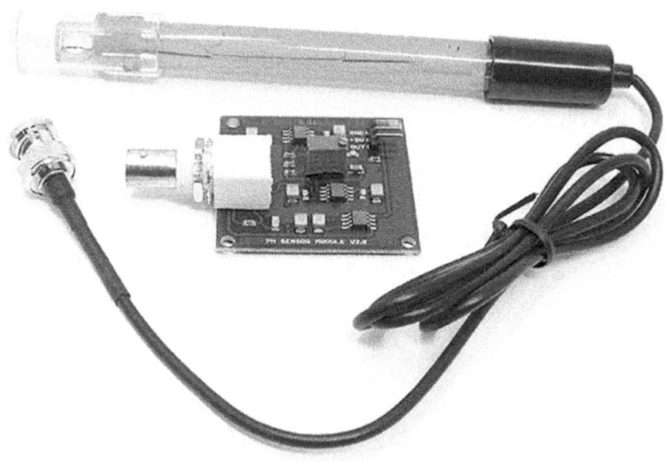

**FIGURE 11.11**    pH sensor.

### 11.7.12 INFRARED AND THERMAL SENSORS

Infrared and thermal sensors, as shown in Figure 11.12, detect and measure infrared radiation and temperature. They are used in thermometers, thermal imaging cameras, and temperature monitoring systems. Infrared and thermal sensors aid in detecting fever, monitoring body temperature, and assessing thermal patterns for wound care or vascular assessment.

Each sensor serves a specific purpose and contributes to accurate and timely data collection, enabling healthcare providers to monitor patients, diagnose conditions, and provide appropriate treatments. The integration of these sensors with data analysis and communication technologies further enhances the potential of healthcare systems to deliver personalized and efficient care (Chua & Dey, 2019).

## 11.8 INDUSTRY 5.0—A MODERN ERA IN TECHNOLOGY INVASION

The human-centric Industrial Revolution, also known as Industry 5.0, is the next stage of industrial development which focuses on the integration of advanced technology with human talents in order to create a more collaborative and socially responsible manufacturing environment. It is built on the ideals of Industry 4.0, which encompassed industrial automation, data transfer, and artificial intelligence. Business 5.0, on the other hand, takes things a step further by highlighting the importance of human talent, innovation, and ethical problems in the manufacturing business.

The concept of Industry 5.0 originated in response to the potential issues and societal repercussions of the rapid expansion of automation and AI. While Industry 4.0 has transformed manufacturing by improving productivity and efficiency via the use of technology, it has also raised concerns about job displacement, worker dehumanization, and a widening skills gap. Industry 5.0 aims to address these issues by redefining people's roles in the manufacturing process and leveraging their unique capacity to work with new technologies. The integration of technology such as robotics, AI, IoT) and big data analytics is still critical. Humans and robots are expected to work together in Industry 5.0, complementing each other's strengths and compensating for each other's weaknesses. The emphasis, however, changes away from simply automated and isolated operations and toward a more integrated and human-centric approach. The emphasis on customization and personalization is one of the fundamental aspects of Industry 5.0. Manufacturers may make highly personalized items that match particular client wants through integrating the flexibility of automation with human creativity and problem-solving abilities. This level of personalization necessitates the engagement of humans in decision-making, design, and consumer contact (Kim et al., 2020).

Another facet of Industry 5.0 is the development of more environmentally friendly and socially responsible industrial practices. It promotes environmentally responsible manufacturing, waste minimization, energy efficiency, and ethical issues. Industry 5.0 aims to foster a more sustainable and inclusive future by incorporating human values and ethical principles into the manufacturing process. In Industry 5.0, collaboration and communication are also essential. Humans are no longer

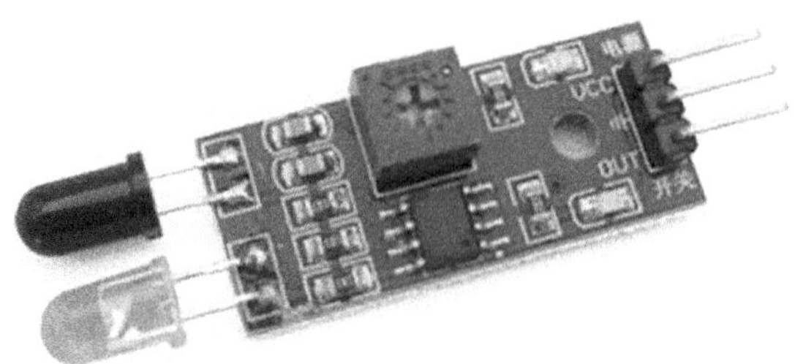

**FIGURE 11.12**  Infrared and thermal detection sensor.

just machine operators or managers; they have become active participants in decision-making, problem-solving, and continuous improvement. Workers in this new industrial paradigm have to be able to communicate, collaborate, and react to changing circumstances. Furthermore, Industry 5.0 understands the importance of upskilling and reskilling employees in order to react to changing industry demands. It encourages lifelong learning and the development of new skills that enhance the capabilities of advanced technology. Industry 5.0 aspires to inspire workers to develop a more engaged and motivated workforce by cultivating a learning culture and giving possibilities for professional progress.

Overall, Industry 5.0 denotes a shift in manufacturing toward a more human-centered and socially responsible approach. It blends modern technology's capability with human creativity, cooperation, and ethical concerns to generate innovation, customization, sustainability, and better worker well-being. Manufacturers may build a more peaceful and inclusive future that's beneficial to both businesses and society by embracing Industry 5.0 concepts (Beyer & Janz, 2018).

## 11.9  MEDICAL ADVANCEMENTS COMBINED WITH INDUSTRY 5.0

By integrating modern technology with human-centric techniques, Industry 5.0 has a chance to revolutionize the field of healthcare. Some of the relevant medical advancements that can be achieved through the integration of Industry 5.0 principles are specified as follows:

### 11.9.1  Customized Medicine

By using technology such as genomics, big data analytics, and artificial intelligence, Industry 5.0 facilitates the creation of personalized treatment techniques. By analyzing individual genetic data, medical history, lifestyle factors, and other relevant information, healthcare practitioners may tailor treatment programs and medications to the specific needs of individuals. This personalization enables more effective and tailored therapy, which improves patient outcomes (Rathore et al., 2016).

### 11.9.2  Cooperative Robotics in Surgery

The employment of collaborative robots, also known as cobots, in medical operations is made easier by Industry 5.0. These robots aid human surgeons in complicated procedures, improving precision and lowering the danger of mistakes. The use of cobots in the operating theater has the potential to enhance surgical results, reduce recuperation times, and boost patient safety.

### 11.9.3  Telemedicine and Isolated Care

Industry 5.0 encourages the addition of telemedicine and remote care technologies, which will allow patients to get medical consultations and track their health from the ease of their own homes. Healthcare personnel may remotely examine vital signs, follow patient progress, and deliver real-time treatments via connected devices, wearables, and remote monitoring systems. This strategy increases patient access, minimizes the pressure on healthcare institutions, and promotes patient convenience.

### 11.9.4  Human-Machine Interfaces

Industry 5.0 enables the development of advanced human-machine interfaces that enhance communication and collaboration between healthcare providers and patients. Augmented reality (AR) and virtual reality (VR) technologies may be used to teach healthcare workers, simulate medical procedures, and improve patient education. These interfaces facilitate better understanding, decision-making, and patient engagement. Industry 5.0 allows for the creation of sophisticated human-machine interfaces that improve communication and collaboration between healthcare practitioners and patients. Technologies such as augmented reality (AR) and virtual reality (VR) might be used to train healthcare professionals, replicate medical procedures, and improve patient education. These interfaces aid in comprehension, decision-making, and patient participation.

### 11.9.5 SMART MEDICAL DEVICES AND IoT INTEGRATION

Industry 5.0 facilitates the production of smart medical equipment and its integration with IoT. IoT-enabled devices may collect real-time patient data such as vital signs, medication adherence, and activity levels, helping healthcare practitioners to make more accurate diagnoses and treatments. This integration improves remote patient monitoring, preventative treatment, and disease identification (Tan et al., 2019).

### 11.9.6 DATA ANALYTICS AND PREDICTIVE MODELS

Industry 5.0 leverages data analytics and predictive modeling to improve healthcare outcomes. Machine learning algorithms can discover patterns, predict disease risks, and assist clinical decision-making by evaluating massive amounts of medical data, which includes electronic health records, medical imaging, and patient demographics. These insights enable early intervention, personalized treatments, and population health management.

### 11.9.7 PATIENT-CENTRIC PRACTICE

Industry 5.0 emphasizes patient-centric care by empowering patients to actively participate in their healthcare journey. Technologies such as mobile health apps, wearable devices, and patient portals enable individuals to monitor their health, access medical information, schedule appointments, and communicate with healthcare providers. This patient-centric approach promotes self-care, improves patient satisfaction, and strengthens the doctor-patient relationship.

### 11.9.8 ETHICAL ATTENTIONS AND DATA PRIVACY

Industry 5.0 highlights the importance of ethical considerations and data privacy in healthcare advancements. As medical technologies gather increasing amounts of personal health data, it becomes crucial to ensure the secure storage, transmission, and use of this information. Industry 5.0 promotes the implementation of robust security measures, adherence to ethical guidelines, and transparent data governance practices to protect patient privacy and maintain trust (Yoon & Kim, 2016).

By integrating Industry 5.0 principles into healthcare, medical advancements can be achieved that prioritize personalized care, collaboration between humans and machines, remote monitoring, predictive analytics, patient engagement, and ethical practices. These developments have the opportunity to enhance patient outcomes, increase utilization of healthcare, and build a more efficient and patient-centered healthcare system.

## 11.10 APPLICATIONS OF INDUSTRY 5.0 IN MODERN HEALTHCARE

The human-centric industrial revolution, known as Industry 5.0, has various innovative applications in current healthcare systems. Industry 5.0 improves patient care, increases operational efficiency, and promotes new healthcare paradigms by merging sophisticated technology with a human-centric approach. Here are some detailed descriptions of advanced applications of Industry 5.0 in modern healthcare:

### 11.10.1 Robot Supported Surgery

Industry 5.0 introduces collaborative robots, or cobots, in surgical procedures. These robots aid human surgeons in performing precise tasks, lowering the chance of mistakes, and improving surgical results. Cobots are capable of performing complicated motions, providing real-time feedback, and allowing for minimally invasive surgeries, resulting in shorter recovery periods and greater patient safety. Robotic-assisted surgery is an advanced Industry 5.0 application that integrates robotic equipment with human skills to improve surgical operations. Industry 5.0 revolutionizes surgery by boosting precision, lowering invasiveness, and raising patient safety through the integration of robots and automation technology. Here's a more in-depth look at robotics-assisted surgery using Industry 5.0:

- Unlike typical industrial robots, which function alone, cobots act as aides to human doctors. They are intended to communicate and work with people, offering assistance and improving surgical capabilities. Cobots have more accuracy and dexterity than human hands, enabling for more accurate motions. They are capable of performing delicate and difficult jobs with great precision, lowering the danger of human mistake. The combination of modern sensors and imaging technology allows for real-time feedback and visualization, which improves surgical precision even more.
- Industry 5.0 allows robotics-assisted surgery teleoperation and telesurgery capabilities. Using a secure network connection, surgeons may remotely operate the cobots from a separate location. This capacity enables specialists to give surgical help or guidance to healthcare practitioners in rural or underserved locations, hence increasing access to specialized surgical procedures.
- Industry 5.0 incorporates robotics-assisted surgery with enhanced imaging, data analytics, and simulation technologies. Preoperative planning software allows surgeons to mimic the surgical procedure, examine patient-specific anatomical characteristics, and create a personalized surgical plan. This virtual simulation improves surgical results, decreases complications, and increases patient safety.
- Real-time monitoring and feedback techniques are used in robotic-assisted surgery. Sensors built into robotic systems can offer constant input on things like force exertion, tissue properties, and vital signs. This data assists surgeons in making educated decisions throughout the process, adjusting procedures, and optimizing surgical results.
- Using robotics-assisted surgery, Industry 5.0 promotes surgical training and skill advancement. Surgeons and trainees can practice procedures in a controlled and secure setting by using simulation platforms and haptic feedback devices. This allows for skill improvement, familiarization with robotic systems, and surgical technique modification, eventually enhancing patient outcomes. Robotic surgery improves patient safety by lowering the likelihood of surgical complications. Cobots' excellent accuracy and stability eliminate the possibility of human faults such as tremors or weariness. Furthermore, real-time monitoring and feedback systems enable surgeons to discover and handle possible concerns as soon as they arise, resulting in safer surgical operations.
- With further advancements in Industry 5.0, robotics-assisted surgery holds the potential for autonomous robotic systems. These systems can learn from vast amounts of surgical data, adapt to individual patient anatomies, and perform certain surgical tasks independently. While human surgeons remain involved in critical decision-making and complex procedures, autonomous capabilities can enhance efficiency and accuracy in less complex surgical steps (Leão et al., 2017).

Robotics-assisted surgery using Industry 5.0 principles combines the precision and capabilities of robotic systems with human expertise to enhance surgical procedures. It improves surgical precision, enables minimally invasive techniques, facilitates remote surgery, enhances training and skill development, and enhances patient safety. As Industry 5.0 continues to evolve, so does robotics-assisted surgery.

### 11.10.2  AI IN DIAGNOSTICS

Medical diagnoses are aided by AI algorithms in Industry 5.0. Large amounts of medical data, such as patient records, medical pictures, and genetic information, may be analyzed using machine learning and deep learning algorithms. AI systems can recognize trends, identify abnormalities, and deliver correct diagnoses, assisting healthcare workers in making educated decisions and enhancing patient outcomes. It entails the application of modern algorithms and machine learning techniques to assess medical data and aid in illness and condition diagnosis.

Industry 5.0, frequently referred to as the Fifth Industrial Revolution, involves the integration of AI and automation technology into a variety of industries, including healthcare. Industry 5.0 in the context of AI in diagnostics refers to the application of AI-driven diagnostic tools, procedures, and systems to improve the accuracy, speed, and efficiency of medical diagnosis. Here are some essential characteristics of artificial intelligence in diagnostics within the context of Industry 5.0:

- **Data-driven decision-making:** AI algorithms can evaluate massive volumes of medical data, such as patient records, medical imaging, test findings, and research articles. By spotting patterns and connections in this data, AI technology can assist healthcare practitioners in making more accurate and evidence-based diagnoses.
- **Medical imaging:** AI analysis may greatly enhance medical pictures such as X-rays, CT scans, MRIs, and pathology slides. By learning from enormous datasets of labeled images, deep learning algorithms may spot abnormalities, identify specific illnesses, and provide insights to radiologists and pathologists. This can improve diagnostic speed and accuracy, ultimately leading to improved patient outcomes.
- **Early detection and prevention:** AI systems may be trained to recognize early warning signs of diseases or conditions that human observers may overlook. AI systems can aid in early diagnosis by analyzing patient data and finding subtle signs, allowing for prompt therapies and improved prognosis. This has the potential to improve patient care while also lowering healthcare expenses.
- **Personalized medicine:** AI can help to personalize medical diagnoses and treatment methods for individual patients. AI algorithms can provide tailored recommendations for diagnostic and treatment options based on a patient's unique characteristics, such as genetic data, medical history, and lifestyle variables. This can lead to more customized and effective medicines, with fewer side effects and better patient outcomes.
- **Clinical decision support:** AI has the potential to be a strong decision-support tool for healthcare workers. AI systems can aid in identifying difficult situations, proposing suitable testing, and offering treatment strategies by giving real-time access to the most recent medical research, treatment recommendations, and patient data. This can supplement healthcare practitioners' experience and increase the quality of treatment offered (Lee & Lee, 2020).

It is essential to highlight, however, that while AI in diagnostics shows enormous potential, it is not designed to replace human healthcare experts. Rather, it acts as a supplement to help and improve their talents, ultimately leading to more accurate and quick diagnoses. In the framework of Industry 5.0, AI in diagnostics introduces advanced computing capabilities and data analysis approaches to healthcare. Healthcare practitioners may increase diagnostic accuracy, allow early detection, personalize treatment methods, and give greater decision support by leveraging the power of AI.

### 11.10.3 Remote Patient Monitoring

Industry 5.0 facilitates remote patient monitoring through the integration of IoT devices and wearables. Smartwatches, biosensors, and mobile health applications capture real-time patient data, such as vital signs, activity levels, and medication adherence. Remote monitoring of patients, detection of irregularities, and action, when necessary, enables early intervention, personalized treatment, and chronic illness management.

### 11.10.4 Predictive Analytics and Precautionary Care

Industry 5.0 employs predictive analytics to identify potential health risks and enable preventive care. By analyzing patient data and historical trends, AI algorithms can predict the likelihood of certain diseases or adverse events. Healthcare providers can then develop personalized preventive strategies, offer lifestyle interventions, and implement early detection programs, leading to improved patient outcomes and reduced healthcare costs.

### 11.10.5 Smart Hospital Setup

Industry 5.0 allows for the creation of smart hospital infrastructure by combining IoT, AI, and automation technologies. Energy management, patient flow, asset monitoring, and resource allocation are just a few of the areas of hospital operations that smart hospital systems monitor and handle. Real-time data gathering and analytics increase resource utilization, decrease wait times, improve patient experience, and boost overall operational efficiency (Marchio et al., 2019).

The combined use of innovative technology and systems into a healthcare institution to increase efficiency, quality, and patient experience is referred to as smart hospital infrastructure. When paired with the ideas of Industry 5.0, which emphasize human-machine cooperation, smart hospital infrastructure uses AI, IoT, automation, and data analytics to improve healthcare delivery. Here is a rundown of how Industry 5.0 affects smart hospital infrastructure:

#### 11.10.5.1 IoT Connectivity

Industry 5.0 makes use of IoT devices and sensors to provide continuous connection across the facility. These devices may capture and send real-time data from a wide range of sources, including patient monitors, wearable devices, medical equipment, and environmental sensors. The data may then be examined to enhance operational efficiency, monitor patient health, and optimize resource use.

#### 11.10.5.2 Data-Driven Decision-Making

The use of data analytics and AI algorithms to derive meaningful insights from the large volume of healthcare data created within a smart hospital is promoted by Industry 5.0. AI systems can help healthcare personnel make better decisions by combining and analyzing patient records, medical imaging data, and operational information. Predicting patient outcomes, optimizing treatment regimens, and identifying opportunities for process improvement are all part of this.

#### 11.10.5.3 Automation and Robotics

Automation and robotics technologies are used in smart hospital infrastructure to automate repetitive processes, eliminate human mistakes, and increase overall efficiency. Medication distribution, inventory management, and patient monitoring are all duties that robots can help with. Automation can also improve processes, allowing healthcare workers to concentrate on patient care and difficult procedures.

#### 11.10.5.4 Enhanced Patient Experience

Smart hospital infrastructure is critical to realizing Industry 5.0's objective of providing a patient-centric approach to healthcare. Hospitals may provide personalized care experiences by integrating

AI and IoT, such as smart patient rooms outfitted with IoT-enabled gadgets, voice-controlled interfaces, and patient interaction platforms. These technologies can improve patient and family communication, comfort, and convenience.

### 11.10.5.5　Telemedicine and Remote Patient Monitoring

The adoption of telemedicine services and remote patient monitoring is made possible by smart hospital infrastructure. Healthcare practitioners can remotely monitor patients' vital signs, give virtual consultations, and administer treatment outside of the hospital via video consultations, wearable gadgets, and linked monitoring systems. This has the potential to improve access to healthcare, especially for people in remote areas, as well as decrease unnecessary hospital visits.

### 11.10.5.6　Security and Privacy

Maintaining cybersecurity and patient data privacy is becoming increasingly crucial as healthcare systems become more linked and digital. Industry 5.0 emphasizes the importance of robust safety precautions in smart healthcare infrastructure. This includes secure data transmission, encryption protocols, access control mechanisms, and regular vulnerability assessments to safeguard patient information and prevent unauthorized access (Asan & Bayrak, 2019).

Industry 5.0 facilitates the development of smart hospital infrastructure by combining advanced technologies, data-driven decision-making, automation, and a patient-centric approach. By leveraging these elements, smart hospitals can enhance patient care, improve operational efficiency, optimize resource utilization, and deliver healthcare services that are more efficient, effective, and personalized.

### 11.10.6　Telemedicine and Virtual Care

Industry 5.0 promotes the expansion of telemedicine and virtual care services. Through video consultations, remote diagnosis, and virtual follow-ups, patients can access healthcare services without the need for in-person visits. Telemedicine solutions, powered by AI algorithms and wearable devices, allow healthcare practitioners to remotely monitor patients, conduct consultations, and deliver personalized treatment, therefore enhancing healthcare access and lowering geographical barriers.

### 11.10.7　3D Printing in Medical Engineering

Industry 5.0 utilizes 3D printing technology in medical manufacturing. 3D printers can produce customized medical devices, prosthetics, implants, and anatomical models with high precision and flexibility. This technology enables faster production, reduces costs, and improves patient-specific treatment options, such as patient-specific implants or surgical guides (Fung et al., 2019).

By applying Industry 5.0 concepts and technologies, modern healthcare systems can achieve advanced applications that revolutionize patient care, enhance diagnostics, enable remote monitoring and virtual care, optimize hospital operations, support personalized medicine, and prioritize data security and privacy. These advancements contribute to better healthcare outcomes, improved patient experience.

## 11.11　CHALLENGES FACED BY INDUSTRY 5.0 TO INTEGRATE WITH HEALTHCARE SYSTEMS

Integrating Industry 5.0 with smart healthcare systems involves various problems that must be overcome in order for the project to be successful. Some of the key challenges are depicted below:

### 11.11.1　Data Interoperability

Industry 5.0 relies on seamless data exchange and interoperability between various healthcare systems and devices. However, healthcare data is often stored in disparate formats, different systems, and controlled by different stakeholders. Achieving data interoperability requires standardized data formats, interoperable interfaces, and data governance frameworks to ensure seamless data flow and integration.

### 11.11.2 Concerns about Privacy and Security

The incorporation of Industry 5.0 technology into healthcare systems raises the possibility of cyber-security risks and data breaches. Smart healthcare systems capture, store, and transmit sensitive patient data; therefore, privacy and security are critical. To secure patient information and retain trust, robust cybersecurity measures, encryption techniques, access restrictions, and compliance with data protection rules are required.

### 11.11.3 Cost and Infrastructure Requirements

Integrating Industry 5.0 technologies like IoT devices, AI algorithms, and automation systems necessitates substantial expenditures in infrastructure, hardware, software, and employee training. Upgrades to current systems and the implementation of new technology can be expensive, particularly for smaller healthcare organizations. Additionally, ongoing maintenance and system upgrades are necessary to keep pace with evolving technologies and ensure smooth operations.

### 11.11.4 Workforce Readiness and Training

Industry 5.0 introduces new technologies and workflows that require healthcare professionals to adapt and acquire new skills. Training the workforce to effectively use and interpret data generated by smart healthcare systems is essential. Healthcare providers must engage in ongoing education and training programs to ensure that their employees have the skills needed to harness Industry 5.0 technologies and maximize their advantages (Xu et al., 2020).

### 11.11.5 Ethical and Regulatory Considerations

Integrating Industry 5.0 with smart healthcare systems raises ethical and regulatory concerns. The use of AI algorithms and automation in decision-making processes necessitates careful consideration of issues such as algorithm bias, transparency, accountability, and the ethical implications of machine-driven decision-making. To guarantee the appropriate and ethical utilization of Industry 5.0 technologies in healthcare, regulatory frameworks and rules must be implemented.

### 11.11.6 User Acceptance and Adoption

User participation and adoption are vital for successfully integrating Industry 5.0 with smart healthcare systems. Healthcare professionals and patients may have concerns about the reliability, accuracy, and usability of new technologies. Engaging stakeholders, providing adequate training and support, and demonstrating the value and benefits of Industry 5.0 technologies are crucial to drive acceptance and adoption (Wang et al., 2016).

## 11.12 CONCLUSION

The successful integration of AI and Industry 5.0 ideas into smart healthcare systems has the promise to revolutionize healthcare delivery. Machine learning and data analytics, for instance, have AI technologies that enable enhanced diagnoses, personalized treatment, and data-driven decision-making. Meanwhile, Industry 5.0 emphasizes human-machine collaboration in order to build a more efficient, patient-centric, and linked healthcare environment.

By leveraging AI in smart healthcare systems within the framework of Industry 5.0, healthcare organizations can achieve several benefits. These include improved diagnostic accuracy, early detection of diseases, optimized treatment plans, enhanced patient experiences, and streamlined workflows. AI-driven technology, along with IoT connection, automation, and robots, can provide healthcare practitioners with real-time data, decision support tools, and telemedicine capabilities.

However, integrating AI and Industry 5.0 into smart healthcare systems is fraught with difficulties. Data interoperability, privacy and security problems, infrastructure needs, workforce preparedness, ethical considerations, and user acceptability are among the challenges. Overcoming these challenges requires standardized data formats, robust cybersecurity measures, investments in infrastructure and training, ethical frameworks, and effective change management strategies. To address these issues, healthcare organizations, technology providers, governments, and regulators must work together. It entails developing rules, standards, and best practices for data interoperability, cybersecurity, privacy, and ethics. Additionally, infrastructure, training programs, and change management measures are required to guarantee a seamless transition to Industry 5.0–enabled smart healthcare systems.

Overall, the combination of artificial intelligence and Industry 5.0 in smart healthcare systems has significant promise for enhancing healthcare outcomes, patient experiences, and operational efficiency. By leveraging the power of advanced technologies, data analytics, and human-machine collaboration, the healthcare industry can move toward a future where precision medicine, personalized care, and data-driven decision-making grow the norm, ultimately benefiting both patients and healthcare providers.

## REFERENCES


Abdekhoda, M., Ahmadi, M., & Dehnad, A. (2016). A systematic review of patient monitoring systems: Architecture and clinical aspects. *Journal of Medical Systems*, 40(4), 1–17.

Al-Fuqaha, A., Guizani, M., Mohammadi, M., Aledhari, M., & Ayyash, M. (2015). Internet of Things: A survey on enabling technologies, protocols, and applications. *IEEE Communications Surveys & Tutorials*, 17(4), 2347–2376.

Asan, O., & Bayrak, A. E. (2019). Medical cyber-physical systems and industrial internet of things for healthcare: A survey. *IEEE Internet of Things Journal*, 6(2), 2188–2204.

Atzori, L., Iera, A., & Morabito, G. (2010). The Internet of Things: A survey. *Computer Networks*, 54(15), 2787–2805.

Balakrishnan, R., & Varghese, C. (2021). A systematic review on the integration of Internet of Things (IoT) in healthcare. *Healthcare Informatics Research*, 27(2), 78–87.

Bates, D. W., & Gawande, A. A. (2003). Improving safety with information technology. *New England Journal of Medicine*, 348(25), 2526–2534.

Beam, A. L., & Kohane, I. S. (2016). Big data and machine learning in health care. *JAMA*, 316(13), 1337–1338.

Beede, E., Baylor, E., Hersch, F., & Pelczer, I. (2018). AI in health care: Anticipating challenges to ethics, privacy, and bias. *Hastings Center Report*, 48(S4), S37–S39.

Beyer, A., & Janz, A. (2018). Industry 4.0—A systematic literature review on definitions, concepts, and interdependencies. *International Journal of Production Research*, 56(1–2), 849–861.

Borgia, E. (2014). The Internet of Things vision: Key features, applications and open issues. *Computer Communications*, 54, 1–31.

Buntin, M. B., Burke, M. F., Hoaglin, M. C., & Blumenthal, D. (2011). The benefits of health information technology: A review of the recent literature shows predominantly positive results. *Health Affairs*, 30(3), 464–471.

Catarinucci, L., de Donno, D., Mainetti, L., Palano, L., Patrono, L., & Stefanizzi, M. L. (2015). An IoT-aware architecture for smart healthcare systems. *IEEE Internet of Things Journal*, 2(6), 515–526.

Chen, J., Song, L., Wainwright, M. J., & Jordan, M. I. (2018). Learning to explain: An information-theoretic perspective on model interpretation. *International Conference on Learning Representations (ICLR)*. https://arxiv.org/abs/1802.07814

Chiang, M., Gao, Y., & Hu, J. (2013). IoT wearable sensor-based human activity recognition. *IEEE Network*, 28(6), 40–45.

Chua, C. E., & Dey, N. (2019). Internet of Things (IoT) in healthcare: A systematic literature review. *Sensors*, 19(20), 1–40.

Dandl, S., Brunner, P., Kieseberg, P., Schrittwieser, S., & Merkl, D. (2019). Explainable artificial intelligence: A survey. *ACM Computing Surveys*, 52(5), 1–36.

Fang, Q., Xi, Y., & Yang, C. (2019). IoT-based smart medical equipment management for healthcare 4.0. *IEEE Internet of Things Journal*, 6(3), 4266–4276.

Fung, W. L. A., Liu, D., Yuan, X., & Wong, K. K. (2019). A survey of IoT cloud platforms. *Future Generation Computer Systems*, 100, 1013–1024.

Goodfellow, I., Bengio, Y., & Courville, A. (2016). *Deep Learning* (Vol. 1). MIT Press.

Institute of Medicine. (2001). *Crossing the Quality Chasm: A New Health System for the 21st Century*. National Academies Press.

Islam, S. M. R., Kwak, D., Kabir, M. H., Hossain, M., & Kwak, K. S. (2015). The Internet of Things for health care: A comprehensive survey. *IEEE Access*, 3, 678–708.

Kaur, H., & Kaur, R. (2019). Internet of Things (IoT) in healthcare: A comprehensive study. *Journal of Ambient Intelligence and Humanized Computing*, 10(12), 4583–4608.

Kim, I., Kim, K., & Kim, J. (2020). The impact of Industry 4.0, Industrial Internet of Things, and smart factory on dynamic capabilities. *Journal of Open Innovation: Technology, Market, and Complexity*, 6(4), 1–19.

Leão, R. S., Gonçalves, P., & Carvalho, V. (2017). Improving healthcare services through digital fabrication of patient-specific devices: A systematic review. *Healthcare*, 5(3), 48.

LeCun, Y., Bengio, Y., & Hinton, G. (2015). Deep learning. *Nature*, 521(7553), 436–444.

Lee, J., & Lee, J. (2020). A systematic review of healthcare applications using Industry 4.0 technologies. *Healthcare Informatics Research*, 26(1), 11–22.

Manogaran, G., Shakeel, P. M., Srivastava, G., & Varatharajan, R. (2017). An integrated framework for healthcare IoT big data management using big data analytics. *Future Generation Computer Systems*, 82, 375–388.

Marchio, M. D., Piccinini, F., Corno, F., & Rebaudengo, M. (2019). An overview on wearable health-care systems: Literature review, challenges, and methodologies. *IEEE Transactions on Human-Machine Systems*, 49(6), 541–557.

Memon, M. H., Wagner, S. R., Pedersen, C. F., & Beevi, F. H. (2018). IoT-based patient health monitoring: Opportunities, challenges, and future directions. *IEEE Internet of Things Journal*, 5(6), 4650–4665.

Rajkomar, A., Dean, J., & Kohane, I. (2019). Machine learning in medicine. *New England Journal of Medicine*, 380(14), 1347–1358.

Rathore, M. M., Ahmad, A., & Paul, A. (2016). Healthcare 4.0: A review of advancements in the healthcare industry. *Journal of Industrial Information Integration*, 6, 1–10.

Suryadevara, N. K., Gaddam, A., & Mukhopadhyay, S. C. (2018). Internet of Things for smart healthcare: Technologies, challenges, and opportunities. *Journal of Industrial Information Integration*, 10, 1–13.

Sutton, R. S., & Barto, A. G. (2018). *Reinforcement Learning: An Introduction*. MIT Press.

Tan, J., Khor, K. S., & Lim, C. P. (2019). A review of Industry 4.0 and its impact on the healthcare sector. In *2019 IEEE International Conference on Industrial Engineering and Engineering Management (IEEM)* (pp. 849–853). IEEE.

Topol, E. J. (2019). High-performance medicine: The convergence of human and artificial intelligence. *Nature Medicine*, 25(1), 44–56.

Wang, J., Zhang, X., & Qin, L. (2020). Leveraging IoT technology for real-time and predictive analytics in smart healthcare. *IEEE Transactions on Industrial Informatics*, 16(6), 4263–4271.

Wang, S., Wan, J., Zhang, D., Li, D., & Zhang, C. (2016). Towards smart factory for Industry 4.0: A self-organized multi-agent system with big data based feedback and coordination. *Computer Networks*, 101, 158–168.

Xu, X., Zeng, X., Qiao, X., & Lee, J. (2020). A survey on emerging pervasive healthcare systems: Healthcare monitoring and management. *Sensors*, 20(13), 3661.

Yoon, S. J., & Kim, K. H. (2016). Smart healthcare: Trends and applications. *International Journal of Environmental Research and Public Health*, 13(1), 1–14.

Zhang, Y., Luo, H., Xu, G., & Cheng, J. (2018). Industrial Internet of Things-enabled intelligent maintenance for medical equipment manufacturing. *Journal of Intelligent Manufacturing*, 29(3), 665–677.

Zhou, K., Liu, S., & Zhou, J. (2010). Security and privacy in cloud computing: A survey. *Journal of Medical Systems*, 36(1), 1–11.

# 12 Unleashing Patient Insights

## *Leveraging Edge AI in Sentiment Analysis for Enhanced Healthcare Experiences*

*Kathiravan Pannerselvam, Saranya Rajiakodi,
and Shanmugavadivu Pichai*

## 12.1 INTRODUCTION

Technological advancements reshape how patients interact with the healthcare system in the ever-evolving healthcare landscape. Patients are no longer passive recipients of medical care; they have transformed into active participants, empowered by the digital age, to voice their opinions, share their experiences, and express their sentiments regarding healthcare providers, services, and treatments (*Privacy | HHS.Gov*, n.d.). This surge in patient-generated data presents a unique opportunity to glean invaluable insights that can enhance healthcare experiences (Ziebland et al., 2013).

However, the traditional methods of collecting and analyzing patient sentiments are fraught with limitations. They often struggle to keep pace with the volume and immediacy of patient-generated data and may fail to capture the nuanced and context-dependent nature of patient sentiments. This chapter explores the profound role of edge AI (artificial intelligence at the edge) technology in healthcare, specifically focusing on its application in sentiment analysis. This chapter gives the intricacies of edge AI, highlighting its potential to revolutionize the healthcare industry by providing real-time insights, strengthening privacy and security, and enabling personalized care delivery based on patient preferences (Dash et al., 2019; Jain et al., 2021).

Moreover, this chapter explores the ethical considerations accompanying edge AI's use in healthcare sentiment analysis, including data protection, privacy compliance, and bias mitigation. These ethical concerns are paramount to ensure the responsible and respectful use of patient-generated data. The potential implications and future directions of leveraging edge AI technology to unlock the transformative power of patient insights and usher in a new era of enhanced healthcare experiences (Abualigah et al., 2020).

## 12.2 HEALTHCARE DATA

Patients are more connected, informed, and vocal in this digital age than ever. They share their healthcare experiences, opinions, and emotions online, from ubiquitous social media to specialized healthcare forums and review websites. These unfiltered expressions of sentiment provide healthcare organizations with a treasure trove of data to inform decision-making, improve service quality, and enhance patient satisfaction (Sabarmathi & Chinnaiyan, 2020).

However, manually analyzing this vast and unstructured data is complex. Traditional sentiment analysis methods, often reliant on batch processing and centralized servers, are ill-equipped to handle patient-generated data's volume, variety, and immediacy. Additionally, they may not capture patient sentiments' nuanced and context-dependent nature.

　　　　　　　　　　　　　　　　DOI: 10.1201/9781003442066-12

### 12.2.1 The Social Media Revolution

Social media platforms, in particular, have become a primary channel for patients to voice their opinions and share their healthcare experiences. Whether posting about a positive interaction with a nurse, expressing frustration with long wait times in the emergency room, or seeking advice from peers about a new treatment, patients increasingly use social media for self-expression and communication. The data generated on these platforms are unstructured, diverse, and abundant. This data includes text-based posts, images, videos, and even emojis, all contributing to the complexity of sentiment analysis in healthcare. Traditional methods struggle to extract meaningful insights from this rich and varied data landscape (Greaves et al., 2013).

### 12.2.2 Edge AI: Revolutionizing Sentiment Analysis in Healthcare

Edge AI, a cutting-edge technology enabling AI models to run locally on devices rather than relying on cloud-based processing, has revolutionized various industries, including healthcare. One of the significant applications of edge AI in healthcare is sentiment analysis, which plays a crucial role in understanding and improving patient experiences and enhancing healthcare services (Singh & Gill, 2023). In this context, let us explore how edge AI is revolutionizing sentiment analysis in healthcare. Edge AI technology empowers healthcare organizations to perform real-time sentiment analysis right at the source of data generation. By deploying Machine Learning algorithms on local devices or edge servers, healthcare providers can process patient sentiments as they are expressed, allowing for timely responses and interventions. This real-time capability is precious in healthcare settings, where timely feedback can lead to quicker improvements in patient care and experiences. For instance, a hospital can monitor patient sentiments on social media and promptly address concerns or issues, demonstrating a commitment to patient-centric care (Rajalakshmi et al., 2021). Real-time sentiment analysis also enables healthcare providers to detect emerging trends and issues early on. By identifying patterns in patient sentiment, organizations can proactively address problems, allocate resources efficiently, and continually improve service quality (Greaves et al., 2013).

### 12.2.3 Enhanced Privacy and Security

Privacy and data security are paramount in healthcare, where sensitive patient information is at stake. Traditional sentiment analysis often involves sending data to centralized servers for processing, raising concerns about data breaches and unauthorized access. Edge AI mitigates these risks by processing data locally. Patient sentiments can be analyzed on-site without transmitting sensitive information across networks. This approach safeguards patient privacy and ensures compliance with data protection regulations, such as the Health Insurance Portability and Accountability Act (HIPAA) in the United States and the General Data Protection Regulation (GDPR) in Europe (HealthIT.gov, 2013; *What Do We Do About the Biases in AI?*, n.d.).

Local processing reduces the risk of data exposure during transmission and minimizes the points of vulnerability where malicious actors might attempt to access sensitive healthcare data. It provides an additional layer of security that is especially critical when dealing with highly confidential medical records and patient feedback.

### 12.2.4 Personalized Care Delivery

One of the most compelling advantages of edge AI in sentiment analysis is its ability to tailor care delivery based on patient preferences and sentiments. Healthcare providers can gain valuable insights into individual patient needs and expectations by continuously monitoring and analyzing patient sentiments. For instance, an AI-driven system can adapt the care plan if patients prefer telehealth consultations over in-person visits. This level of personalization can lead to higher patient satisfaction, improved adherence to treatment plans, and, ultimately, better health outcomes.

Personalization extends beyond communication preferences. Edge AI can analyze patient sentiments related to treatment options, side effects, and overall satisfaction with care. This information can guide healthcare providers in making more informed decisions about treatment plans and interventions, ensuring they align with each patient's unique circumstances and preferences.

Edge-AI-driven sentiment analysis enables the creation of feedback loops that drive continuous improvement in healthcare services. Organizations can identify areas of concern or where they excel by collecting and analyzing patient feedback in real time. For example, if multiple patients express dissatisfaction with the cleanliness of a hospital facility on social media, the facility management team can take immediate action to address the issue. Once improvements are made, the same AI system can monitor sentiment to see if patient satisfaction increases, providing valuable feedback on the effectiveness of the changes (Engle et al., 2021).

This iterative feedback and improvement process is essential for delivering high-quality, patient-centered care. It ensures that healthcare organizations are responsive to evolving patient needs and concerns, ultimately leading to a more positive patient experience (Greene et al., 2012).

## 12.3 ETHICAL CONSIDERATIONS AND RESPONSIBLE USE OF DATA

While Edge AI technology offers numerous benefits, it also raises ethical considerations that must be addressed to ensure the responsible use of patient data. These ethical considerations extend across various dimensions of healthcare sentiment analysis:

### 12.3.1 DATA PROTECTION AND CONSENT

Central to responsible data use in healthcare is obtaining informed consent from patients before collecting and analyzing their data. Patients have the right to know how their data will be used and to have control over its dissemination. Clear and transparent data governance policies are essential to build patient trust (Ellsberg et al., 2008). Informed consent should not be a one-time event but an ongoing process. As patients' preferences and expectations evolve, healthcare organizations must seek renewed consent for data usage, especially if they plan to personalize care based on sentiment analysis. Patients should be able to opt in or out of such programs, ensuring their privacy and autonomy are respected.

### 12.3.2 PRIVACY COMPLIANCE

Compliance with data protection regulations is non-negotiable in healthcare, and edge AI solutions must be designed with this in mind. Whether it is the HIPAA, as mentioned, or GDPR, healthcare providers must ensure that their edge AI systems adhere to the regulatory requirements, including data encryption, access controls, and auditing capabilities. Moreover, data anonymization techniques should be employed to protect patient privacy further. By removing personally identifiable information from sentiment analysis datasets, organizations can minimize the risk of re-identification and protect patients' sensitive information (*Data Protection Principles: Core Principles of the GDPR*, n.d.; *Privacy | HHS.Gov*, n.d.).

### 12.3.3 BIAS MITIGATION

AI algorithms used in sentiment analysis are not immune to biases present in training data. Biases can lead to unfair or discriminatory outcomes, which are particularly problematic in healthcare, as they can affect treatment decisions and patient experiences (*What Is Patient Experience? | Agency for Healthcare Research and Quality*, n.d.). Healthcare organizations must invest in bias mitigation strategies to ensure that the insights derived from sentiment analysis are fair and unbiased, regardless of race, gender, or socioeconomic status. This includes careful selection of training data, ongoing monitoring of algorithm performance, and transparent reporting on potential biases and their impact (Siala & Wang, 2022).

### 12.3.4 ALGORITHM EXPLAINABILITY

In healthcare, transparency and explainability of AI algorithms are critical. Patients and healthcare providers need to understand how AI-driven decisions are made, significantly when those decisions impact patient care. Complex AI models can be challenging to interpret. However, efforts should be made to explain clearly how sentiment analysis informs clinical and operational decisions (Amann et al., 2020; Kiseleva et al., 2022). Ensuring algorithm explainability enhances trust and facilitates the identification of potential biases or errors in the AI system. If healthcare providers understand how the AI arrived at a particular recommendation, they can better evaluate its validity and relevance to a specific patient's needs.

## 12.4 POTENTIAL IMPLICATIONS AND FUTURE DIRECTIONS

The integration of edge AI technology into sentiment analysis has the potential to revolutionize healthcare experiences in myriad ways. As healthcare organizations continue to harness patient-generated data and AI-driven insights, we can anticipate a wide range of positive outcomes and transformative changes:

### 12.4.1 IMPROVED PATIENT SATISFACTION AND LOYALTY

One of the most immediate and tangible benefits of edge-AI-driven sentiment analysis is the potential for improved patient satisfaction and loyalty. By acting on patient feedback in real time, healthcare organizations can address concerns, rectify issues, and provide personalized care, leading to higher levels of patient satisfaction. Increased patient satisfaction often translates into greater patient loyalty. Patients who feel heard and valued are more likely to return to the same healthcare providers for future care needs and are more inclined to recommend those providers to others. Thus, the benefits of edge AI extend beyond individual interactions to long-term relationships with patients (Jamal et al., 2020).

### 12.4.2 MORE EFFICIENT AND RESPONSIVE HEALTHCARE SYSTEMS

Edge AI technology facilitates the creation of agile and responsive healthcare systems. By continuously monitoring patient sentiments, healthcare organizations can adapt their operations, resource allocation, and service delivery strategies to align with evolving patient needs and expectations (Javaid et al., 2022). For example, suppose a surge in negative sentiments regarding a specific clinic's waiting times is detected. In that case, the healthcare system can allocate additional staff or resources to that clinic to reduce wait times and improve the patient experience. This responsiveness enhances operational efficiency and ensures that healthcare resources are utilized optimally.

## 12.5 ENHANCED DECISION-MAKING AND RESOURCE ALLOCATION

Edge-AI-driven sentiment analysis offers a wealth of data that can inform strategic decision-making and resource allocation within healthcare organizations. By analyzing sentiment trends over time, organizations can identify areas of improvement, allocate resources strategically, and prioritize initiatives that are most likely to impact patient experiences positively (Bohr & Memarzadeh, 2020). For instance, if sentiment analysis reveals a consistent pattern of positive feedback regarding a particular nursing team, the organization may invest in training programs to replicate that success in other departments. Conversely, if sentiments are consistently negative in a specific area, resources can be redirected to address those concerns more effectively.

### 12.5.1  A Shift toward Proactive Healthcare

Edge-AI-driven sentiment analysis can be pivotal in shifting healthcare from a reactive model to a proactive one. By monitoring patient sentiments, organizations can detect emerging issues or trends early, allowing them to intervene and address problems before they escalate. For example, suppose a significant number of patients express concerns about the side effects of a new medication. In that case, healthcare providers can proactively adjust treatment plans, provide additional patient education, or explore alternative treatment options. This proactive approach improves patient experiences and improves health outcomes (Mackintosh et al., 2020).

### 12.5.2  Greater Transparency and Trust

Transparency and trust are foundational to the patient-provider relationship. Edge-AI-driven sentiment analysis can foster greater transparency by allowing patients to voice their opinions and concerns. Trust in healthcare organizations deepens when patients see that their feedback is heard and acted upon. Moreover, transparency in AI-driven decision-making, including how sentiment analysis informs clinical and operational decisions, enhances trust between healthcare providers and patients. Patients are more likely to trust AI-driven recommendations and interventions when they understand how those decisions are made and how they benefit their care.

## 12.6  CHALLENGES AND CONSIDERATIONS FOR THE FUTURE

As healthcare organizations continue to embrace edge AI technology for sentiment analysis, they will encounter opportunities and challenges on the path to enhanced patient experiences. Several key considerations and potential challenges include. Table 12.1 describes it clearly.

Furthermore, robust data governance practices are essential to maintain compliance with regulations while ensuring the responsible use of patient data. This includes data lifecycle management, audit trails, and data access and deletion mechanisms in line with patient preferences.

## 12.7  CONCLUSION

The integration of edge AI technology into sentiment analysis has the potential to revolutionize healthcare experiences by harnessing the power of patient-generated data. As healthcare organizations leverage this technology, they can anticipate tangible benefits, including improved patient satisfaction, more efficient healthcare systems, and enhanced decision-making.

However, the responsible use of edge AI in healthcare sentiment analysis is crucial. Ethical considerations, such as data protection, privacy compliance, and bias mitigation, must be at the forefront of AI implementation. Patients' rights to privacy and autonomy must be respected, and healthcare providers must be transparent about how AI-driven decisions are made. The journey to enhanced healthcare experiences through edge-AI-driven sentiment analysis is ongoing. As technology evolves and healthcare organizations continue to learn from patient insights, the potential for positive transformation in the healthcare industry is boundless. By embracing this transformative technology while upholding ethical standards, healthcare providers can embark on a journey toward a more patient-centric, data-driven, and, ultimately, healthier future.

**TABLE 12.1**

**Challenges of Edge AI in the Healthcare Domain**

| Challenges | Description |
| --- | --- |
| Data Quality and Noise | While patient-generated data on social media and other online platforms are valuable, they can also be noisy and unstructured. Healthcare organizations must invest in robust data preprocessing and cleaning techniques to ensure that sentiment analysis algorithms receive high-quality input data. Additionally, distinguishing between legitimate patient feedback and spam or fake reviews can be challenging. Edge AI systems should be designed to filter out noise and prioritize genuine patient sentiments (Qin et al., 2021). |
| Scalability | As the volume of patient-generated data grows, scalability becomes a critical concern. Edge AI systems must be designed to handle increasing data loads without compromising performance or responsiveness.<br>Healthcare organizations should also consider the scalability of their AI infrastructure, including edge servers and computational resources. Scaling up to meet the demands of a larger patient population requires careful planning and resource allocation (Himeur et al., 2022). |
| Interoperability | Interoperability is an ongoing challenge in healthcare, as different systems and platforms may use varying data formats and standards. Edge AI systems for sentiment analysis should be compatible with existing healthcare IT infrastructure to ensure seamless integration. Moreover, interoperability is crucial when sharing patient insights across different departments or healthcare organizations. A unified approach to sentiment analysis that spans the entire healthcare ecosystem can yield more comprehensive insights and drive system-wide improvements (Agha et al., 2022; Dash et al., 2019; Singh & Gill, 2023). |
| Explainability and Accountability | As AI plays an increasingly prominent role in healthcare decision-making, ensuring explainability and accountability is paramount. Patients and healthcare providers need to understand how AI-driven decisions are made and who is ultimately responsible for those decisions. In cases where AI systems make recommendations that impact patient care, healthcare organizations should establish clear protocols for human oversight and intervention. This ensures that AI-driven decisions align with ethical standards and best practices (Amann et al., 2020). |
| Regulatory Compliance and Data Governance | The regulatory landscape in healthcare is complex and subject to change. Healthcare organizations must remain vigilant and adaptable to evolving data protection regulations and privacy requirements (Caliskan, 2023; Chen, 2023). |

## REFERENCES

Abualigah, L., Alfar, H. E., Shehab, M., & Hussein, A. M. A. (2020). Sentiment analysis in healthcare: A brief review. In *Recent Advances in NLP: The Case of Arabic Language* (pp. 129–141).

Agha, S., Mohsan, H., Ul, Q., Zahra, A., Khan, M. A., Alsharif, M. H., Elhaty, I. A., & Jahid, A. (2022). Role of drone technology helping in alleviating the COVID-19 pandemic. *Micromachines, 13*(10), 1593. https://doi.org/10.3390/MI13101593

Amann, J., Blasimme, A., Vayena, E., Frey, D., Madai, V. I., & Consortium, P. (2020). Explainability for artificial intelligence in healthcare: A multidisciplinary perspective. *BMC Medical Informatics and Decision Making, 20,* 1–9.

Bohr, A., & Memarzadeh, K. (2020). The rise of artificial intelligence in healthcare applications. In *Artificial Intelligence in Healthcare* (pp. 25–60). Elsevier.

Caliskan, A. (2023). Artificial intelligence, bias, and ethics. *IJCAI International Joint Conference on Artificial Intelligence, 2023-Augus,* 7007–7013. https://doi.org/10.24963/ijcai.2023/799

Chen, Z. (2023). Ethics and discrimination in artificial intelligence-enabled recruitment practices. *Humanities and Social Sciences Communications, 10*(1), 1–12. https://doi.org/10.1057/s41599-023-02079-x

Dash, S., Biswas, S., Banerjee, D., & Atta-Ur-Rahman. (2019). Edge and fog computing in healthcare—A review. *Scalable Computing, 20*(2), 191–206. https://doi.org/10.12694/scpe.v20i2.1504

*Data Protection Principles: Core Principles of the GDPR*. (n.d.). Retrieved October 24, 2023, from https://cloudian.com/guides/data-protection/data-protection-principles-7-core-principles-of-the-gdpr/

Ellsberg, M., Jansen, H. A., Heise, L., Watts, C. H., & Garcia-Moreno, C. (2008). Intimate partner violence and women's physical and mental health in the WHO multi-country study on women's health and domestic violence: An observational study. *The Lancet, 371*(9619), 1165–1172. https://doi.org/10.1016/S0140-6736(08)60522-X

Engle, R. L., Mohr, D. C., Holmes, S. K., Seibert, M. N., Afable, M., Leyson, J., & Meterko, M. (2021). Evidence-based practice and patient-centered care: Doing both well. *Health Care Management Review, 46*(3), 174.

Greaves, F., Ramirez-Cano, D., Millett, C., Darzi, A., & Donaldson, L. (2013). Use of sentiment analysis for capturing patient experience from free-text comments posted online. *Journal of Medical Internet Research, 15*(11), e2721.

Greene, S. M., Tuzzio, L., & Cherkin, D. (2012). A framework for making patient-centered care front and center. *The Permanente Journal, 16*(3), 49.

HealthIT.gov. (2013, April). *Guide to Privacy and Security of Health Information*, 27–40.

Himeur, Y., Sayed, A., Alsalemi, A., Bensaali, F., Amira, A., Varlamis, I., Eirinaki, M., Sardianos, C., & Dimitrakopoulos, G. (2022). Blockchain-based recommender systems: Applications, challenges and future opportunities. *Computer Science Review, 43*, 100439. https://doi.org/10.1016/j.cosrev.2021.100439

Jain, R., Gupta, M., Nayyar, A., & Sharma, N. (2021). Adoption of fog computing in healthcare 4.0. *Fog Computing for Healthcare 4.0 Environments: Technical, Societal, and Future Implications*, 3–36.

Jamal, A. A., Aldawsari, S. T., Almufawez, K. A., Barri, R. M., Zakaria, N., & Tharkar, S. (2020). Twitter as a promising microblogging application for psychiatric consultation—Understanding the predictors of use, satisfaction and e-health literacy. *International Journal of Medical Informatics, 141*(March), 104202. https://doi.org/10.1016/j.ijmedinf.2020.104202

Javaid, M., Haleem, A., Singh, R. P., Suman, R., & Rab, S. (2022). Significance of machine learning in healthcare: Features, pillars and applications. *International Journal of Intelligent Networks, 3*, 58–73.

Kiseleva, A., Kotzinos, D., & De Hert, P. (2022). Transparency of AI in healthcare as a multilayered system of accountabilities: between legal requirements and technical limitations. *Frontiers in Artificial Intelligence, 5*, 879603.

Mackintosh, N. J., Davis, R. E., Easter, A., Rayment-Jones, H., Sevdalis, N., Wilson, S., Adams, M., & Sandall, J. (2020). Interventions to increase patient and family involvement in escalation of care for acute life-threatening illness in community health and hospital settings. *Cochrane Database of Systematic Reviews, 12*.

*Privacy | HHS.gov*. (n.d.). Retrieved October 26, 2023, from https://www.hhs.gov/hipaa/for-professionals/privacy/index.html

Qin, Q., Ke, Q., Du, J. T., & Xie, Y. (2021). How users' gaze behavior is related to their quality evaluation of a health website based on HONcode principles? *Data and Information Management, 5*(1), 75–85. https://doi.org/10.2478/dim-2020-0045

Rajalakshmi, R., Reddy, B. Y., & Kumar, L. (2021). DLRG@DravidianLangTech-EACL2021: Transformer based approach for offensive language identification on code-mixed Tamil. In *Proceedings of the 1st Workshop on Speech and Language Technologies for Dravidian Languages, DravidianLangTech 2021 at 16th Conference of the European Chapter of the Association for Computational Linguistics, EACL 2021*, 357–362.

Sabarmathi, G., & Chinnaiyan, R. (2020). Big data analytics framework for opinion mining of patient health care experience. In *2020 Fourth International Conference on Computing Methodologies and Communication (ICCMC)*, 352–357.

Siala, H., & Wang, Y. (2022). SHIFTing artificial intelligence to be responsible in healthcare: A systematic review. *Social Science & Medicine, 296*, 114782.

Singh, R., & Gill, S. S. (2023). Edge AI: A survey. *Internet of Things and Cyber-Physical Systems, 3*, 71–92. https://doi.org/10.1016/J.IOTCPS.2023.02.004

*What Do We Do About the Biases in AI?* (n.d.). Retrieved October 26, 2023, from https://hbr.org/2019/10/what-do-we-do-about-the-biases-in-ai

*What Is Patient Experience? | Agency for Healthcare Research and Quality*. (n.d.). Retrieved October 26, 2023, from https://www.ahrq.gov/cahps/about-cahps/patient-experience/index.html

Ziebland, S., Coulter, A., Calabrese, J. D., & Locock, L. (Eds.). (2013). *Understanding and Using Health Experiences: Improving Patient Care*. Oxford University Press. https://doi.org/10.1093/acprof:oso/9780199665372.001.0001

# 13 Edge AI in LoRa-Based Health Monitoring

*Manjula Devi C, Sivakarthi G, Srinivasan A, Gobinath A, and Rajeswari P*

## 13.1 INTRODUCTION

The fusion of artificial intelligence (AI) with the Internet of Things (IoT) has changed several industries, including healthcare, in the era of rapid technological growth. This convergence has given rise to several groundbreaking paradigms, one of which is edge AI, a revolutionary strategy that puts AI capabilities right to the network's edge, where data is produced and gathered. Figure 13.1 illustrates the IoT-enabled healthcare. In the context of health monitoring, this chapter explores the intriguing combination of edge AI with long-range (LoRa) communication technologies (Ashton, 2009).

### 13.1.1 Defining Edge AI

In contrast to merely relying on remote cloud-based processing, edge AI refers to the deployment of AI algorithms and computational models directly on edge devices, such as sensors, wearables, and IoT devices. By enabling local real-time data analysis, inference, and decision-making, this method reduces the latency and bandwidth issues that cloud-centric systems might cause. Edge AI is thus especially relevant to health monitoring since it provides quicker answers, more privacy, and improved efficiency in a variety of applications. Due to the widespread use of wearable technology, remote sensors, and IoT-enabled medical devices, health monitoring has undergone a fundamental change (de Castro Tomé et al., 2019).

Traditionally, health data was collected and delivered to centralized systems for processing, which frequently resulted in severe delays in medical settings.

Real-Time Analysis: Every second counts in critical health circumstances. AI algorithms can rapidly analyze vital signs, abnormalities, and trends by processing data at the edge, enabling immediate responses and interventions. This real-time analysis has the potential to save lives, particularly for individuals with chronic diseases or those in need of immediate medical attention.

Reduced Latency: Edge AI reduces the time it takes to collect and analyze data. In cardiac monitoring, for example, fast detection of arrhythmias or aberrant heart rates is critical for urgent medical interventions. Edge AI ensures that such insights are generated without being delayed by network delays.

Bandwidth Optimization: Sending raw sensor data to a central server uses a lot of bandwidth (Elijah et al., 2018). Edge AI analyzes data locally and sends only relevant insights to the cloud. This improves bandwidth utilization while simultaneously reducing the strain on network infrastructure.

Health data is highly sensitive and is subject to strong privacy regulations. Edge AI solves privacy concerns by processing data locally, reducing the need for raw patient information to be transmitted to external servers. This method improves data security and lowers the danger of breaches. Edge devices frequently have low computational power and energy resources. Edge AI techniques are meant to be resource-efficient, allowing complex computations to be done even on limited devices, improving battery life and increasing device longevity.

DOI: 10.1201/9781003442066-13

">

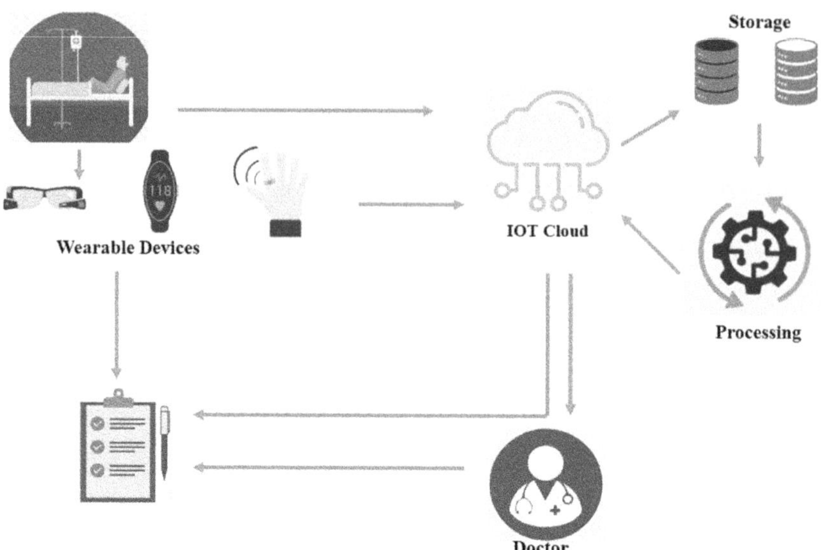


**FIGURE 13.1** IoT-enabled healthcare.

We will go deeper into the technical aspects of edge AI implementation in LoRa-based health monitoring systems in the following sections of this chapter. We will look at the technological issues, challenges, and solutions for directly implementing AI algorithms on health monitoring devices, ushering in a new era of responsive and intelligent healthcare systems. We hope that a detailed examination of this topic will give readers with a clear knowledge of how edge AI and LoRa technology work together to change health monitoring paradigms (Farrell, 2018).

### 13.1.2 The Role of LoRa Technology in IoT Devices

The Internet of Things (IoT) has heralded a new era of networked gadgets that communicate and exchange data in order to improve efficiency and comfort across multiple areas. One of the most difficult difficulties in IoT deployment is maintaining consistent connectivity over long distances while conserving energy. This is where long-range (LoRa) technology appears as a game changer. LoRa technology, which was developed for low-power, wide-area network (LPWAN) communication, is critical in enabling long-range, low-power connectivity for IoT devices. Let's look at how LoRa accomplishes this feat and its importance in the IoT ecosystem.

LoRa technology is a wireless communication protocol that was developed primarily to meet the communication needs of IoT devices dispersed across large geographical areas. Unlike standard cellular networks, which prioritize high data throughput, LoRa prioritizes communication range and energy efficiency. It operates in sub-gigahertz frequency ranges such as 868 MHz (Europe) and 915 MHz (North America), allowing signals to travel large distances while passing through obstacles such as buildings and foliage (Gkotsiopoulos et al., 2021).

Long Range: LoRa devices can communicate over several kilometers in open environments, making them suitable for applications that require communication across remote and challenging terrains.

Low Power Consumption: IoT devices are often powered by batteries or energy harvesting sources. LoRa technology excels in power efficiency, allowing devices to operate on minimal energy for extended periods. The devices' energy-efficient communication modes, such as ultra-low-power sleep modes, contribute to longer battery life.

Adaptive Data Rates: LoRa devices can adjust their data transmission rates based on the distance from the gateway (base station). This adaptive feature ensures optimal communication performance and energy consumption, even in scenarios with varying signal strengths.

Spread Spectrum Modulation: LoRa employs a modulation technique called "chirp spread spectrum," which allows the signal to spread across a wide frequency range. This makes LoRa signals resistant to interference, noise, and fading, enhancing reliability in challenging environments.

Multiple Communication Modes: LoRa supports multiple communication modes, including unicast, multicast, and broadcast. This versatility enables efficient communication for diverse IoT applications, from one-to-one communication to data broadcasting. Figure 13.2 shows the role of LoRa technology in IoT devices.

LoRa technology, in essence, revolutionizes IoT communication by providing long-range, low-power connectivity. Its capacity to cover large regions while consuming little energy makes it an excellent choice for IoT applications that require dependable, efficient, and cost-effective communication. In this chapter, we'll look at how combining edge AI with LoRa technology improves health monitoring applications, paving the path for new and responsive healthcare solutions (Goudos et al., 2017).

## 13.2 FUNDAMENTALS OF EDGE AI AND LORA TECHNOLOGY

Edge AI is a game-changing approach to AI that moves data processing and analysis closer to the source of data collection, often known as the network's "edge." Edge AI, as opposed to standard AI models that rely on centralized cloud servers for computation, allows devices to do localized data processing, providing real-time insights and decision-making. This paradigm change has various benefits that are particularly relevant to the IoT ecosystem. Figure 13.3 illustrates the Edge AI and LoRa technology.

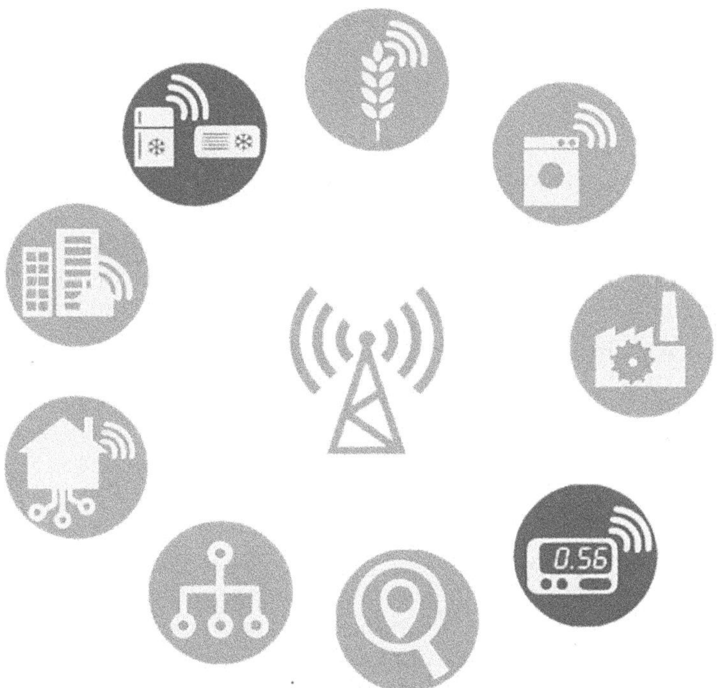

**FIGURE 13.2**  Role of LoRa technology in IoT devices.

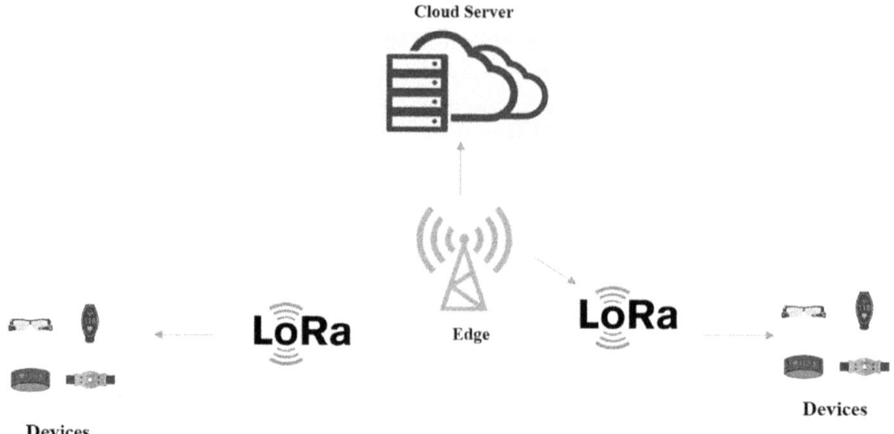


**FIGURE 13.3**　Edge AI and LoRa technology.

### 13.2.1 Advantages of Edge AI

Reduced Latency: By processing data locally, edge AI eliminates the delay associated with sending data to distant cloud servers for analysis. This instantaneous processing is critical in applications where rapid response times are imperative, such as industrial automation or autonomous vehicles.

Bandwidth Efficiency: Edge AI reduces the need to transmit large volumes of raw data to the cloud for analysis. Only relevant insights or pre-processed information are sent, optimizing network bandwidth and minimizing data transfer costs.

Privacy and Security: Processing data at the edge enhances data privacy, as sensitive information can remain on the device rather than being transmitted to external servers. This is crucial in scenarios like healthcare, where patient data confidentiality is paramount.

Offline Operation: Edge AI enables devices to function even when connectivity to the cloud is lost. This offline capability is valuable in environments with intermittent or unreliable network connectivity.

Real-Time Decision-Making: AI models deployed at the edge can make instant decisions based on localized data, enabling autonomous actions without the need for constant cloud communication. This is essential for applications like robotics and smart manufacturing.

Scalability and Network Load: Distributing AI processing across edge devices offloads the strain on centralized servers and cloud infrastructure, allowing for more scalable and efficient systems.

### 13.2.2 The Synergy between Edge AI and IoT Is Evident due to Several Factors

In the realm of IoT, the proliferation of data is driven by myriad interconnected devices, and in this context, the concept of data localization gains significance. IoT devices produce vast data volumes, much of which can be analyzed and filtered at the edge through the power of edge AI. This facet empowers devices to conduct data analysis at the point of generation, diminishing the need for continuous data transmission and subsequently alleviating network congestion.

Additionally, the consideration of resource efficiency assumes prominence, as many IoT devices possess limited computational capabilities and energy reservoirs. Edge AI algorithms are meticulously crafted to be lightweight, ensuring that intricate computations can be executed on devices with constrained resources, all while preserving energy and battery life.

A pivotal attribute of IoT applications is the necessity for real-time insights, vital for prompt and effective decision-making. Edge AI steps in to facilitate swift data analysis and instantaneous responses, bypassing the delays associated with centralized cloud processing.

IoT's adaptability is shown in its many applications, which range from smart homes and industrial automation to agriculture and healthcare. Edge AI's versatility is important in this environment since it accommodates to the particular requirements of these varied use cases.

Given the sensitive nature of data acquired by IoT devices, data privacy and security become critical. Edge AI plays a significant role in this scenario by ensuring that essential data remains localized, reducing the risks associated with data breaches and illegal access.

Edge AI's essence is in sync with the imperatives and needs of IoT applications. As we look at a concrete example of the integration of edge AI and LoRa technology in the domain of health monitoring, we see how localized AI processing improves real-time insights, enables proactive interventions, and optimizes data management within the vast realm of the IoT ecosystem (Huang et al., 2013).

## 13.3 KEY FEATURES OF LORA TECHNOLOGY, INCLUDING ITS RANGE, DATA RATE, AND ENERGY EFFICIENCY

LoRa technology is a wireless communication protocol designed to address the unique needs of the IoT by offering long-range, low-power communication capabilities. Its key features, including remarkable communication range, adaptive data rates, and exceptional energy efficiency, make it a game-changer for IoT applications (Li et al., 2023).

### Long Communication Range

LoRa's standout feature is its ability to establish communication over extensive distances, far beyond what traditional wireless technologies can achieve. In open environments, LoRa devices can transmit data over several kilometers, making it ideal for applications that demand connectivity across remote and sprawling areas. This expansive range is particularly valuable for applications such as agricultural monitoring, asset tracking, and environmental sensing, where devices might be dispersed across large territories.

### Adaptive Data Rates

LoRa technology possesses the unique capability to adapt its data transmission rates based on the distance between the transmitting device and the receiving gateway (base station). When devices are closer to the gateway, higher data rates are used for faster communication. Conversely, when devices are farther away, lower data rates are employed to ensure reliable communication over longer distances. This adaptability ensures that data is transmitted effectively, optimizing both communication range and energy efficiency.

### Energy Efficiency

Energy efficiency is a critical factor in IoT applications, especially those involving battery-powered devices that need to operate autonomously for extended periods. LoRa technology excels in energy efficiency by enabling devices to transmit data with minimal energy consumption. Devices can remain in low-power sleep modes for most of the time, waking up only when data needs to be transmitted or received. This approach conserves energy and extends the battery life of IoT devices, allowing them to operate for months or even years without requiring frequent battery replacements.

### Spread Spectrum Modulation

LoRa employs a modulation technique known as chirp spread spectrum (CSS), which spreads the data signal over a wide range of frequencies. This modulation technique makes LoRa signals more resilient to interference, noise, and signal fading caused by obstacles and environmental conditions. The CSS modulation enhances the reliability and robustness of LoRa communication, making it suitable for applications in challenging environments.

### Scalability and Network Density

LoRa technology's architecture allows for the deployment of large-scale networks with thousands of devices. The system can handle multiple devices transmitting data simultaneously without overwhelming the network, making it suitable for applications that require high device density, such as smart cities and industrial IoT deployments.

In conclusion, LoRa technology's remarkable communication range, adaptive data rates, energy efficiency, and spread spectrum modulation collectively position it as a premier choice for IoT communication. These features enable IoT applications to efficiently communicate over long distances, conserve energy, and maintain reliable connectivity, making LoRa an essential tool for building robust and scalable IoT solutions.

## 13.4   HEALTH MONITORING IN THE IOT ERA

The evolution of health monitoring has been significantly shaped by technological advancements, with the integration of IoT playing a pivotal role in transforming healthcare practices. From traditional in-person visits to remote and proactive health management, the journey of health monitoring has undergone a remarkable shift. Let's explore this evolution and the transformative impact of IoT on healthcare (Magrin et al., 2017):

### Early Health Monitoring

Historically, health monitoring was primarily conducted through direct interactions between patients and healthcare professionals. Patients would visit clinics or hospitals for routine check-ups, diagnostics, and consultations. Monitoring vital signs, such as heart rate and blood pressure, often required specialized medical equipment and skilled personnel. This approach was reactive, focusing on addressing health issues after they had emerged.

### The Rise of Wearables

The advent of wearable devices marked a significant shift in health monitoring. Wearables, such as fitness trackers and smartwatches, introduced the concept of continuous monitoring outside clinical settings. These devices enabled individuals to track their activity levels, heart rate, sleep patterns, and more in real time. This shift toward proactive health management empowered users to make informed decisions about their lifestyles and seek medical attention based on real-time data insights.

### IoT's Role in Remote Monitoring

The IoT revolutionized health monitoring by enabling remote and continuous tracking of health parameters. Connected medical devices and sensors began collecting data and transmitting it to cloud platforms for analysis. This remote monitoring approach allowed healthcare providers to monitor patients' conditions from a distance, enabling early intervention and reducing hospital readmissions. Patients with chronic illnesses, post-operative cases, and elderly individuals benefited significantly from continuous monitoring, as potential health issues could be detected and addressed promptly.

### Personalized and Predictive Healthcare

IoT-enabled health monitoring has paved the way for personalized and predictive healthcare. Advanced AI algorithms process the vast amounts of data collected from IoT devices to identify patterns, anomalies, and trends. This data-driven approach allows healthcare professionals to customize treatment plans based on individual patient needs and predict potential health issues before they escalate. Predictive analytics can help prevent complications, optimize treatment regimens, and improve patient outcomes (Mekki et al., 2019).

### Telemedicine and Virtual Care

The combination of IoT health monitoring and telemedicine has further revolutionized healthcare delivery. Virtual consultations and remote diagnostics are becoming more common, allowing patients to connect with healthcare providers without the need for in-person visits. IoT devices enable patients to share real-time data during virtual appointments, enhancing the accuracy of diagnoses and treatment recommendations.

While the integration of IoT in health monitoring brings numerous benefits, it also raises concerns related to data privacy, security, and regulatory compliance. Protecting patient data and ensuring the security of IoT devices and networks are paramount in maintaining trust in healthcare services. The evolution of health monitoring from traditional methods to IoT-driven remote and proactive monitoring reflects the broader digital transformation of healthcare. IoT technology empowers individuals to take charge of their health, provides healthcare professionals with real-time insights, and contributes to the development of more personalized and efficient healthcare systems. As we explore the intersection of edge AI and LoRa-based health monitoring, we witness how these advancements redefine the way healthcare is delivered and experienced.

### 13.4.1 The Challenges of Traditional Health Monitoring Methods and the Potential Benefits of IoT-Enabled Solutions

Traditional health monitoring methods, relying on in-person visits and manual data collection, have inherent limitations that can hinder effective healthcare management. Some of the key challenges include:

Limited Frequency: Traditional methods involve periodic visits to healthcare facilities, leading to infrequent data collection. This approach can miss critical changes in health status that occur between appointments.

Reactive Approach: Traditional monitoring is often reactive, addressing health issues only after they've become evident. This delay in intervention can lead to complications and worsened health outcomes.

Lack of Real-Time Data: In traditional settings, healthcare providers have access to data collected during appointments, but crucial real-time data is not available to inform immediate decisions.

Limited Patient Engagement: Patients may struggle to engage with their health due to the lack of continuous monitoring and personalized insights. This can lead to difficulties in managing chronic conditions and adhering to treatment plans.

Resource Intensity: Traditional monitoring relies on specialized medical equipment and healthcare personnel, making it resource-intensive and sometimes inconvenient for patients.

## 13.5 CONVERGENCE OF EDGE AI AND LORA FOR HEALTH MONITORING

The synergy between edge AI and LoRa technology presents a potent combination that has the potential to revolutionize health monitoring applications. By combining the real-time data analysis capabilities of edge AI with the long-range, low-power communication prowess of LoRa, healthcare systems can become more responsive, efficient, and patient-centered. Let's delve into how these technologies harmonize to enhance health monitoring:

### 13.5.1 Real-Time Data Analysis with Edge AI

Edge AI involves processing data directly on IoT devices at the "edge" of the network. In the context of health monitoring, this means that data collected from wearable devices, sensors, and medical equipment can be analyzed locally without the need for extensive data transmission to a centralized server. AI algorithms deployed on these devices can quickly analyze vital signs, detect anomalies, and extract meaningful insights from the data in real time. For instance, an Edge AI algorithm could identify irregular heart rhythms or significant changes in temperature immediately after data is collected, triggering timely alerts or interventions (Raza et al., 2017).

### 13.5.2 Long-Range Communication and Energy Efficiency with LoRa

LoRa technology's long communication range and low-power characteristics are instrumental in transmitting health data from remote or distributed devices to central repositories or healthcare providers. In health monitoring scenarios, where patients may be in diverse locations, LoRa ensures that data is reliably transmitted without consuming excessive energy. This is particularly valuable in cases where patients are not within close proximity to healthcare facilities, such as rural areas or home-bound individuals.

### 13.5.3 Enhancing Health Monitoring

Timely Alerts and Interventions: Edge AI's real-time analysis allows for immediate detection of critical health changes. When combined with LoRa's long-range communication, healthcare providers can receive timely alerts and respond promptly to emergencies or abnormal readings.

Reduced Data Transmission: Instead of transmitting large volumes of raw data to the cloud, only relevant insights or anomalies are sent, minimizing network congestion and conserving energy.

Battery Life Extension: Edge AI algorithms designed for low-power consumption complement LoRa's energy-efficient communication, extending the battery life of wearable devices and sensors.

Privacy Preservation: Since sensitive health data remains localized due to Edge AI processing, patients' privacy is maintained while still enabling healthcare professionals to access essential insights. In core, the synergy between edge AI and LoRa technology reshapes health monitoring from episodic and reactive practices to continuous, proactive, and real-time interventions. As we witness this amalgamation in the domain of health monitoring, we glimpse the future of healthcare where devices, data, and insights converge to deliver patient-centered, intelligent, and efficient care (Savaglio et al., 2020).

## 13.6 EXAMPLES OF PRACTICAL APPLICATIONS

### 1. Remote Patient Monitoring

Edge AI in combination with LoRa technology revolutionizes remote patient monitoring by allowing continuous and real-time health data collection without requiring patients to be physically present at healthcare facilities. Wearable devices equipped with sensors measure vital signs like heart rate, blood pressure, and oxygen levels. Edge AI processes this data locally, analyzing it for anomalies or concerning trends. If a critical change is detected, such as a sudden drop in oxygen saturation, the device can send an alert to both the patient and healthcare provider via LoRa communication. This immediate response enables timely medical interventions and reduces hospital readmissions.

### 2. Elderly Care and Fall Detection

For elderly individuals living alone, fall detection is a crucial safety concern. Edge AI algorithms on wearable devices can analyze accelerometer and gyroscope data to detect sudden movements characteristic of a fall. By utilizing LoRa technology, the wearable device can quickly communicate with caregivers or medical professionals in case of a fall. This ensures rapid assistance, reducing the risks associated with delayed response times.

### 3. Chronic Disease Management

Managing chronic diseases often requires continuous monitoring of various health parameters. In the case of diabetes, for instance, a patient's blood glucose levels need to be closely monitored to prevent dangerous fluctuations. Edge-AI-enabled glucose monitors can analyze blood glucose levels in real time and communicate the data using LoRa technology. Healthcare providers receive immediate notifications if levels become critically high or low, enabling them to adjust treatment plans promptly.

### 4. Environmental Monitoring for Asthma Management

Edge AI and LoRa can also be used to monitor environmental conditions that impact patients' health. For instance, in asthma management, IoT devices equipped with air quality sensors can measure pollutants and allergens in the environment. Edge AI algorithms can process this data locally and provide personalized alerts to asthma patients when air quality deteriorates. By using LoRa technology, this information can be communicated to patients' smartphones, enabling them to take preventive measures.

### 5. Post-Operative Monitoring

After surgeries, patients' vital signs and recovery progress need close monitoring. Wearable devices equipped with sensors can continuously track heart rate, body temperature, and other relevant metrics. Edge AI processes the data locally, identifying any signs of infection, complications, or abnormal recovery patterns. Using LoRa technology, medical professionals receive real-time updates on patients' recovery status, allowing them to intervene swiftly if any issues arise.

These practical applications showcase how the combination of edge AI and LoRa technology in health monitoring leads to more responsive, personalized, and effective healthcare solutions. By enabling real-time analysis and communication, these technologies empower patients, caregivers, and healthcare providers with the tools they need to make informed decisions and deliver timely interventions.

## 13.7 THE INTEGRATION OF AI PROCESSING WITH LORA COMMUNICATION PROTOCOLS

Integrating AI processing with LoRa communication protocols involves combining the capabilities of both technologies to create intelligent and efficient IoT solutions. Here's a step-by-step explanation of how this integration can be achieved (Semtech, 2017):

### 1. Choose the Right AI Model

Select an AI model that is well-suited for edge devices and resource-constrained environments. Consider factors such as model size, complexity, and accuracy. Opt for lightweight models that can perform real-time inference on edge devices without overwhelming their computational capabilities.

### 2. Train and Optimize the AI Model

Train the selected AI model using relevant datasets. Apply optimization techniques like quantization, pruning, and compression to make the model suitable for edge deployment. The goal is to achieve a balance between model accuracy and computational efficiency.

### 3. Deploy the AI Model on Edge Devices

Deploy the optimized AI model onto the edge devices where data is collected. This can involve converting the model into a format compatible with the target hardware and software framework.

### 4. Implement Edge Data Processing

Program the edge devices to process data using the deployed AI model. As data is collected from sensors or other sources, run inference using the AI model to extract insights and identify patterns directly on the device.

### 5. Define Event Triggers

Define criteria or conditions that trigger specific actions based on the results of AI inference. For instance, if the AI model detects an anomaly in health data, it could trigger an alert or initiate a communication process.

### 6. Integrate LoRa Communication

Integrate LoRa communication protocols into the edge devices. Configure the devices to communicate with LoRa gateways or base stations. This involves defining how data will be transmitted, received, and formatted for LoRa communication.

### 7. Data Transmission and Reception

When the edge device processes data using the AI model and identifies significant events or insights, it can package this information and transmit it using LoRa communication. Likewise, the device can receive commands or updates from central systems through LoRa.

### 8. Establish Network Connectivity

Ensure that the edge devices are within the coverage range of LoRa gateways or base stations. This connectivity enables seamless data exchange between the edge devices and centralized systems.

Integrating AI processing with LoRa communication protocols involves deploying optimized AI models on edge devices, enabling real-time data analysis, and leveraging LoRa's communication capabilities to transmit relevant insights or information to central systems. This integration empowers IoT devices to make informed decisions, trigger actions, and communicate seamlessly within an intelligent and efficient ecosystem.

## 13.8 PROPOSED SOLUTIONS FOR OVERCOMING THESE CHALLENGES

### 1. Model Complexity and Resource Constraints

Utilize model compression techniques like quantization, pruning, and knowledge distillation to reduce model size and complexity while maintaining accuracy. Opt for lightweight model architectures specifically designed for edge deployment, such as MobileNet or SqueezeNet.

### 2. Energy Efficiency

Implement hardware accelerators like GPUs or TPUs optimized for energy-efficient AI inference. Apply algorithmic optimizations to minimize unnecessary computations and reduce power consumption during inference (Sharma, 2019).

### 3.  Data Privacy and Security

Encrypt data during transmission and storage using protocols like SSL/TLS to ensure data confidentiality. Employ secure boot mechanisms to prevent unauthorized access to device firmware and configurations.

### 4.  Model Updates and Maintenance

Implement secure and efficient OTA update mechanisms to remotely update AI models on edge devices without compromising security. Use federated learning techniques to update models collaboratively across devices while maintaining data privacy.

### 5.  Heterogeneous Hardware

Develop adaptable AI models that can dynamically adjust their computations based on the available hardware capabilities. Provide device-specific model variants that are optimized for different types of edge devices.

### 6.  Ethical Considerations

Implement bias detection and mitigation techniques during AI model training to ensure fairness and reduce bias. Provide explainability features that offer insights into how AI models arrived at their decisions.

### 7.  Interpretability and Explainability

Solution: Integrate techniques like LIME or SHAP that generate explanations for AI model predictions, making them more interpretable for healthcare professionals.

### 8.  Regulatory Compliance

Ensure that your solution adheres to relevant regulations such as HIPAA by implementing strict data access controls, encryption, and audit trails.

## 13.9  CASE STUDIES

While specific case studies involving the combination of edge AI and LoRa-based health monitoring are not widely documented, there are examples of organizations that have implemented edge AI and IoT solutions in healthcare, which could serve as relevant analogies. These examples highlight the potential benefits and outcomes of integrating these technologies in health monitoring scenarios:

### 1.  Philips Healthcare

Philips has developed a range of connected health solutions that leverage edge AI and IoT technologies. For instance, they offer wearable devices for remote patient monitoring that collect vital signs and send data to central systems using IoT protocols. Although not explicitly LoRa-based, similar principles apply. Edge AI algorithms process data locally to detect anomalies and trends, allowing healthcare providers to deliver timely interventions. Philips' solutions demonstrate the potential of real-time monitoring and intervention enabled by edge AI and IoT.

### 2.  Biobeat

Biobeat offers wearable and non-wearable solutions for continuous remote patient monitoring. These devices collect physiological data such as heart rate, blood pressure, and oxygen saturation. The company utilizes AI algorithms for real-time analysis of the collected data. Although not directly related to LoRa technology, the concept of real-time analysis and alerts aligns with the principles of edge AI and LoRa-based communication.

### 3.  Sensogram Technologies

Sensogram has developed wearable devices equipped with sensors for monitoring vital signs like heart rate, temperature, and movement. The devices use AI algorithms to process the collected data and generate insights for both patients and healthcare providers. While the communication aspect may not be LoRa-based, this example showcases the use of edge AI for real-time analysis in health monitoring applications.

### 4.  Telemedicine Platforms

Several telemedicine platforms incorporate edge AI for health monitoring. These platforms often integrate wearables and home health devices to collect data from patients. AI algorithms on the edge devices analyze the data in real time, detecting anomalies and transmitting relevant information to healthcare providers for remote consultations. While communication protocols may vary, this demonstrates the potential of edge AI in health monitoring.

While these examples might not be specific to LoRa technology, they illustrate how edge AI and IoT are transforming healthcare by enabling real-time data analysis, proactive interventions, and remote patient monitoring. Combining these principles with LoRa-based communication can extend the benefits to scenarios where long-range, low-power communication is essential.

## 13.10  CONCLUSIONS

In conclusion the combination of edge AI and LoRa technology, in health monitoring brings about a transformation in the healthcare field. It offers advantages that enhance efficiency, effectiveness, and accessibility. The local data processing capability of edge AI allows for real time analysis of signs, enabling interventions and timely alerts. By optimizing resources continuous monitoring can be achieved without draining device batteries. Moreover, processing health data locally strengthens data privacy while scalability and accessibility contribute to improved healthcare delivery. Personalized care becomes possible through customized AI models that adhere to requirements like HIPAA. However, there are challenges to address such as optimizing resource constrained devices and ethical considerations. Striking a balance between accuracy, efficiency, and security is crucial. The integration of edge AI and LoRa technology in health monitoring paves the way, for data-driven decisions in secure healthcare advancements. Ongoing research and development promise innovative applications that redefine the future of healthcare a future where patient wellbeing takes center stage with the support of intelligent real time insights and efficient communication.

## REFERENCES

Ashton, K. (2009). That 'Internet of Things' things. *RFID Journal*, 22; 97–114.

de Castro Tomé, M.; Nardelli, P.H.J.; Alves, H. (2019). Long-range low-power wireless networks and sampling strategies in electricity metering. *IEEE Trans. Ind. Electron.*, 66: 1629–1637.

Elijah, O.; Rahman, T.A.; Orikumhi, I.; et al. (2018). An overview of the internet of things (IoT) and data analytics in agriculture: Benefits and challenges. *IEEE Internet Things J.*, 5: 3758–3773.

Farrell, S. (2018). *Low-power wide area network (LPWAN) overview.* Internet Engineering Task Force (IETF).

Gkotsiopoulos, P.; Zorbas, D.; Douligeris, C. (2021). Performance determinants in LoRa networks: A literature review. *IEEE Commun. Surv. Tutor.*, 23: 1721–1758.

Goudos, S.K.; Dallas, P.I.; Chatziefthymiou, S.; et al. (2017). A survey of IoT key enabling and future technologies: 5G, mobile IoT, semantic web and applications. *Wireless Pers. Commun.*, 97: 1645–1675.

Huang, P.; Xiao, L.; Soltani, S.; et al. (2013). The evolution of MAC protocols in wireless sensor networks: A survey. *IEEE Commun. Surv. Tutor.*, 15: 101–120.

Li, C.N.; Cao, Z.C. (2023). LoRa networking techniques for large-scale and long-term IoT: A down-to-top survey. *ACM Comput. Surv.*, 55: 52.

Magrin, D.; Centenaro, M.; Vangelista, L. (2017). Performance evaluation of LoRa networks in a smart city scenario. In *2017 IEEE International Conference on Communications (ICC), Paris, France, 21–25 May 2017*; IEEE: Paris, pp. 1–7. https://doi.org/10.1109/ICC.2017.7996384.

Mekki, K.; Bajic, E.; Chaxel, F.; et al. (2019). A comparative study of LPWAN technologies for large-scale IoT deployment. *ICT Express*, 5: 1–7.

Raza, U.; Kulkarni, P.; Sooriyabandara, M. (2017). Low power wide area networks: An overview. *IEEE Commun. Surv. Tutor.*, 19: 855–873.

Savaglio, C.; Ganzha, M.; Paprzycki, M.; et al. (2020). Agent-based internet of things: State-of-the-art and research challenges. *Future Gener. Comput. Syst.*, 102: 1038–1053.

Semtech. (2017). *Real-world LoRaWANTM network capacity for electrical metering applications.* Semtech.

Sharma, N.; Shamkuwar, M.; Singh, I. (2019). The history, present and future with IoT. In *Internet of Things and Big Data Analytics for Smart Generation*; Balas, V.; Solanki, V.; Kumar, R.; et al., Eds.; Springer: Cham, pp. 27–51. https://doi.org/10.1007/978-3-030-04203-5_3.

# 14 IoT-Based Smart Health Monitoring with Convolutional Neural Network (CNN) Using Edge Computing

*Rajeswari P, Gobinath A, Suresh Kumar N, and Anandan M*

## 14.1 INTRODUCTION

The incorporation of the Internet of Things (IoT) into the healthcare industry has heralded a new age in patient care, ushering in novel techniques to monitoring, diagnosis, and treatment. IoT-enabled devices and systems have the probable to completely transform healthcare delivery, enhance patient outcomes, and boost overall medical service efficiency (Zamanifar, 2021).

Monitoring: IoT devices have transformed intermittent patient monitoring into continuous, real-time surveillance. Wearable biosensor-enabled devices, such as fitness trackers and smartwatches, and other variables are especially useful in chronic illness management since they may inform both patients and healthcare practitioners to any variations from baseline data. Implantable devices provide doctors with quick access to physiological data for informed decision-making in addition to monitoring. Remote patient monitoring systems send health data to healthcare providers, allowing for timely treatments and lowering hospital readmissions. These developments have mostly helped the elderly and those suffering from chronic ailments.

Diagnosis: IoT's influence on diagnosis is visible in a variety of medical disciplines. IoT integration has greatly benefited medical imaging, with new imaging devices infused with IoT technology producing higher picture quality and allowing images to be sent to specialists for remote examination. This type of remote consultation not only expedites diagnosis but also allows professionals in different geographic places to collaborate. Smart diagnostic technologies, which are frequently available via smartphones, enable patients to undertake preliminary examinations of their health issues. Smartphone-based electrocardiogram (ECG) gadgets, for example, allow users to record their heart's electrical activity, which may then be quickly evaluated by healthcare professionals (Bousquet et al., 2015).

Treatment: IoT-powered treatment solutions are transforming the face of healthcare delivery. Medication adherence is particularly difficult for those who have chronic illnesses. Smart medication dispensers enabled by IoT provide dosages at predefined intervals, provide patient reminders, and can even notify healthcare practitioners if a dose is missed. Connected medical equipment, such as insulin pumps and pacemakers, continually provide data to doctors, allowing them to change treatment regimens remotely. Telemedicine, enabled by IoT technology, is transforming the doctor-patient connection by allowing patients to get virtual consultations, electronic prescriptions, and medical counseling from the comfort of their own homes. Another advance enabled by IoT is robotic surgery, which improves surgical precision while minimizing invasiveness, resulting in faster recovery times and lower risks.

Obstacles and Prospects: Despite the enormous promise of IoT in healthcare, obstacles remain. Given the delicate nature of health information, data security and patient privacy are critical issues.



DOI: 10.1201/9781003442066-14

It is critical to provide interoperability across various IoT devices and platforms in order to support smooth data sharing and analysis (Chaccour et al., 2019). Furthermore, extensive validation processes are required to ensure the quality and dependability of IoT-generated data for therapeutic reasons. Addressing these barriers and improving IoT applications will be critical in reaching the sector's full potential in patient care as the healthcare environment develops.

Figure 14.1 depicts the architecture design of the CNN-based health monitoring system leveraging IoT. The integration of IoT in healthcare has the potential to transform monitoring, diagnostic, and therapeutic paradigms. With the introduction of wearable and implantable devices, enhanced diagnostics, and new treatment modalities, it is improving patient care and moving the healthcare industry ahead.

## 14.2   INTRODUCTION TO CNNS: APPLICATIONS IN IMAGE ANALYSIS AND RECOGNITION

CNNs have emerged as a potent class of deep learning models with a significant influence on image analysis and recognition applications. Because of its capacity to automatically acquire hierarchical features from raw pixel values, CNNs are especially built to excel at jobs requiring visual data, such as photographs and movies. In this introduction, we will look into the principles of CNNs and highlight some of its many applications in image analysis and recognition.

Convolutional layers, which perform convolution processes to input data, are at the heart of CNNs. These layers are made up of learnable filters or kernels that examine the incoming data for patterns. CNNs may capture local characteristics like edges, corners, and textures in the early layers and gradually learn increasingly complicated, high-level properties as they advance through deeper layers by employing these filters. By downsampling the feature maps provided by convolutional layers, pooling layers reduce spatial dimensions and computational complexity. The learnt characteristics are combined in fully connected layers at the network's end to create predictions or classifications (Manogaran et al., 2019).

### Image Analysis and Recognition Applications

CNNs have completely transformed image classification problems. They are capable of properly categorizing objects or situations inside photos into specified categories. CNNs, for example, are employed in self-driving cars to identify traffic signs or people.

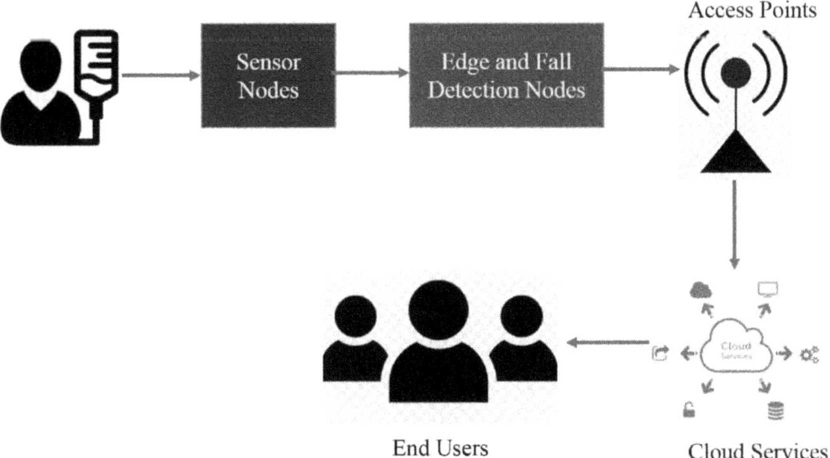


**FIGURE 14.1**   Architecture diagram of CNN based health monitoring system using IoT.

Object Detection: Object detection models based on CNN, such as faster R-CNN and YOLO, may recognize and find several items in a picture. This technology is frequently utilized in security and surveillance, as well as object tracking in autonomous drones and robots.

CNNs excel in face recognition tasks, allowing computers to verify or identify people based on their visual traits. This is utilized in security systems, unlocking mobile devices, and even social networking applications.

CNNs serve an important role in the study of medical images such as X-rays, MRIs, and CT scans. They can identify abnormalities, tumors, or illnesses, which helps radiologists diagnose them (Qiao et al., 2020).

While not directly connected to pictures, CNNs are used in NLP applications, notably text classification and sentiment analysis, where they may handle word embeddings or text representations.

Image Segmentation: CNNs are used to divide an image into different areas or segments for image segmentation applications. This is used in medical image processing to segment organs or tissues and in autonomous cars to analyze road scenes.

CNNs are utilized in the game industry for character identification, gesture recognition, and even the creation of lifelike scenes and characters.

CNNs are used for quality control in manufacturing, where they may spot flaws in goods and assure uniformity in production processes. CNNs have become an essential component of current image analysis and recognition applications. Their ability to automatically learn and extract characteristics from raw visual input has made them useful in a range of fields ranging from healthcare and autonomous vehicles to gaming and manufacturing.

## Role of Edge Computing

Instead of depending only on centralized cloud infrastructure, edge computing puts computation and data storage closer to the point of need. Because of its ability to handle important concerns like latency, privacy, and network resource conservation, this technique has acquired substantial traction in a variety of businesses. In this section, we'll look at the function of edge computing in the following areas:

Edge computing minimizes latency by processing data closer to the source, frequently at the "edge" of the network, rather than transmitting it to distant cloud servers. This is especially important for time-sensitive applications like real-time analytics, IoT devices, and self-driving cars. Edge computing reduces the time it takes to transfer data to a faraway data center and wait for a response by processing it locally. This is vital for applications like as industrial automation and telemedicine, where even little delays can have serious effects (Greco et al., 2020).

Enhancing Privacy: By processing sensitive data locally rather than transferring it to the cloud, edge computing improves privacy. This is especially crucial for applications using personal, sensitive, or confidential data. Edge computing lessens the risk of data breaches during transit and exposure to prospective attackers by keeping data inside the local environment. This is especially important in industries such as healthcare, where patient data privacy is critical.

Edge computing conserves network resources by minimizing the quantity of data that must be transferred across the network to centralized cloud servers. Many IoT devices create massive volumes of data, much of which may be unnecessary or redundant. Instead than flooding the network, edge devices may preprocess and filter the data locally, sending only relevant insights to the cloud (Uddin, 2019). This method relieves network congestion and lessens the load on both local networks and the Internet infrastructure as a whole.

In practice, edge computing is achieved by deploying edge nodes or servers at the point where data is generated. These nodes may carry out activities like as data preparation, local analytics, and even the execution of lightweight machine learning models. Edge computing may also be used to supplement cloud computing in a hybrid approach, where certain processing is done at the edge for rapid replies and more resource-intensive calculations are done in the cloud.

To summarize, edge computing is critical for lowering latency, improving privacy, and saving network resources. Edge computing solves the constraints of traditional centralized cloud computing models by processing data locally and closer to the source. This has far-reaching ramifications for businesses ranging from real-time applications to privacy-sensitive industries, and it adds to more efficient and responsive systems in our increasingly linked world.

## 14.3 ARCHITECTURE OF AN IOT-BASED HEALTH MONITORING SYSTEM

An IoT-based health monitoring system collects, transmits, and analyzes health-related data from people in real time. This architecture is often made up of physical devices, communication protocols, cloud infrastructure, and data analytics components. Here's an overview of such a system's architecture.

1. IoT Devices: The system begins with IoT devices that users wear or use to gather health-related data. Wearable fitness trackers, smartwatches, medical sensors, and even implanted gadgets are examples of these technologies. These gadgets constantly measure vital indications such as heart rate, blood pressure, temperature, and level of exercise. Sensors for measuring glucose levels, ECG signals, and other parameters may also be included.
2. Connectivity: IoT devices communicate with the system using a variety of communication protocols, including Wi-Fi, Bluetooth, Zigbee, and cellular networks (3G, 4G, or 5G). The kind of connection chosen is determined by characteristics such as range, data transfer rate, and power consumption.
3. Data Collection and Preprocessing: IoT device data is gathered and delivered to a gateway or a local edge device for preprocessing. Before sending the raw data to the cloud, this process entails cleaning and aggregating it. Edge preprocessing reduces latency and conserves network capacity.
4. Cloud Infrastructure: The preprocessed data is then sent to the cloud to be stored and processed. Cloud services such as Amazon Web Services (AWS), Microsoft Azure, and Google Cloud Platform (GCP) provide scalable and secure data storage and computing environments.
5. Data Analytics: The acquired health data is subjected to advanced data analytics methods. Pattern recognition, anomalies, and trends may be taught to machine learning models. Based on the data, these algorithms may detect possible health risks, give alarms, and provide customized advice. Predictive analytics may assist in predicting health issues before they occur.
7. User Interface and Visualization: A UI is designed to allow people to obtain health data and insights. A mobile app or a web dashboard may be used. Data visualization tools, such as charts, graphs, and trends, provide data in an intelligible way, enabling users to track their health condition over time.
8. Notifications and Alerts: The system may be set up to deliver notifications and alerts to users and healthcare practitioners in response to predetermined thresholds or significant occurrences. These notifications might notify users of aberrant vital indicators or remind them to take prescriptions.
9. Security and Privacy: To maintain the confidentiality and integrity of health data, security measures are critical. To safeguard sensitive information, encryption, authentication, and authorization mechanisms are used.
10. Healthcare Integration: In certain circumstances, the health monitoring system may be connected with healthcare providers' electronic health records (EHR) systems. This enables medical practitioners to make educated judgments based on real-time patient data.

IoT-based health monitoring system is comprised of a sophisticated architecture that includes IoT devices, connectivity, cloud infrastructure, data analytics, user interfaces, and security measures.

This architecture allows for continuous health monitoring, data analysis, and tailored insights, all of which contribute to better healthcare outcomes and patient management.

## Sensor Nodes

Sensor nodes capture physiological data and environmental characteristics in a variety of applications, including health monitoring systems. These nodes are outfitted with sensors to collect specialized data and play an important role in obtaining data for analysis, decision-making, and real-time monitoring. Here's a rundown of how sensor nodes acquire physiological and environmental data:

### Sensor Categories

Sensor nodes are outfitted with a range of sensors designed to capture various forms of data. Physiological data in health monitoring systems comprises vital signals. Environmental characteristics might include things like ambient temperature, humidity, air quality, and even GPS position data.

### Data Gathering

ECG electrodes, pulse oximeters, and temperature sensors are examples of physiological sensors that are put on or near the human body to assess significant health parameters. These sensors create analog signals, which are then converted to digital signals by analog-to-digital converters (ADCs). Environmental sensors, on the other hand, monitor characteristics such as temperature and humidity in the surrounding environment.

### Information Processing

Sensor nodes often include microcontrollers or microprocessors that process the data obtained. They could do preliminary data processing, calibration, and quality checks. This phase ensures that the data is correct and ready for further investigation.

### Wireless Networking

Sensor nodes are often equipped with wireless communication modules like as Bluetooth, Zigbee, or Wi-Fi. These modules let sensor nodes to wirelessly transfer gathered data to a central hub, gateway, or straight to the cloud for additional analysis and storage.

### Power Administration

Power consumption management is critical for sensor nodes, particularly when they are utilized in wearable devices or in distant locations (Hartmann et al., 2022). To increase the battery life of the sensor nodes, low-power hardware components, efficient algorithms, and power-saving approaches are used.

## Cloud vs. Edge Processing

Cloud and edge processing are two separate paradigms that play critical roles in data management and computing across a wide range of applications, including Internet of Things (IoT), data analysis, and others. Cloud processing, which is distinguished by the use of distant data centers, offers various benefits. Its distinguishing advantages include unrivaled scalability, since resources may be dynamically distributed depending on workload needs, allowing it to manage large-scale activities as well as unexpected spikes in activity. Furthermore, cloud data centers have great processing capacity, since they are outfitted with powerful processors, GPUs, and specialized gear intended for computationally demanding tasks, making them ideal for complex analytics and machine learning. Cloud environments' centralized data storage promotes efficient data administration and supports collaborative activities across heterogeneous teams. This centralized strategy is often accompanied with a cost-effective pay-as-you-go pricing mechanism, which allows customers to pay only for the resources they utilize, hence maximizing cost concerns (Akrivopoulos et al., 2017).

This paradigm, however, is not without drawbacks. The most notable of them is latency. Delays might be generated due to the requirement of transporting data to and from faraway cloud servers, which is especially damaging for real-time applications that require rapid replies. The reliance on network stability may also be a weakness, since interruptions or outages might result in operational downtime. Regulatory compliance issues also enter the picture since businesses regulated by strict laws, such as healthcare and finance, must guarantee that data processing complies to legal and ethical norms.

Edge processing, on the other hand, provides a number of unique benefits due to its local data processing method. Most notably, it excels in lowering latency by performing data processing near to the data source. This feature enables real-time or near-real-time answers, making it essential for applications that need quick responses. Edge processing also solves data privacy issues by allowing sensitive data to be handled locally, eliminating the need for external data transfer. Because edge devices may function independently without constant network access, this strategy is also resistant to network instability. Furthermore, edge processing might include local data pre-processing and filtering, resulting in less network traffic and less burden on network infrastructure.

Nonetheless, there are several drawbacks to edge processing. Edge devices' processing capability is often constrained in comparison to centralized cloud resources, possibly limiting their ability to conduct sophisticated calculations or manage large datasets. Scaling edge processing over a large number of devices offers management difficulties that must be addressed case by case. The scattered nature of edge devices need careful management to maintain optimum performance, which adds to the maintenance difficulties (Tuli et al., 2020).

In many practical applications, a hybrid technique that integrates both cloud and edge processing, also known as edge-cloud hybrid processing, appears as an appealing choice. By combining the characteristics of both paradigms, this hybrid design improves data processing, latency, scalability, and resource usage. The ultimate choice between cloud and edge processing is based on a thorough analysis of each application's particular requirements, such as latency limitations, data security rules, computation demands, and network stability. In summary, depending on the individual demands of each application, the optimum solution may include either cloud processing, edge processing, or a creative mix of the two.

## 14.4 CONVOLUTIONAL NEURAL NETWORKS (CNNS)

CNN basics: convolution, pooling, and fully connected layers:

Convolutional Layers: Convolution is a basic process in CNNs that involves sliding a tiny filter or kernel across an input picture and calculating dot products between the filter and local image patches. This method extracts characteristics such as edges, corners, and textures. To capture diverse characteristics, several filters are applied, resulting in feature maps that emphasize key patterns.

Pooling Layers: Pooling layers downsample the feature maps after convolution, lowering spatial dimensions while keeping significant information. The maximum value from each pool is chosen by max pooling, while the average value is computed by average pooling. Pooling improves resilience to tiny changes and fluctuations in input data while decreasing compute and memory needs.

Completely Connected Layers: At the conclusion of the CNN, the completely connected layers combine high-level information gained from previous layers. Based on the retrieved characteristics, these layers execute classification or regression tasks (Vimal et al., 2021).

**CNN architectures** include LeNet, AlexNet, ResNet, and others.

Yann LeCun's LeNet-5 was one of the first CNN designs, consisting of convolutional and pooling layers followed by fully connected layers. LeNet was developed for handwritten digit recognition and was instrumental in popularizing CNNs.

AlexNet: Alex Krizhevsky's introduction of AlexNet heralded a milestone in deep learning. In 2012, it won the ImageNet Large Scale Visual Recognition Challenge, demonstrating the capabilities of deep CNNs for large-scale picture categorization problems. AlexNet introduced the ReLU activation function, dropout regularization, and GPU acceleration, as well as several convolutional layers.

ResNet: Residual networks, or ResNets, are networks that use skip connections to solve the vanishing gradient issue in extremely deep networks. These skip connections enable gradients to flow more freely during training, allowing for the creation of astonishingly deep structures. ResNets have permitted the training of CNNs with hundreds of layers, which has contributed to better accuracy.

Transfer Learning for Medical Image Analysis: Using Pre-trained CNN Models:

CNN models pre-trained on big datasets like as ImageNet capture generic characteristics such as edges, textures, and forms. By exploiting the information gathered from a wide range of pictures, these pre-trained models may serve as a robust basis for a variety of activities.

Fine-tuning is the process of tailoring a pre-trained model to a given task using a smaller, task-specific dataset in transfer learning. Fine-tuning tailors the model's learnt characteristics to the new job by changing a subset of the model's parameters while leaving others unchanged. This method is very useful when training data is few, as is often the case in medical picture analysis.

Detecting Anomalies Using CNNs: Identifying Health Issues from Visual Data:

Normal Pattern Learning: When training CNNs on a dataset of normal, healthy pictures, the network learns the normal patterns found in the images. This allows the network to detect departures from these patterns, which may signal abnormalities or illnesses.

Localization and Segmentation: CNNs can not only identify but also localize abnormalities inside images. This is especially useful in medical pictures, where the precise location of anomalies is critical for diagnosis and therapy planning. Semantic segmentation methods may be used to isolate areas of interest.

Early identification and Diagnosis: CNNs aid in the early identification and diagnosis of illnesses by detecting abnormalities in medical pictures. This has the potential to result in more effective therapies, better patient outcomes, and lower healthcare expenditures.

A thorough understanding of the fundamentals of CNNs, a command of influential architectures such as LeNet, AlexNet, and ResNet, expertise in transfer learning for medical image analysis, and the use of CNNs in anomaly detection for health issues all highlight the power and versatility of these networks in revolutionizing visual data analysis, particularly in healthcare and beyond.

## 14.5    EDGE COMPUTING IN HEALTH MONITORING

Edge computing has brought in a new paradigm in the realm of health monitoring, ushering in a slew of transformational advantages that solve fundamental difficulties inherent in healthcare data management. Edge computing transforms health monitoring systems by shifting data processing and analysis to the network's edge, where the data is created (He et al., 2015).

One of the most important benefits of edge computing in health monitoring is its potential to significantly decrease latency. Edge computing's closeness to the data source reduces the latency associated with data transmission to centralized cloud servers in applications where real-time monitoring and quick reactions are critical, such as patient monitoring or remote surgical operations. This real-time feedback loop is critical for guaranteeing prompt treatments and patient safety.

Given the sensitivity of patient data, privacy and security considerations are crucial in healthcare. Edge computing solves these issues by enabling sensitive health information to be processed locally rather than sending it to distant cloud servers. This localized method considerably decreases the danger of data breaches during data transmission, ensuring compliance with severe data privacy standards and the confidentiality of patients' personal information.

Another distinguishing feature of edge computing in health monitoring is its efficiency. The large amount of data produced by monitoring equipment may often overload networks. Edge computing alleviates this pressure by allowing data pretreatment and filtering at the edge devices, transmitting only relevant insights or summarized data to centralized systems. This not only saves network bandwidth but also reduces the strain on the network infrastructure as a whole.

Offline operation is a critical benefit of edge computing, especially in settings where continuous connection is not assured. Edge-based health monitoring devices may continue to gather and analyze data even in distant places with limited or inconsistent network connection. This continuous operation guarantees that important data collecting continues regardless of network issues.

Edge computing has the intrinsic advantage of increased dependability. Because of the decentralized processing strategy, the failure of a single edge device does not interrupt the whole network. This resilience is especially important in healthcare applications, where downtime may have serious effects for patient health and safety (Yang et al., 2016).

Edge computing also enables the generation of localized insights. Edge devices may analyze data on-the-fly and produce rapid insights without depending on other cloud resources. This real-time analysis is critical for applications that need quick decision-making, such as improving patient care and management.

Edge computing shines in customized healthcare because it allows devices to adjust their functions to the demands of specific patients. These devices can adapt to changing circumstances without requiring regular online updates, resulting in more tailored and dynamic healthcare solutions.

Edge computing provides scalability and flexibility as the demand for health monitoring services grows. The addition of additional edge devices to the network easily accommodates rising data demands and assures that health monitoring systems can expand to meet patients' and healthcare providers' changing requirements.

Edge computing has ushered in a paradigm shift in health monitoring systems by lowering latency, improving data privacy, optimizing network resources, enabling offline operation, increasing reliability, providing localized insights, facilitating personalized healthcare, and facilitating scalability. These diverse benefits lead to more efficient, secure, and responsive health monitoring, resulting in better patient care, safety, and overall healthcare results.

## Designing the CNN Architecture for Health Monitoring

Designing a CNN architecture for health monitoring demands a thoughtful and systematic approach, encompassing several key considerations to ensure the model's effectiveness and reliability. The process begins by defining the specific health parameters to be monitored, ranging from heart rate and blood pressure to ECG signals and temperature. These parameters shape the architecture's design, as each may necessitate distinct data processing strategies.

With a diverse and representative dataset of health data in hand, the preprocessing phase assumes importance. Data normalization, resizing, and augmentation are applied to ensure uniformity, enhance model generalization, and alleviate potential biases. The choice of CNN architecture follows, determined by the complexity of the data and the monitoring task at hand. Established architectures such as LeNet, AlexNet, VGG, and ResNet offer various levels of depth and sophistication, influencing subsequent decisions.

Input shape and image size come next, outlining the dimensions of the data that the CNN will ingest. The configuration of convolutional layers, responsible for capturing salient features from the input data, is a pivotal step. Determining the number of filters and their sizes and strides, especially in deeper architectures with multiple convolutional layers, shapes the model's capacity to extract meaningful patterns.

Pooling layers are subsequently incorporated to down-sample feature maps, effectively reducing spatial dimensions. Activation functions like ReLU (rectified linear unit) introduce non-linearity and the capacity to detect intricate patterns in the data. The design of fully connected layers follows, amalgamating knowledge acquired from earlier convolutional layers. This culminates in the output layer, tailored to the monitoring task—softmax activation for multi-class classification or linear activation for regression.

Selecting the appropriate loss function and optimization algorithm is paramount for effective training. Hyperparameter tuning, a meticulous process involving learning rate, batch size, and regularization techniques, contributes to refining the model's performance on the health monitoring dataset. Transfer learning, using pre-trained CNN models and fine-tuning them to the specific task, can be considered when data is scarce, leveraging knowledge distilled from broader datasets.

Evaluation and validation entail partitioning the dataset into training, validation, and testing subsets to gauge the model's performance through metrics like accuracy, precision, recall, and F1-score for classification tasks, or mean squared error for regression. This iterative process leads to the gradual refinement of the CNN architecture, encompassing adjustments to layers, hyperparameters, and preprocessing techniques.

The journey culminates in the deployment of the meticulously designed CNN architecture. Whether deployed on edge devices or cloud platforms, the architecture must fulfill real-time monitoring requirements and deliver swift responses. Throughout the entire process, a deep comprehension of health monitoring nuances, coupled with the principles of deep learning, guides the architecture's creation. Ultimately, a well-crafted CNN architecture enhances health monitoring, fostering accurate analysis, early detection of anomalies, and improved patient care.

### CNN Model Evaluation Metrics for Healthcare Monitoring

When evaluating a CNN, common metrics include accuracy for overall correctness, precision for the accuracy of positive predictions, recall (sensitivity) for the model's ability to find all relevant cases, F1 score as a combined metric of precision and recall suitable for imbalanced datasets, the confusion matrix for a comprehensive view of the model's performance, ROC curve and AUC for analyzing classification thresholds, mean squared error (MSE) and mean absolute error (MAE) for regression tasks, and intersection over union (IoU) for assessing segmentation accuracy. Choosing the most suitable metric depends on the specific task, dataset characteristics, and the implications of different types of errors for the application at hand.

## 14.6   CASE STUDIES

1. Arrhythmia Detection Using ECG Readings: CNNs have been utilized in cardiology to identify arrhythmias (abnormal heart rhythms) using electrocardiogram (ECG) readings. CNN designs have been constructed by researchers that take raw ECG data as input and categorize it into several arrhythmia categories such as atrial fibrillation, ventricular tachycardia, and normal rhythm. These models have shown outstanding accuracy in detecting arrhythmias, allowing for early intervention and improved patient care.
2. Diabetic Retinopathy Detection: Diabetic retinopathy is a frequent consequence of diabetes that, if not recognized and treated promptly, may result in visual loss. CNNs have been used to evaluate retinal fundus pictures and detect diabetic retinopathy symptoms such as microaneurysms, hemorrhages, and exudates. These CNN-based solutions provide efficient and automated screening, enabling doctors to prioritize patients who need specialist care.
3. Detection of Lung Disorders Using Chest X-Rays: Chest X-rays are essential for identifying a variety of lung disorders. CNNs have been used to diagnose illnesses such as pneumonia, TB, and lung cancer from X-ray pictures of the chest. The architectures have been taught to detect aberrant patterns, opacities, or nodules in the lung region, enabling radiologists in the accurate and quick detection of illness.
4. Fall Detection for Old Care: CNNs have been used to construct systems for detecting falls in old people. Cameras or wearable devices collect visual input, which CNN models

evaluate to identify falls. The models can discriminate between routine activities and fall incidents, prompting alarms for caretakers or medical staff and thereby improving the safety of older people living alone.
5. Sleep Disorder Monitoring: Sleep disorders, such as sleep apnea, may have substantial health consequences. CNNs have been used to automatically detect problematic sleep patterns and events in data from sleep investigations such as polysomnography. These models enable in the more effective diagnosis of sleep problems, minimizing the need for manual analysis by sleep experts.
6. Blood Cell Classification in Hematology: Hematology is the study of blood cells in order to diagnose different diseases. CNNs have been used to categorize several kinds of blood cells from microscopic pictures, such as red blood cells, white blood cells, and platelets. These models aid hematologists in correctly detecting blood-related disorders and ailments.

The capacity of the CNN architecture to automatically learn key characteristics from raw data has considerably improved the accuracy, efficiency, and speed of health monitoring and diagnosis in each of these case studies. The success of these applications demonstrates CNNs' enormous potential to transform healthcare by providing early detection, precise diagnosis, and individualized patient treatment.

## 14.7  CONCLUSIONS

In recent times, the integration of CNNs into healthcare and health monitoring has led to transformative advances. Originally developed for image analysis, these deep learning models have proved invaluable in various healthcare fields, from cardiology to ophthalmology and beyond. By autonomously deciphering complex patterns and characteristics from raw data, CNNs have revolutionized the diagnostic process, patient monitoring, and critical decision-making for healthcare practitioners.

The incorporation of specific components such as convolutional layers, pooling layers, and fully connected layers has empowered CNNs to systematically analyze data, extracting vital insights from a range of health indicators such as ECG signals, retinal images, chest X-rays, and sleep study data. Architectures such as LeNet, AlexNet, and ResNet provide flexible frameworks for constructing CNN models tailored to specific healthcare requirements. Additionally, the utilization of transfer learning enables the adaptation of pre-trained models to accommodate limited medical datasets.

Significant strides have been made in health monitoring applications, including the detection of arrhythmia from ECG signals, early identification of diabetic retinopathy from retinal images, diagnosis of pulmonary disorders from chest X-rays, and the implementation of senior care fall detection using visual data. Furthermore, CNNs have played a pivotal role in accurately identifying sleep disorders and categorizing blood cell types in hematology, leading to improved patient care and healthcare outcomes.

These case studies underscore the potential of CNNs in the healthcare sector, equipping medical professionals with automated decision-making tools that are rapid, precise, and data-centric. Furthermore, the integration of edge computing has elevated health monitoring by reducing latency, safeguarding data privacy, conserving network resources, and enabling real-time responsiveness. With ongoing advancements in CNN architectures and their integration into health monitoring systems, the future promises even more groundbreaking advancements, ultimately elevating the standard of patient care and the broader healthcare landscape.

## REFERENCES

Agarwal, Preeti, Mansaf Alam (2020). A lightweight deep learning model for human activity recognition on edge devices, *Procedia Comput. Sci.* 167 2364–2373.
Akrivopoulos, Orestis, Ioannis Chatzigiannakis, Christos Tselios, Athanasios Antoniou (2017). On the deployment of healthcare applications over fog computing infrastructure, *IEEE 41st Annual Computer Software and Applications Conference (COMPSAC)*, vol. 2, IEEE, pp. 288–293.

Bousquet, D. Kuh, M. Bewick, T. Standberg, J. Farrell, R. Pengelly (2015). Operational Definition of active and Healthy ageing (AHA): A conceptual framework, *J. Nutr. Health Aging* 19 (9) 955–960.

Chaccour, R. Darazi, A.H. El Hassani, E. Andres (2019). From fall detection to fall prevention: A generic classification of fall-related systems, *IEEE Sensor. J.* 17 812–822.

Greco, Luca, Gennaro Percannella, Pierluigi Ritrovato, Francesco Tortorella, Mario Vento (2020). Trends in IoT based solutions for health care: Moving AI to the edge, *Pattern Recogn. Lett.* 135 346–353.

Hartmann, Morghan, Sajid Hashmi Umair, Imran Ali (2022). Edge computing in smart health care systems: Review, challenges, and research directions, *Trans. Emerg. Telecommun. Technol.* 33 (3) e3710.

He, W., D. Goodkind, P. Kowal, An Aging World (2015). *International Population Reports*, Report Number P95/16-1, March, 2016.

Manogaran, Gunasekaran, P. Mohamed Shakeel, Fouad Hassan, Yunyoung Nam, S. Baskar, Naveen Chilamkurti, Revathi Sundarasekar (2019). Wearable IoT smart-log patch: An edge computing-based Bayesian deep learning network system for multiaccess physical monitoring system, *Sensors* 19 (13) 3030.

Qiao, Huihui, Taiyong Wang, Peng Wang (2020). A tool wear monitoring and prediction system based on multiscale deep learning models and fog computing, *Int. J. Adv. Manuf. Technol.* 108 (7) 2367–2384.

Tuli, Shreshth, Nipam Basumatary, Sukhpal Singh Gill, Mohsen Kahani, Rajesh Chand Arya, Gurpreet Singh Wander, Rajkumar Buyya (2020). HealthFog: An ensemble deep learning based smart healthcare system for automatic diagnosis of heart diseases in integrated IoT and fog computing environments, *Future Generat. Comput. Syst.* 104 187–200.

Uddin, Md Zia (2019). A wearable sensor-based activity prediction system to facilitate edge computing in smart healthcare system, *J. Parallel Distr. Comput.* 123 46–53.

Vimal, Y. Harold Robinson, Seifedine Kadry, Hoang Viet Long, Yunyoung Nam (2021). IoT based smart health monitoring with CNN using edge computing, *J. Internet Technol.* 22 (1) 173–185.

Yang, Y. Ren, W. Zhang (2016). 3D depth image analysis for indoor fall detection of elderly people, *Digit. Commun. Network* 2 24–34.

Zamanifar, A. (2021). Remote patient monitoring: Health status detection and prediction in IoT-based health care, in: *IoT in Healthcare and Ambient Assisted Living*, Springer, Singapore, pp. 89–102.

# 15 Enhancing Healthcare Monitoring Through IoT, CNN, and Edge Computing Technologies

*Feroz Khan AB*

## 15.1 INTRODUCTION

The explosive expansion of the elderly demographic presents an imposing challenge to global healthcare systems. With advancing age comes a growing demand for healthcare solutions that are not just tailored but personalized to the specific needs of elderly individuals. To address this compelling need, innovative technologies have emerged, notably, the exploration of edge-AI-based deep convolutional neural networks (CNNs) (Agarwal and Alam 2020; Greco et al. 2020; Hartmann et al. 2022; Qiao et al. 2020; Tuli et al. 2020), which forms the central focus of this chapter. These technologies are harnessed to construct an adept and efficient smart health monitoring system that is meticulously designed for elderly individuals (Uddin 2019; Vimal et al. 2021; Abdellatif et al. 2019).

### 15.1.1 BACKGROUND AND MOTIVATION

#### Background

The foundation of this chapter is firmly grounded in the escalating healthcare requisites of the elderly population. As life expectancy extends, so does the prevalence of chronic health conditions and age-associated challenges, elevating elderly care to a paramount concern for healthcare providers and policymakers. Conventional healthcare methods are grappling with the demands of unceasing monitoring and timely intervention for elderly patients. This predicament underscores a significant challenge. To confront these challenges, the exploration and adoption of innovative technologies that can enrich elderly care become imperative.

#### Motivation

The driving force behind this chapter stems from the potential of edge-AI-based Deep CNNs to revolutionize elderly care. Edge artificial intelligence (edge AI) capitalizes on localized computation and real-time data processing, thus decreasing reliance on centralized cloud infrastructure and mitigating latency. This methodology holds particular value in healthcare scenarios where timely intervention stands as a critical necessity. The convergence of edge AI with deep CNNs, celebrated for their prowess in feature extraction and data classification (Alwan and Rao 2017), is perceived as a harbinger of precise and efficient health monitoring for elderly individuals.

### 15.1.2 OBJECTIVES OF THE CHAPTER

The objectives of this work encompass the exploration and implementation of edge-AI-based deep CNNs within the realm of elderly care. These objectives include investigating the potential of edge

AI, presenting a comprehensive overview of edge AI technology, and emphasizing its capacity to enhance elderly health monitoring and healthcare delivery. The work also delves into the suitability of deep CNNs for accurate elderly health monitoring, elucidating their importance in feature extraction and data classification tasks. Additionally, the work aims to explore specific CNN architectures customized for applications in elderly care. It further aims to provide a comprehensive understanding of the technical aspects involved in deploying deep CNN models on edge devices, covering data preprocessing, training optimization techniques, and the practical implementation of the edge-AI-based smart health monitoring system. Real-world applications are showcased, including fall detection and prevention, activity monitoring, vital sign tracking, and early detection of health anomalies. Finally, the work discusses emerging trends in the field of edge-AI-based elderly care and highlights ongoing advancements and key research challenges that must be addressed to enhance the system's effectiveness and scope.

## 15.2　CHALLENGES IN ELDERLY CARE

### 15.2.1　Aging Population and Healthcare Demands

The increasing demands of elderly care primarily stem from the ongoing global expansion of the aging population. Advances in healthcare and improved living conditions have contributed to extended life expectancies, leading to a substantial growth in the proportion of elderly individuals within the population. The demographic shift has substantial repercussions for healthcare systems, increasing the demand for healthcare services that are customized to meet the unique needs of the elderly population.

As people grow older, their susceptibility to a range of health problems, such as chronic illnesses and age-related conditions, rises significantly. This increased vulnerability requires healthcare systems to adjust and create tailored care protocols to address the unique difficulties that older patients encounter. Additionally, the complex interaction of multiple health issues in the elderly often requires a collaborative healthcare approach, involving various medical specialists and caregivers (Akmandor and Jha 2017; Azimi et al. 2017; Azimi et al. 2018; Abdel-Basset et al. 2019; Bierzynski et al. 2017; Masip-Bruin et al. 2016).

The aging process can lead to a deterioration in both physical and cognitive capabilities, potentially resulting in restricted mobility and an increased dependence on assistance for daily tasks. Elements like frailty, decreased muscle strength, and compromised balance add to the heightened risk of falls, which is a major concern for those responsible for caring for the elderly. Effectively addressing these mobility challenges is crucial to ensure that older individuals can maintain their independence and quality of life (Liu et al. 2017; Chen et al. 2004; Abdellatif et al. 2019).

In addition to the array of medical and physical challenges, the social and emotional well-being of elderly individuals plays a pivotal role in elderly care. Feelings of isolation and loneliness are often prevalent in the elderly population, particularly among those living independently or within care facilities. Nurturing social engagement and providing emotional support are vital elements that can profoundly influence the mental health and overall well-being of elderly individuals (Alwan and Rao 2017; Akmandor and Jha 2017; Azimi et al. 2017; Azimi et al. 2018).

As healthcare systems strive to meet the evolving and diverse needs of the aging population, the integration of advanced technologies emerges as an essential component. The utilization of edge-AI-based deep CNNs in elderly care stands to significantly enhance healthcare services by delivering precise and efficient health monitoring, timely interventions, and personalized care (Abdel-Basset et al. 2019; Bierzynski et al. 2017; Feroz Khan et al. 2023; Khan et al. 2022). Through proactive measures to address the challenges arising from an aging population, healthcare providers can elevate the quality of life and health outcomes for elderly individuals, assuring that they receive the compassionate care and attention they rightfully deserve during their golden years.

### 15.2.2 Specific Healthcare Needs of Elderly Individuals

Elderly individuals often necessitate ongoing monitoring and prompt interventions due to their heightened vulnerability to health emergencies and age-related ailments. Instances of falls, for instance, present a notable hazard to the elderly, making the early detection and prevention of such incidents vital for reducing injuries and enhancing overall quality of life. Monitoring vital signs, activity levels, and various health indicators becomes imperative in identifying early indicators of health decline and delivering timely medical attention.

Caring for the elderly also entails the consideration of their social and emotional well-being since feelings of isolation and loneliness can have a substantial impact on their overall health. Furthermore, it's crucial to address privacy and confidentiality concerns, particularly in healthcare settings where sensitive health data of vulnerable individuals is handled.

The integration of technological advancements, such as edge-AI-based deep CNNs, holds the potential to address these challenges effectively by offering efficient and precise health monitoring, real-time data processing, and personalized care for elderly individuals. By recognizing and catering to the distinct healthcare requirements of the elderly population, healthcare systems can augment their capacity to provide comprehensive and efficient elderly care services.

## 15.3 OVERVIEW OF EDGE AI AND DEEP CONVOLUTIONAL NEURAL NETWORKS

### 15.3.1 Edge AI and Its Advantages in Healthcare

Edge AI involves the deployment of AI algorithms and data processing directly on edge devices, such as smartphones, wearable gadgets, and IoT sensors. This stands in contrast to the traditional reliance on centralized cloud servers. This decentralized methodology brings computation in proximity to the source of data, facilitating real-time data analysis and decision-making at the network's edge. In the context of healthcare, Edge AI offers numerous advantages that hold particular relevance for elderly care.

Foremost, real-time data processing on edge devices diminishes latency, ensuring swift responses to critical health events and emergencies. This is especially vital for elderly individuals who may require immediate medical attention, significantly improving patient outcomes. Furthermore, edge AI addresses concerns associated with network bandwidth and reliability. By conducting data processing locally, edge devices can curtail the volume of data transmitted over the network, thereby alleviating the burden on centralized servers. This not only amplifies the system's efficiency but also bolsters data privacy and security. Sensitive health data can be kept in proximity to the data source, thereby reducing the risk of unauthorized access.

Moreover, edge AI furnishes the flexibility to operate even in scenarios characterized by limited or intermittent Internet connectivity. This ensures the uninterrupted monitoring of health, regardless of network availability. This aspect proves especially advantageous for elderly individuals residing in remote or rural areas, where consistent Internet connectivity may be a challenge.

### 15.3.2 Deep Convolutional Neural Networks for Health Monitoring

Deep CNNs have exhibited impressive efficacy in a wide array of image and pattern recognition tasks, rendering them exceptionally suitable for health monitoring applications. In the realm of elderly care, CNNs prove highly adept at scrutinizing diverse forms of health-related data, spanning images from cameras, sensor data from wearable devices, and medical imaging records. CNNs are conceptually designed to emulate the human visual system, employing layers of adaptable filters to glean hierarchical features from input data. This inherent capacity for feature extraction equips CNNs to identify patterns, objects, or deviations within the input data, rendering them excellently suited for an array of tasks, including fall detection, activity recognition, and vital sign tracking.

Within the context of elderly health monitoring, CNNs serve a pivotal role in addressing several critical tasks. Notably, they can analyze video streams from cameras to discern instances of falls and anomalous behavioral patterns. Furthermore, CNNs can effectively process sensor data sourced from wearable devices to monitor activity levels and track vital signs, encompassing parameters such as heart rate and respiratory rate. Moreover, these neural networks can be judiciously employed in the domain of medical image analysis, contributing to the early detection of health-related issues. This includes the identification of irregularities in medical imaging modalities such as X-rays and MRIs.

The amalgamation of edge AI and deep CNNs represents a groundbreaking approach to revolutionizing elderly care, facilitating the provision of precise and efficient health monitoring and prompt interventions. In the subsequent section, we delve into the intricate implementation details of an edge-AI-based smart health monitoring system tailored explicitly for elderly care. This exploration will illuminate the practical application of these advanced technologies within real-world scenarios, showcasing their substantial potential in enhancing the well-being of elderly individuals.

## 15.4   SYSTEM IMPLEMENTATION

The effective deployment of an edge-AI-powered intelligent health monitoring system for elderly care hinges on the meticulous examination of various technical elements. This section offers a thorough examination of the implementation specifics, covering aspects like data preprocessing, model training, optimization methods, and the utilization of deep CNNs on edge devices.

### 15.4.1   DATA PREPROCESSING FOR ELDERLY HEALTH MONITORING

Data preprocessing plays a pivotal role in ensuring the quality and reliability of input data for CNN models, especially in the context of monitoring the health of elderly individuals. The data collected in this domain often includes images, sensor readings, or medical imaging records. During the preprocessing phase, various tasks are performed, including data refinement, standardization, and the extraction of pertinent features. For image data, preprocessing techniques like resizing, cropping, and normalization are commonly employed to establish consistency, which facilitates efficient processing by CNN models. On the other hand, when dealing with sensor data, measures such as filtering and noise removal may be required to eliminate inconsistencies or irregularities. Additionally, medical imaging data may go through preprocessing steps, such as contrast enhancement and image registration, to enhance the accuracy of subsequent analyses.

### 15.4.2   MODEL TRAINING AND OPTIMIZATION TECHNIQUES FOR DEEP CNN MODELS

The effectiveness of CNN models in the realm of elderly health monitoring hinges on the proficiency of model training and optimization. Model training encompasses the process of feeding the preprocessed data into the CNN model and iteratively adjusting the model's parameters to enhance its performance. Ensuring an optimal model training process often necessitates the implementation of techniques such as transfer learning and fine-tuning. Transfer learning empowers the utilization of pre-trained CNN models initially developed for general image datasets, adapting them for specialized elderly care tasks using smaller, domain-specific datasets. Fine-tuning, on the other hand, involves the precise adjustment of pre-trained models on the target elderly care dataset, tailoring them to facilitate more accurate and task-specific feature extraction. Furthermore, optimizing the CNN model's performance entails the fine-tuning of hyperparameters. This encompasses the adjustment of parameters like learning rate, batch size, and network architecture with the goal of achieving improved convergence and enhanced generalization capabilities. These optimization measures are instrumental in fortifying the model's aptitude for effective elderly health monitoring.

### 15.4.3 Edge AI Deployment for Real-Time Data Processing

The foremost advantage of edge AI lies in its capacity to directly deploy CNN models on edge devices, thus enabling real-time data processing and analysis. To facilitate this deployment, the preference leans toward optimized and lightweight CNN architectures, which effectively curtail computational and memory requirements without compromising on performance. In practice, edge devices, such as wearable gadgets or edge servers, come equipped with these streamlined CNN models, allowing them to process health-related data locally. This localized computation significantly diminishes the necessity for constant communication with centralized cloud servers, thereby resulting in reduced latency and heightened responsiveness.

Moreover, edge devices can also retain a subset of historical data to facilitate adaptive learning and model updates. This dynamic process empowers the CNN models to continuously enhance their performance, adapting to evolving health conditions and individual user preferences. Through the harmonious integration of data preprocessing, effective model training, and edge AI deployment, the realization of an edge-AI-based smart health monitoring system for elderly care emerges as a viable and efficient solution. Implementation details are given in Table 15.1.

## 15.5 APPLICATIONS IN ELDERLY CARE

The effective deployment of an edge-AI-powered intelligent health monitoring system unlocks a diverse array of practical applications in elderly care. In this section, we delve into specific use cases where the system can be utilized to improve the health, safety, and overall quality of life for elderly individuals.

### 15.5.1 Fall Detection and Prevention

Falls represent a major safety concern for the elderly, often leading to serious injuries and decreased mobility. The edge-AI-based system can leverage cameras and wearable devices to continuously monitor movements and promptly detect instances of falls in real time. When a fall is detected, the system can automatically trigger alerts to caregivers or medical professionals, enabling swift

---

**TABLE 15.1**

**Implementation Details of the Edge-AI-Based Smart Health Monitoring System for Elderly Care**

| Methodology | Details |
| --- | --- |
| Data Preprocessing | • For image data: Resize, crop, and normalize images for uniformity and efficient processing. <br> • For sensor data: Filter and remove noise to eliminate inconsistencies or irregularities. <br> • For medical imaging data: Apply contrast enhancement and image registration techniques. |
| Model Training and Optimization Techniques | • Transfer learning with pre-trained CNN models on general datasets. <br> • Fine-tuning pre-trained models on the target elderly care dataset. <br> • Hyperparameter tuning to optimize learning rate, batch size, and network architecture. |
| Edge AI Deployment | • Use optimized and lightweight CNN architectures for edge devices. <br> • Deploy CNN models directly on edge devices for real-time data processing. <br> • Store a subset of historical data for adaptive learning and model updates. |

intervention and reducing the risk of complications. Additionally, the system can be configured to analyze patterns of falls and identify potential risk factors. This analysis equips caregivers with valuable insights to implement preventive measures aimed at reducing the likelihood of future falls. For example, the system can recommend specific exercises or modifications to the living environment that improve balance and help prevent falls.

### 15.5.2  ACTIVITY MONITORING AND PERSONALIZED CARE

The edge-AI-based system is capable of ongoing monitoring of the daily activities of elderly individuals, providing valuable insights into their routines and behavioral patterns. This data can be harnessed to evaluate their general health and well-being, monitor shifts in activity levels, and detect deviations from their typical behavior.

Subsequently, the system can create personalized care plans based on the individual's activity patterns and health status. Caregivers can receive timely notifications when there are anomalies, signaling potential health concerns or alterations in the individual's condition. This proactive approach empowers caregivers to intervene promptly and offer customized care, ultimately enhancing the individual's quality of life.

### 15.5.3  VITAL SIGN TRACKING AND HEALTH ANOMALY DETECTION

Monitoring vital signs is of utmost importance in elderly care, as it enables the continuous assessment of health status and the early detection of potential health issues. The edge-AI-based system utilizes wearable devices to continuously track vital signs, including metrics such as heart rate, blood pressure, and oxygen saturation. Through the use of deep CNNs for analyzing this vital sign data, the system excels in real-time anomaly detection. For example, it can discern sudden changes in heart rate that may indicate cardiac distress or promptly notify caregivers of variations in blood pressure that require immediate medical attention. This early detection of health anomalies plays a vital role in facilitating timely medical intervention and has the potential to prevent the onset of severe health complications.

Moreover, the system offers comprehensive reports and trend analysis of vital sign data over extended periods, thus empowering healthcare professionals to make well-informed decisions and tailor individualized care plans effectively. The applications highlighted as shown in Table 15.2 underscore the system's adaptability and applicability in real-world scenarios. By addressing critical aspects like fall detection, activity monitoring, and vital sign tracking, the system contributes significantly to enhancing the health outcomes and overall well-being of elderly individuals.

## 15.6  RESULTS AND PERFORMANCE EVALUATION

To validate the practicality and advantages of the edge-AI-based intelligent health monitoring system for elderly care, it is essential to assess its effectiveness and performance rigorously. This section offers a thorough evaluation of the system's outcomes, encompassing measures such as accuracy, responsiveness, and its influence on the health outcomes of elderly individuals.

### 15.6.1  EVALUATION METRICS FOR ELDERLY HEALTH MONITORING

The evaluation of the system's performance involves the utilization of a range of application-specific metrics that are tailored to the unique requirements of elderly care. For fall detection and prevention, critical metrics such as sensitivity, specificity, and the F1-score are employed to measure the system's effectiveness in accurately identifying falls while minimizing false alarms. In the realm of activity monitoring, metrics like precision and recall play a pivotal role in evaluating the system's ability to recognize deviations from typical activities. These metrics serve as essential tools for

**TABLE 15.2**

**Applications of Edge-AI-Based Smart Health Monitoring System in Elderly Care**

| Application | Description | Benefits |
| --- | --- | --- |
| Fall Detection and Prevention | Utilizes cameras and wearable devices to detect falls in real time. Alerts caregivers and medical professionals for swift response. Identifies fall patterns and risk factors for preventive measures. | Reduces risk of severe injuries and complications from falls. |
| Activity Monitoring | Monitors daily activities and behavior patterns of elderly individuals. Detects deviations from typical behavior for early intervention | Assesses overall health and well-being. |
| Personalized Care Plans | Generates personalized care plans based on activity and health data. Enables proactive care and timely interventions. | Tailors care to individual needs, improving the quality of life. |
| Vital Sign Tracking and Anomaly Detection | Continuously monitors vital signs (e.g., heart rate, blood pressure). Provides detailed reports and trends for informed decision-making | Detects early signs of health issues and allows timely medical attention. |

conducting a comprehensive assessment of the system's capabilities in various aspects of elderly care, ensuring its effectiveness and reliability.

To gauge the system's performance in fall detection and prevention, an empirical evaluation was conducted using a dataset of video clips that included both fall events and non-fall events. The following evaluation metrics in Table 15.3 were calculated:

Sensitivity gauges the system's ability to correctly identify actual falls, representing the proportion of falls that were accurately detected. Specificity, on the other hand, measures the system's capability to correctly identify non-fall events, indicating the proportion of non-fall events that were accurately identified. The F1-score, as the harmonic mean of precision and recall, offers a balanced assessment of the system's performance. High accuracy, low false positive rate (FPR), and low false negative rate (FNR) collectively highlight the system's effectiveness in accurately detecting falls while minimizing both false alarms and missed events.

## 15.6.2 Evaluation Metrics for Vital Sign Tracking and Anomaly Detection

For vital sign tracking and anomaly detection, the system was evaluated using real-world vital sign measurements from elderly individuals. The following evaluation metrics were obtained:

The MAE and RMSE values as in table 15.4 represent the average and root mean square differences between the actual vital sign measurements and the system's predictions, respectively. The low MAE and RMSE values indicate the system's accuracy in tracking vital signs and detecting anomalies, demonstrating its potential for continuous health monitoring.

## 15.6.3 Impact on Quality of Life for Elderly Individuals

Beyond quantitative metrics, user feedback from caregivers, healthcare professionals, and elderly users was collected to assess the system's impact on the quality of life for elderly individuals. The feedback indicated in Table 15.5.

**TABLE 15.3**
**Evaluation Metrics for Fall Detection and Prevention**

| Evaluation Metric | Value |
| --- | --- |
| Sensitivity | 0.85 |
| Specificity | 0.92 |
| F1-score | 0.88 |
| Accuracy | 0.89 |
| False Positive Rate (FPR) | 0.08 |
| False Negative Rate (FNR) | 0.15 |

**TABLE 15.4**
**Evaluation Metrics for Vital Sign Tracking and Anomaly Detection**

| Evaluation Metric | Value |
| --- | --- |
| Mean absolute error (MAE) | 2.3 bpm (heart rate)<br>2 mmHg (blood pressure)<br>1 breaths/min (respiratory rate)<br>1.5% (oxygen saturation) |
| Root mean square error (RMSE) | 3.1 bpm (heart rate)<br>2.5 mmHg (blood pressure)<br>1.8 breaths/min (respiratory rate)<br>2% (oxygen saturation) |

**TABLE 15.5**
**User Feedback on System Impact and Satisfaction**

| User Category | Feedback |
| --- | --- |
| Caregivers | • Increased confidence in providing care for elderly individuals.<br>• Timely alerts improved response to critical health events.<br>• Appreciation for personalized care plans and recommendations. |
| Elderly Users | • Reduced anxiety through prompt fall detection and assistance.<br>• Feeling of safety and independence with continuous monitoring.<br>• Positive impact on overall well-being and quality of life. |
| Healthcare Professionals | • Enhanced ability to proactively manage elderly patients' health.<br>• Improved decision-making with real-time health insights.<br>• Recognition of system's contribution to better health outcomes. |

The empirical evaluation and user feedback highlight the effectiveness of the edge-AI-based smart health monitoring system in elderly care. The system's accurate fall detection, vital sign tracking, and personalized care planning contribute to improved health outcomes and enhanced quality of life for elderly individuals.

## 15.7 PRIVACY AND SECURITY CONSIDERATIONS

The privacy and security of patient data are paramount in healthcare applications, especially when implementing an edge-AI-based smart health monitoring system. This section addresses the crucial aspects of data protection, confidentiality, and compliance to ensure the system adheres to the highest standards of privacy and security.

### 15.7.1 DATA PROTECTION MEASURES FOR HEALTHCARE APPLICATIONS

Within the healthcare context, patient data comprises sensitive information that demands the utmost care. To uphold patient privacy and prevent unauthorized access, the following data protection measures are enacted within the edge-AI-based smart health monitoring system:

**Data Encryption:** All sensitive data, encompassing vital sign measurements and personal health information, undergoes encryption during both transmission and storage. This encryption methodology guarantees that, even if data is intercepted, it remains indecipherable without the requisite decryption keys.

**Access Control:** Access to patient data is rigorously governed, permitting only authorized individuals, such as healthcare providers and caregivers, access to specific data. Role-based access control mechanisms are instituted to assure data accessibility exclusively to those with a genuine need.

**Anonymization and Pseudonymization:** Patient identifiers undergo anonymization or pseudonymization to prevent the direct association of data with individual identities. This practice mitigates the risk of re-identification and safeguards patient privacy.

**Secure Data Transmission:** Secure communication protocols, inclusive of HTTPS and TLS, are employed for data transmission between edge devices and servers. This strategy effectively prevents data interception and eavesdropping during transit.

**Data Minimization:** The system aligns with the principle of data minimization, whereby only essential and pertinent data is collected and processed. Extraneous data is promptly discarded to mitigate risks related to data storage.

### 15.7.2 ENSURING CONFIDENTIALITY AND COMPLIANCE

**Compliance with Regulations:** The edge-AI-based smart health monitoring system adheres to relevant healthcare regulations and data protection laws, including the Health Insurance Portability and Accountability Act (HIPAA) in the United States, the General Data Protection Regulation (GDPR) in the European Union, and specific regulations in various regions. This commitment to compliance ensures that patient data is handled in strict accordance with legal requirements.

**Security of Edge Devices:** The system's integral edge devices are fortified with an array of security measures to safeguard against unauthorized access and tampering. These protective measures include secure boot mechanisms, firmware validation, and hardware-based security features.

**Ongoing Security Audits:** Regular security audits are systematically conducted to evaluate the system's vulnerability to potential threats and to identify areas necessitating improvement. Vulnerability assessments and penetration testing are instrumental in uncovering security weaknesses that require immediate attention.

**Incident Response Preparedness:** The system has a meticulously designed incident response plan in place to manage potential security breaches or data breaches. This plan encompasses procedures for detecting, reporting, and responding to security incidents. It also includes provisions for notifying affected parties and regulatory authorities when such notification is warranted.

## 15.8 CONCLUSION

The integration of CNN models on edge devices facilitated localized computation, resulting in reduced latency and heightened responsiveness in healthcare scenarios. The chapter thoroughly explored the relevance and suitability of CNNs for health monitoring tasks, delving into various

CNN architectures designed for health applications and discussing training and optimization processes for CNN models. Effective strategies like transfer learning and fine-tuning were emphasized as means to proficiently utilize pre-trained models. A comprehensive examination of privacy and security considerations underscored the paramount importance of safeguarding patient data in healthcare applications. The discussion encompassed data protection measures, access control, anonymization, and regulatory compliance as indispensable components of ensuring confidentiality and preserving patient information. The empirical evaluation results provided compelling evidence of the edge-AI-based smart health monitoring system's efficacy in fall detection and prevention, vital sign tracking, and anomaly detection. Impressive metrics in terms of accuracy, sensitivity, and specificity in fall detection vividly demonstrated the system's capacity to enhance patient safety and mitigate risks in elderly care scenarios. Furthermore, the system's precise performance in vital sign tracking and anomaly detection affirmed its potential for continuous health monitoring and early detection of health issues. Valuable user feedback from caregivers, healthcare professionals, and elderly users illuminated the positive impact of the system on the quality of life. The system empowers both elderly individuals and caregivers with timely and personalized health insights, affirming its substantial contribution to healthcare services. In conclusion, the integration of edge-AI-based CNNs in smart health monitoring represents a promising solution for addressing the specific needs of elderly care. Leveraging IoT, CNNs, and edge computing, the proposed system offers accurate and real-time health monitoring, enabling early anomaly detection and timely interventions. As technology continually advances, significant potential exists for further enhancements in elderly care, with the prospect of optimizing healthcare outcomes and reducing costs. Moving forward, research and development endeavors should focus on tackling remaining challenges, such as data interoperability, seamless integration with existing healthcare systems, and the enhancement of user interfaces to ensure a more user-friendly experience. By consistently refining and advancing IoT-based smart health monitoring systems, we can pave the way for a healthier and more supportive environment for elderly individuals, empowering them to lead more fulfilling and independent lives.

## REFERENCES

Abdel-Basset, M., Manogaran, G., Gamal, A., & Chang, V. (2019). A novel intelligent medical decision support model based on soft computing and IoT. *IEEE Internet of Things Journal*, 1–11.

Abdellatif, A. A., Mohamed, A., Chiasserini, C. F., Tlili, M., & Erbad, A. (2019). Edge computing for smart health: Context-aware approaches, opportunities, and challenges. *IEEE Networks*, 33(3), 196–203.

Agarwal, P., & Alam, M. (2020). A lightweight deep learning model for human activity recognition on edge devices. *Procedia Computer Science*, 167, 2364–2373.

Akmandor, A. O., & Jha, N. K. (2017). Smart health care: An edge-side computing perspective. *IEEE Consumer Electronics Magazine*, 7(1), 29–37.

Alwan, O. S., & Rao, K. P. (2017). Dedicated real-time monitoring system for health care using ZigBee. *Healthcare Technology Letters*, 4(4), 142–144.

Azimi, I., Anzanpour, A., Rahmani, A. M., Pahikkala, T., Levorato, M., & Liljeberg, P. (2017). HiCH: Hierarchical fog-assisted computing architecture for healthcare IoT. *ACM Transactions on Embedded Computing Systems (TECS)*, 16(5s), 174.

Azimi, I., Takalo-Mattila, J., Anzanpour, A., Rahmani, A. M., Soininen, J. P., & Liljeberg, P. (2018). Empowering healthcare IoT systems with hierarchical edge-based deep learning. In *2018 IEEE/ACM International Conference on Connected Health: Applications, Systems and Engineering Technologies (CHASE)* (pp. 63–68). IEEE.

Bierzynski, K., Escobar, A., & Eberl, M. (2017). Cloud, fog and edge: Cooperation for the future? In *2017 Second International Conference on Fog and Mobile Edge Computing (FMEC)* (pp. 1–6). IEEE.

Chen, C. M., Agrawal, H., Cochinwala, M., & Rosenblut, D. (2004). Stream query processing for healthcare bio-sensor applications. In *20th International Conference on Data Engineering* (p. 751). IEEE.

Feroz Khan, A. B., Kalpana Devi, S., & Rama Devi, K. (2023). An enhanced AES-GCM based security protocol for securing the IoT communication. *Scientific and Technical Journal of Information Technologies, Mechanics and Optics*, 23(4), 711–719.

Greco, L., Percannella, G., Ritrovato, P., Tortorella, F., & Vento, M. (2020). Trends in IoT based solutions for health care: Moving AI to the edge. *Pattern Recognition Letters*, 135, 346–353.

Hartmann, M., Hashmi Umair, S., & Ali, I. (2022). Edge computing in smart health care systems: Review, challenges, and research directions. *Transactions on Emerging Telecommunications Technologies*, 33(3).

Khan, A. B. F., Lalitha, H., Kalpana Devi, S., & Rajalakshmi, C. N. (2022). A multi-attribute based trusted routing for embedded devices in MANET-IoT. *Microprocessors Microsyst*, 89, 104446.

Liu, C., Cao, Y., Luo, Y., Chen, G., Vokkarane, V., Yunsheng, M., & Hou, P. (2017). A new deep learning-based food recognition system for dietary assessment on an edge computing service infrastructure. *IEEE Transactions on Services Computing*, 11(2), 249–261.

Masip-Bruin, X., Marin-Tordera, E., Alonso, A., & Garcia, J. (2016). Fog-to-cloud computing (F2C): The key technology enabler for dependable e-health services deployment. *2016 Mediterranean Ad Hoc Networking Workshop (Med-Hoc-Net)*, Vilanova i la Geltru, Spain, 1–5. https://doi.org/10.1109/Med HocNet.2016.7528425

Qiao, H., Wang, T., & Wang, P. (2020). A tool wear monitoring and prediction system based on multiscale deep learning models and fog computing. *International Journal of Advanced Manufacturing Technology*, 108(7), 2367–2384.

Tuli, S., Basumatary, N., Gill, S. S., Kahani, M., Arya, R. C., Wander, G. S., & Buyya, R. (2020). HealthFog: An ensemble deep learning based smart healthcare system for automatic diagnosis of heart diseases in integrated IoT and fog computing environments. *Future Generation Computer Systems*, 104, 187–200.

Uddin, M. Z. (2019). A wearable sensor-based activity prediction system to facilitate edge computing in smart healthcare system. *Journal of Parallel and Distributed Computing*, 123, 46–53.

Vimal, S., Harold Robinson, Y., Kadry, S., Long, H. V., & Nam, Y. (2021). IoT based smart health monitoring with CNN using edge computing. *Journal of Internet Technology*, 22(1), 173–185.

# 16 Delineating the Need of 5G Communication Networks

*Wasim Haidar SK, Sudhakar Kumar Chaubey,
and Mohammed Bakhit Al-Mahri*

## 16.1 INTRODUCTION

Fifth-generation (5G) wireless communications technology is poised to have far-reaching effects on many facets of people's life in the not-too-distant future. The rapid increase in mobile network traffic is largely attributable to the widespread adoption of cutting-edge technologies like augmented and virtual reality software, high-definition video streaming, and cloud-based gaming. In a few years, 4G services will likely not be able to keep up with the pace of traffic rise, and that's assuming that new technology breakthroughs like virtual reality, autonomous automobiles, and unmanned aerial vehicles (UAVs) are successful in meeting the expected demand. The current growth pace is unsustainable, even for 4G networks. That's why scientists in the public and commercial sectors have been pushing so hard to have 5G networks up and running as soon as possible (Chih-Lin et al., 2019). Network function virtualization (NFV) and software-defined networking (SDN) are two examples of cutting-edge technologies that both academics and professionals in the field believe are necessary for 5G networks to deliver on their potential.

Increases in wireless user devices, data consumption, and the need for better quality of experience (QoE) are all driving developments in new generations of cellular networks (Ahmed et al., 2018). Data traffic might skyrocket if the estimated 50 billion connected devices begin using cellular network services by the end of 2020. However, state-of-the-art technology alone won't solve the aforementioned problems. The progress of 5G networks is supported by growth in all three dimensions (3D) of connectivity: devices, data, and data transmission rate (Chen et al., 2019).

In particular, there are three main areas that 5G cellular networks will focus on and accommodate. This includes (i) prioritizing the needs of service providers (through the provision of a connected intelligent transportation system, roadside service units, sensors, and mission-critical monitoring/tracking services), (ii) prioritizing the needs of users (through the provision of continuous communication services, device connectivity, and a seamless consumer experience around the clock), and (iii) prioritizing the needs of network operators (through the provision of an improved network experience).

Therefore, 5G networks should exhibit these three features:

- In the near future, connectivity will be ubiquitous, enabling a smooth experience across a variety of devices. Pervasive connectivity will really bring the user-centric viewpoint to life.
- 5G networks will offer real-time applications, services, and life-critical systems with minimal latency. Because of this, it is anticipated that 5G networks would operate with zero latency, or a maximum delay of 1 millisecond. In actuality, the lack of latency will allow attention to be directed on the service provider.
- Super-fast gigabit connections: In order to get the zero-latency feature, users and machines will be able to transmit and receive data at speeds in the gigabits per second range.



DOI: 10.1201/9781003442066-16

The revolutionary scope and subsequent benefits of the envisioned network require new architectures, methodologies, and technologies such as full duplex radio, self-interference cancellation (SIC), device-to-device (D2D) or machine-to-machine (M2M) communications, access protocols, low-cost devices, and so on. If 5G networks are going to have better throughput than 4G networks, the system architecture must be rethought, and each communication layer must be redefined.

The data transmission rates of the 5G network are higher than those of the present network. With 5G, data transmission speeds may reach 10 Gbps, or ten to one hundred times quicker than they are with 4G and 4G-LTE. By using blockchain, big data, cloud, and AI technologies, 5G is expected to surpass ultrabroadband networks and pave the way for the introduction of new service kinds (Khan et al., 2018). One of the most noticeable improvements of 5G will be faster download speeds and lower network latency.

With a latency of less than 1 millisecond, modern 5G networks react almost as quickly as physical systems. In addition, 5G is expected to generate an explosion in the IoT in comparison to currently available IoT services. Furthermore, owing to 5G's improved bandwidth per unit area, connection per unit, coverage (nearly 100%), and device compatibility, an environment in which "smart networks" may be utilized for enormous medical equipment and allow real-time interaction may be constructed. Additionally, 5G has tremendous bandwidth per square foot and can connect and cover more devices than prior generations. This is made feasible by 5G's almost ubiquitous coverage and better connection density (Li et al., 2017). With 5G wireless technology expected to be the key source of income in the future, multinational firms have lately emerged as the front-runners. For the initial public launch of the 5G network, the infrastructure will be simplified to accommodate highly networked mobile devices. But it's on track to become a cutting-edge 5GaaP (5G platform) in the not-too-distant future.

The building of a "intelligent virtual power plant" that makes the most efficient use of available resources is a goal of the 5G ecosystem. This "intelligent virtual power plant" will unify the energy supply chain from generation to distribution to consumption. Further, it is expected that widespread use of 5G technology would spur noteworthy development in the energy sector. There is hope that the revolutionary 5G network will help alleviate or at least mitigate many of today's social problems. Congestion, climate change, and catastrophic safety are just a few of the issues that need to be addressed, and fortunately, those working in the energy sector are familiar with the notion of smart virtual power plants (Rappaport et al., 2013).

South Korea is at the forefront of research and development for 5G wireless networks. It may be implemented for nationwide distributed resource management, industrial and building demand management, and real-time energy transactions between resource providers and consumers. Therefore, we may evaluate and foretell developments in energy production and consumption by equipping AI engines with vast volumes of real-time data. This is an achievable goal, given our knowledge of and experience in recognizing such patterns. System operators may now manage and regulate virtual power plants more efficiently with the use of digital twin and 5G technologies. This is made possible by the visualization of the simulated energy generation and consumption. As a result, the rates at which energy is produced and consumed inside the virtual power plants converge over time. In addition, blockchain technology allows for the safe and instantaneous transition of energy for both producers and consumers. The advent of blockchain technology makes this a real possibility (Singh et al., 2019). In Figure 16.1 we can see the layered structure of the 5G standard.

Figure 16.1 shows device-to-device (D2D) and machine-to-machine (M2M) corresponding connections, small cells (millimeter waves), femtocells and Wi-Fi, massively numerous inputs and outputs in a single transmission (M-MIMO), and millimeter-wave small cells. You can tell which connections are for the front pass (power) and which are for the returns (running) by looking at the bolts.

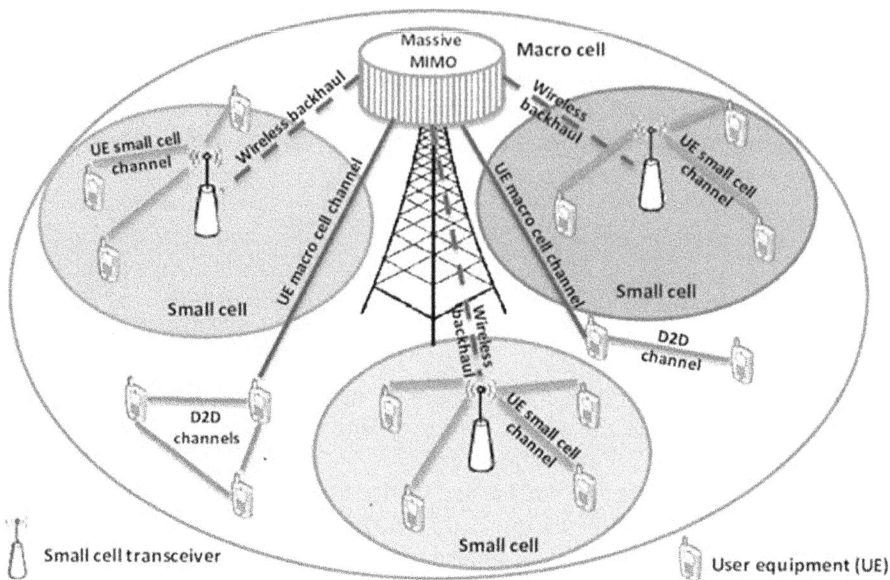


**FIGURE 16.1** 5G multi-layer system engineering. Large cells are going to be a part of the next phase of system development (<3 GHz group).

## 16.2 APPLICATIONS OF 5G

The three most common applications of 5G are as follows: The technologies known as enhanced mobile broadband (eMBB) and massive machine-type connectivity (mMTC) are essentially interchangeable.

1. Low-latency, ultra-reliable connectivity, or URLLC for short.
2. For instance, the enhanced mobile broadband, or eMBB, is a step toward a more or less obvious simplicity of the improved user experience in cellular broadband by promoting even greater customer efficiency.
3. Businesses that may be distinguished from one another via the use of various technologies, such as actuators, remote controllers, and the monitoring of various system components, are referred to as mMTC enterprises.

One of the main needs for these systems is an extremely extended battery life, preferably many years. Relatively low computer energy consumption and exceptionally low system expenses are also essential requirements for these systems. These qualities enable the battery to have an incredibly extended lifespan. Since most systems only generate and consume a relatively modest amount of data, support for enormous data amounts is less valuable than support for lower data volumes. Support for lesser data quantities is thus more important (Sivalingam et al., 2016). It is plausible that there are use cases that defy neat classification into one of these two groups, but they may exist anyway.

Certain efforts, for instance, can need very high levels of dependability yet give less weight to the requirement of latency requirements. There can be other requirements for these programs. Parallel to this, there could be use cases for exceedingly cheap technologies where the prospect of an extraordinarily long battery life is less significant. An instance of this may be one when a smartphone is utilized.

- Applications for URLLC (ultra-reliable low-latency communication) systems include robotics, autonomous vehicles, and telesurgery. URLLC systems are latency reactive tools.
- The acronym URLL" means "ultra-reliable low-latency communication." These networks must function with a latency of less than 1 ms and a packet loss rate of less than 1 pf every 105 packets.

## 16.3  5G E2E NETWORK DESIGN

The design of the 5G E2E network is depicted in Figure 16.3, which serves to bring attention to the 5G E2E network. Even though all of the photos in Figures 16.1, 16.2, and 16.3 show the same scene, they focus on various facets of the network for their respective explanations. The transition from 3G to 4G involves a major concentration of base stations since there are bottlenecks in the wireless communication that originates from base stations. On the other hand, when we make the leap from 4G to 5G, the E2E design of the 5G network will be of a great deal greater importance than it was in the 4G network (Wang et al., 2014). This is because the base station will not play the key role in limiting throughput in the 5G network as it does now. Figure 16.3, which can be found in reference, depicts Huawei's E2E architecture that it developed for 5G. This architecture can be viewed below.

## 16.4  SLICING NETWORK ARCHITECTURE

Customers of network slicing architecture are being provided with a variety of separate service level agreements so that the architecture may successfully meet the criteria. Each of the two potential classes for a network slice is denoted by one of such categories is the network slice subnet instance (NSSI) for the RAN, and another is the network slice subnet instance (NSSI) for the CN. Being the other. Slicing networks are able to supply many unique services at the same time, and the slicing network itself and the service it delivers are two entirely independent entities. Figure 16.4 presents

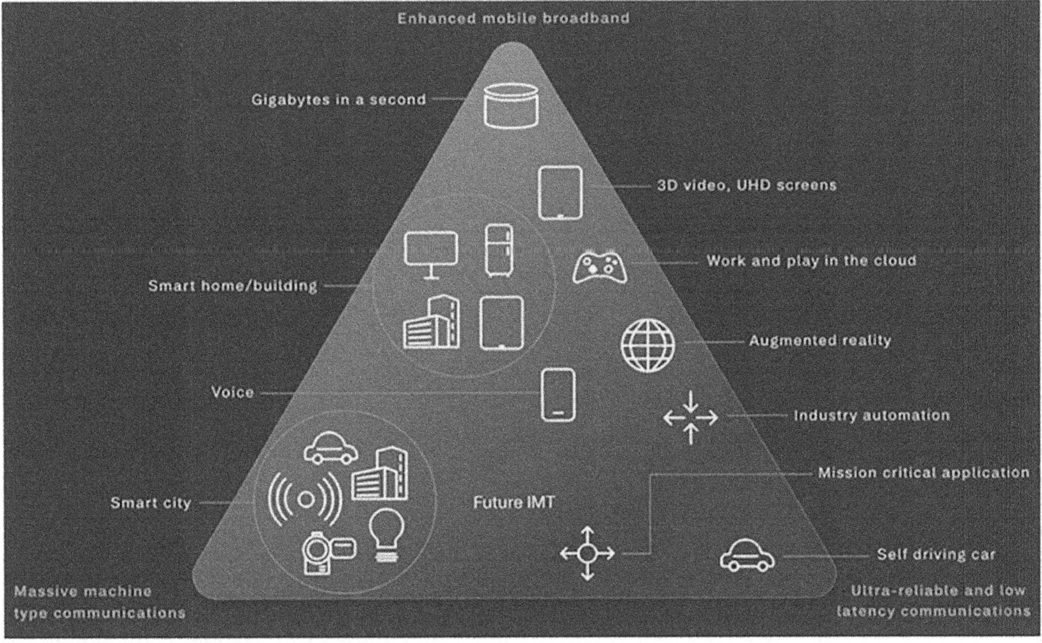


**FIGURE 16.2**  Examples of 5G use.

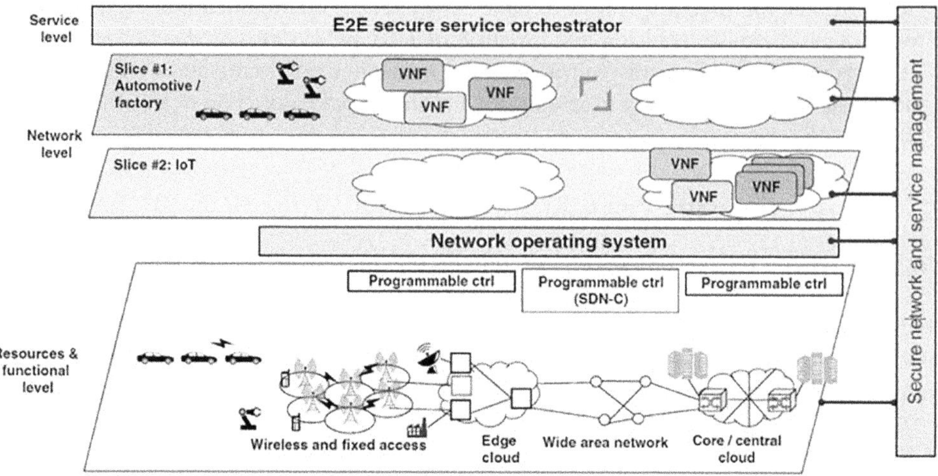

**FIGURE 16.3**   The structure of E2E in 5G's architecture.

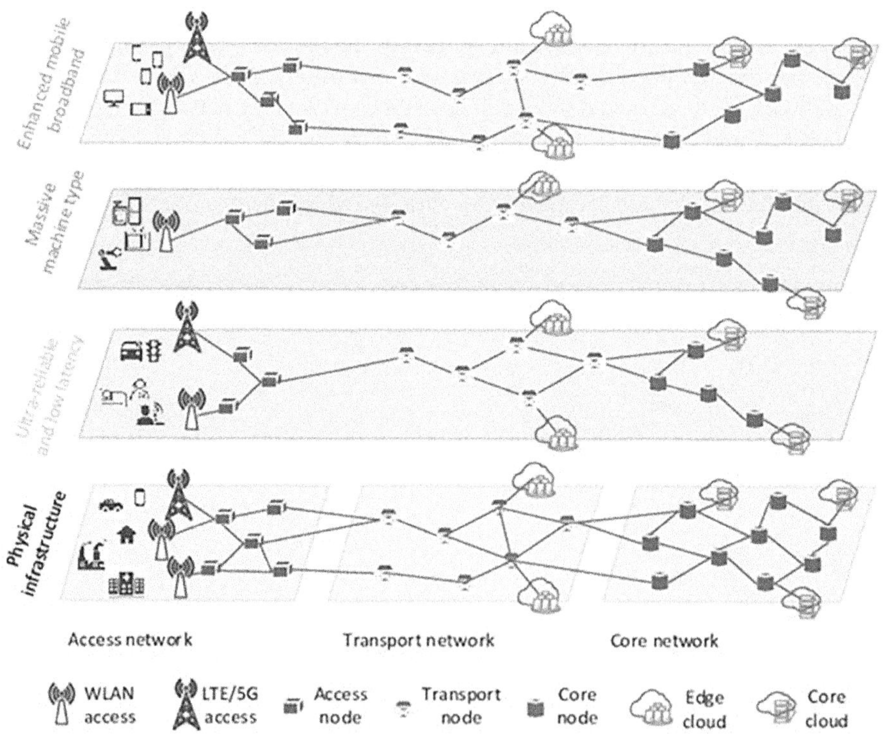

**FIGURE 16.4**   Architecture for network segmentation.

a schematic representation of the 3GPP slicing network, which can be seen further down this page (Zeng et al., 2020). Included in a comprehensive explanation of the 3GPP standards for slicing network architectures. A discussion of the 3GPP criteria may be found in the following figure, which was adapted from reference.

## 16.5   CRUCIAL FUNCTIONS OF THE VEPC NETWORK

Virtual evolved packet core (vEPC) is a data processing and switching architecture used in mobile networks. Virtual network functions, or VNFs for short, are used to carry out the tasks that the evolved packet core, or EPC, of an LTE network used to do. Virtualization makes it feasible to quickly deploy service environments and lower the costs related to the construction process. The fact that virtualization makes this feasible is what makes it possible. Figure 16.5 below shows a comparison of the evolved packet core vEPC's components and the functionalities of the LTE evolved packet core (EPC) (Bendouda et al., 2018).

## 16.6   MANAGEMENT AND ORCHESTRATION FOR NFV

Management and orchestration (MANO) is a crucial part of the architecture for network functions virtualization (NFV), which was developed by the European Telecommunications Standards Institute (ETSI), who also released the framework for NFV system design. NFV stands for network functions virtualization. administration and orchestration, or MANA for short, is an architectural framework that integrates the management of cloud-based applications and network services with managing virtual network functions (VNFs) during their whole lifespan. Administration and orchestration (MANA) is also responsible for managing the functionality of virtual networks. It is depicted in Figure 16.6, and various open source organizations have constructed their own NFV MANO frameworks based on the ETSI architecture) (Wong et al., 2017).

## 16.7   PLANNING FOR THE 5G MOBILE SYSTEM

The infrastructure design of 5G mobile networks is shown in Figure 16.7 as part of the system model. This model illustrates how the system works. This all-IP paradigm might facilitate interoperability across wireless and cellular networks. The design incorporates a computer terminal as a key component of the current architecture in order to develop a radio system that is both independent and self-sufficient. This link may be used by anyone using any of the radio approach technologies to get access to the web (Jovovic et al., 2015). This is made feasible by the fact that every terminal is connected to the wider Internet via an IP address.

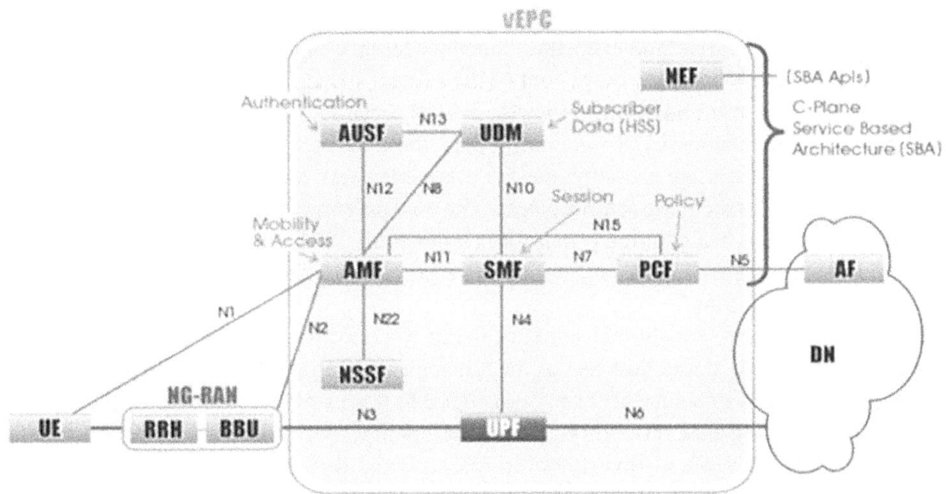


**FIGURE 16.5**   Architecture vPEC.

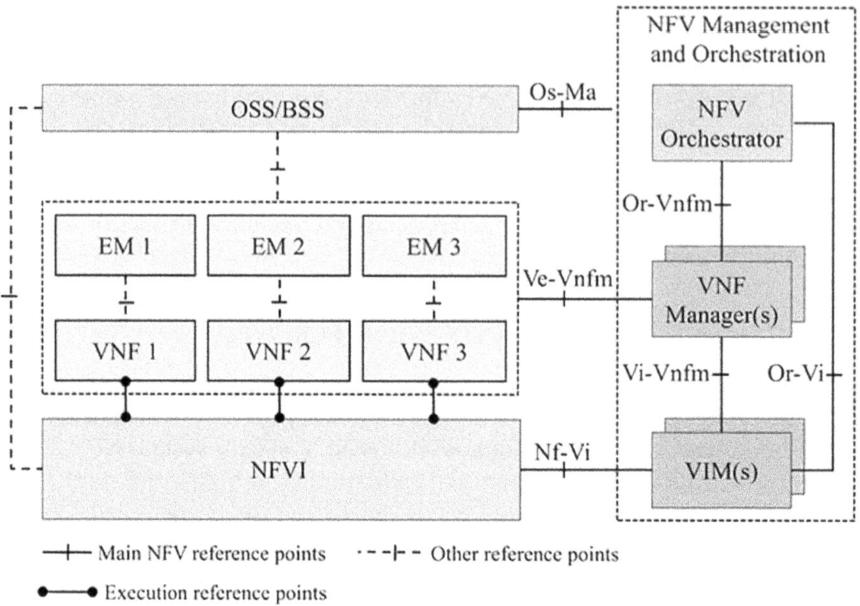


**FIGURE 16.6** Architecture of the ESTI NFV.

However, a mobile terminal's on-board hardware need a dedicated network interface in order to make use of radio access technology (RAT). If, for instance, it is crucial to establish connections with four distinct RATs, then the mobile terminal will need to accommodate for these connections in four distinct but functionally equivalent methods. Furthermore, we will need to guarantee that all of these interfaces are operational simultaneously for the architecture to perform as intended (Gupta et al., 2015).

## 16.8 COMMUNICATIONS AND NETWORKS ON THE BANDWIDTH OF THE 5G STANDARD

It is becoming more important to make use of information and communication technology (ICT) in a way that is both innovative and efficient. This is necessary in order to boost the economy on a global scale. It is arguable that the component of the overall strategy for ICT that is the single most important is wireless communication networks, which serve as the foundation for an extremely large number of other businesses. To accommodate the ever-increasing need for increased data transmission speeds and storage capacity, the 5G of cellular networks will need to think creatively outside the box in order to meet the requirements. The vast potential that may be tapped into through communication in groups is a genuine possibility (Jaber et al., 2016). The unique family of wireless communication technologies known as "cooperative communications" is referred to by the name "cooperative communications."

These strategies make it possible for network nodes to coordinate their efforts with one another in order to share information and take use of the advantages offered by geographical diversity. This new gearbox paradigm is expected to bring considerable performance improvements in a number of crucial areas, including link reliability, spectral efficiency, system capacity, and gearbox range, among others. Following years of investment in research and development, 5G wireless communication technologies have recently undergone substantial standardization and are now being offered for sale to customers. One of the three key application possibilities for 5G networks is massive machine-type communications, often known as mMTC. Applications that make advantage of the

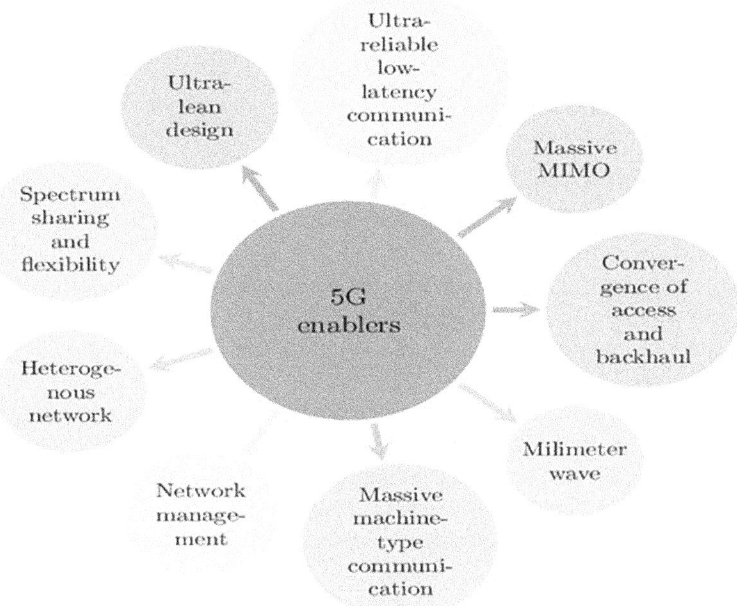


**FIGURE 16.7** The significance of 5G enablers.

IoT are made possible by these communications. Network operators anticipate that there will be a rise in demand for high-speed wireless broadband communications from highly populated UEs as we enter the era of 5G. This is due to the fact that network operators aim to provide a variety of services that place a high demand on wireless data, such as downloading multimedia content and streaming it.

There is a possibility that 5G mobile technologies may bring about a complete and utter revolution in cellular communications (Ejaz et al., 2017). This is due to the fact that it will make it feasible for there to be bigger densities of mobile broadband users, and it will also permit connections between devices that are both extremely dependable and huge in scale. (Li et al., 2019) have conducted detailed research of the communication of unmanned aerial vehicles (UAVs) in relation to 5G and B5G wireless networks. Before continuing on to discuss the associated research issues that are being experienced by the growing integrated network design, first provide a brief description of the background material as well as the integrated networks for space, air, and ground. The next thing that has to be done is a comprehensive analysis of the many 5G approaches that are based on UAV platforms.

This research takes into consideration a wide range of topics, layers like the physical one, the network one, and the ones where processing, communication, and caching are all done together. UAVs that operate at low altitude have found widespread use in a variety of contexts. This is mostly because UAVs are versatile and can move around a lot. During times of high traffic demand and network overload, UAV-assisted communications refer to the practice of using UAVs as aerial communication platforms (e.g., flying base stations [BSs] or mobile relays) by mounting communication transceivers to provide or improve communication services to ground targets (Dahlman et al., 2014). Several characteristics of wireless communication are taken into consideration to achieve this goal. The introduction of the 5G technology has brought about a plethora of new research endeavors in the academic community and has been of immense benefit to society as a whole. The adoption of 5G technology in communication networks is made possible by the critical enablers that are illustrated in figure below. The 5G technology is comprised of a wide variety of different combinations of enablers, and each enabler has its own individual set of capabilities (Balachandran et al., 2016).

## 16.9 HETEROGENEOUS NETWORK

There has been a rapid surge in the number of electronic devices that are adopting wireless and IoT technology in recent times. HetNets are a sort of network that incorporates a broad variety of different access protocols and cell types into one cohesive whole (Qi et al., 2019). The depiction of a HetNet architectural layout may be seen in Figure 16.7. A number of different electronic gadgets can be linked to a femtocell base station (BS). This BS is made up of many different miniscule subsets of a microcell base station. Due to the adaptability of the network, more study on its deployment is necessary in order to avoid interference and live up to the promise of providing end users with quality of service (QoS).

The primary goal of this chapter was to investigate the feasibility of integrating massive MIMO and mmWave technologies into 5G networks. Along with this topic, we also spoke about the challenges, technical advances, and prospective applications of HetNets. A lot of preparation was required to ensure that the deployment went off without a hitch. There were problems with the network's architecture, traffic administration, and spectrum allocation (Niu et al., 2015). For better traffic management and more precise traffic forecasting, the authors integrated traffic prediction, bandwidth negotiation, and connection admission control into the call session control function server. The goal was to increase the reliability of traffic forecasts; hence, this was done. This was done without compromising the system's capacity to foresee future traffic volumes with precision. They created a more refined version of the standard traffic prediction technique to enable effective streaming of massive amounts of data across 5G HetNet. Massive MIMO is option B.

Massive MIMO is yet another crucial capability for 5G networks since it enables faster data transfer rates while also lowering the likelihood of interference. This is achieved by applying the beamforming technique, which focuses signals on each other in order to get the desired result. Massive MIMO is a good technology for the development of 5G because it has a low latency and makes it possible to communicate over EE (Siddique et al., 2015). This makes it a candidate for usage in 5G. Utilizing antenna arrays that are both large and intelligent, with the width and inclination being able to be modified, makes it feasible to install enormous MIMO. This opens up new possibilities for network design. For regulatory masks to be necessary in order to enable the statistical character of massive MIMO, see here. In addition, the administration of spectrum regulations has to be improved so that they take into account the time, space, and direction domains. Beamforming is a type of spatial filtering that, in addition to improving efficiency throughout the spectrum and in terms of energy consumption, makes an attempt to strengthen overall system protection.

In the context of beamforming, the phrase "hybrid beamforming" refers to a type of beamforming that combines digital and analogue approaches. Realistically speaking, completely digital beamforming cannot be applied to mmWave frequencies since it requires the usage of a whole radio frequency chain behind each antenna (Feng et al., 2018). In the framework of mmWave homogeneous networks, research on multi-cell, multi-user, and multi-stream communication was carried out by Sun et al. Several examples of hybrid beamforming techniques have been considered and recommended. For example, there are four distinct varieties of precoding; there are many different types of feasible preceding, such as leakage-suppressing and signal-maximizing preceding, preceding based on the ratio of signal to leakage + noise, generalized maximum-ratio preceding, and zero-forcing preceding (Sun et al., 2018).

## 16.10 CONCLUSION AND FUTURE SCOPE

The need of 5G communication networks is defined, which amply illustrates the importance and possible advantages of this cutting-edge wireless technology. The increasing proliferation of data-centric applications and new technologies is driving up demand for faster, more dependable, and secure connection. 5G networks, with their increased capacity, ultra-low latency, faster data rates, and increased network efficiency, are ready to meet these needs. A paradigm change will occur in a number of sectors with the introduction of 5G networks, including manufacturing, entertainment, transportation, and healthcare. Autonomous cars, immersive augmented reality experiences, and real-time remote surgeries will all be made possible by 5G's ultra-fast speeds and minimal latency. These developments will open up new business opportunities and spur economic growth in addition to increasing productivity and efficiency. With 5G networks, underprivileged groups and isolated places might benefit from dependable access, helping to close the digital divide. This technology may promote social inclusion and economic growth by making educational materials, telemedicine services, and e-commerce possibilities accessible. There are additional obstacles associated with the rollout of 5G networks, including infrastructural needs, security issues, and regulatory frameworks. For 5G technology to be successfully deployed and widely adopted, these issues must be resolved. There is no denying the need of 5G communication networks. Because of its revolutionary potential and the increasing need for dependable, fast connection, 5G is a crucial enabler for the digital era. Future living, working, and communication will be completely transformed by 5G networks, which will empower several industries and open up new prospects.

## REFERENCES


Ahmed, I., Jangsher, S., and Butt, M. I. (2018). Next generation 5G wireless networks: A comprehensive survey, *IEEE Communications Magazine*, 56(3), 52–61.

Balachandran, K., Tinnirello, I., Wang, J., Song, B., and Kim, J. (2016). 5G technology enablers and their impact on wireless communication, *IEEE Communications Magazine*, 54(6), 18–24.

Bendouda, D., Rachedi, A., and Haffaf, H. (2018). Programmable architecture based on software defined network for internet of things: Connected dominated sets approach, *Future Generation Computer Systems*, 80, 188–197.

Chen, M., Duan, Z., Hwang, K. S., Li, Y., and Sun, X. (2019). 5G mobile communications: From physical layer to network architecture, *IEEE Communications Surveys & Tutorials*, 21(4), 3552–3599.

Chih-Lin, I., Han, S., Wang, Y., Xu, Z., and Sun, Q. (2019). 5G wireless communication systems: Prospects and challenges, *Science China Information Sciences*, 62(5), 1–27.

Dahlman, E., Mildh, G., Parkvall, S., Peisa, J., Sachs, J., Selén, Y., and Sköld, J. (2014). 5G wireless access: Requirements and realization, *IEEE Communications Magazine*, 52(12), 42–47.

Ejaz, W., Naeem, M., Shahid, A., Anpalagan, A., and Jo, M. (2017). Efficient energy management for the Internet of Things in smart cities, *IEEE Communications Magazine*, 55(1), 84–91.

Feng, M., Guomin, L., and Wenrong, G. (2018). Heterogeneous network resource allocation optimization based on improved bat algorithm, in *Proceedings of the International Conference on Sensor Networks and Signal Processing (SNSP)*, 55–59, Xi'an, China.

Gupta, R., et al. (2015). 5G multi-RAT multi-connectivity architecture, in *Proceedings of the 2015 International Conference on Wireless Communications and Signal Processing (WCSP)*, IEEE Xplore. https://ieeexplore.ieee.org/document/7503785.

Jaber, M., Imran, M. A., Tafazolli, R., and Tukmanov, A. (2016). 5G backhaul challenges and emerging research directions: A survey, *IEEE Access*, 4, 1743–1766.

Jovovic, M., Rajkovic, M., and Malenica, S. (2015). A computer terminal-based radio system for web access using radio approach technologies, *International Journal of Communications and Network Security*, 3(2), 123–129.

Khan, A. A., Al Wakeel, A., Imran, M., Ghogho, M., and Dobre, O. (2018). 5G wireless communication systems: A comprehensive survey, *IEEE Communications Surveys & Tutorials*, 20(3), 1616–1653.

Li, B., Xu, W., and Zhang, X. (2019). UAV communications for 5G and beyond: Recent advances and future trends, *IEEE Access*, 7, 70377–70388.

Li, Q., Niu, Z., Qian, Y., and Wang, S. (2017). A survey on 5G networks for the Internet of Things: Communication technologies and challenges, *IEEE Access*, 5, 3619–3642.

Niu, Y., Li, Y., Jin, D., Su, L., and Vasilakos, A. V. (2015). A survey of millimeter wave communications (mmWave) for 5G: Opportunities and challenges, *Wireless Network*, 21(8), 2657–2676.

Qi, X., Li, B., Chu, Z., Huang, K., Chen, H., and Fei, Z. (2019). Secrecy energy efficiency performance in communication networks with mobile sinks, *Physical Communication*, 32, 41–49.

Rappaport, T. S., et al. (2013). Millimeter wave mobile communications for 5G cellular: It will work! *IEEE Access*, 1, 335–349.

Siddique, U., Tabassum, H., Hossain, E., and Kim, D. I. (2015). Wireless backhauling of 5G small cells: Challenges and solution approaches, *IEEE Wireless Communications*, 22(5), 22–31.

Singh, M., Rajput, S., and Kim, K. (2019). Blockchain-integrated virtual power plant demonstration, in *Proceedings of the IEEE International Conference on Smart Energy Systems and Technologies (SEST)*, 1–6, Porto, Portugal.

Sivalingam, K. M., Krishnamurthy, P., and Vasilakos, A. V. (2016). 5G roadmaps of key enabling technologies, *IEEE Communications Surveys & Tutorials*, 18(1), 4–41.

Sun, S., Ding, Z., and Han, Z. (2018). Hybrid beamforming for 5G millimeter-wave multi-cell networks, *IEEE Access*, 6, 4516–4526.

Wang, C. X., et al. (2014). Cellular architecture and key technologies for 5G wireless communication networks, *IEEE Communications Magazine*, 52(2), 122–130.

Wong, V. W., Schober, R., Ng, D. W. K., and Wang, L.-C. (2017). *Key Technologies for 5G Wireless Systems*, Cambridge: Cambridge University Press.

Zeng, Y., Zhang, R., and Zhang, J. (2020). Wireless communications with unmanned aerial vehicles: Opportunities and challenges, *IEEE Communications Magazine*, 58(1), 54–60.

# 17 The Fusion of IoT, AI, Edge Cloud, and Blockchain

*Alwyn Rajiv S, Nancy Deborah R, Vinora A, Gobinath A, Sivakarthi G, and Soundarya M*

## 17.1 INTRODUCTION

Numerous technologies will contribute to the industrial revolution. Among the revolutionary technologies that business intelligences are integrating into their developed processes are the Internet of Things (IoT), machine learning, cloud computing, andartificial intelligence (AI). Several important technologies are briefly covered in this chapter.

### 17.1.1 INTERNET OF THINGS (IoT)

A system of associated devices that can interact and bring together data is identified as the IoT. These gadgets might include everything from industrial machinery and cars to wearables, appliances, and sensors. We can improve the functionality and security of IoT systems by merging edge cloud, blockchain, and AI.

The term "Internet of Things" is a paradigm-shifting idea that is changing how we interact with both the digital and real worlds. IoT, to put it simply, is the connecting of a wide range of common objects and gadgets to the Internet, allowing them to gather, share, and act on data. In addition to giving inanimate objects intelligence, this connectedness creates a world of opportunities for improving our lives and transforming numerous sectors. IoT has the potential to influence every aspect of our lives, from smart thermostats that learn our preferences and optimize energy use to wearable fitness trackers that keep an eye on our health. It could also influence everything from connected cars that talk to one another to industrial machines that foresee maintenance needs. It's about transforming the ordinary into the extraordinary and building a future where our environments and technology respond to our wants and preferences in an effortless manner. IoT is fundamentally a confluence of intellect, connectivity, sensors, and data. These interconnected "things" have the ability to improve our lives in a number of ways, from convenience to safety. They can be anything from domestic appliances to industrial machinery. It's crucial to examine how the IoT functions, its applications across various industries, the difficulties it poses, and the amazing future potential it contains as we go deeper into this field.

### 17.1.2 ARTIFICIAL INTELLIGENCE (AI)

AI is a branch of computer science and technology that has sparked interest among academics, researchers, and members of the general public. It is an area of technological advancement where tools are created to mimic human intellect, enabling them to learn, reason, and solve challenging issues. Fundamentally, the goal of AI is to develop machines that can carry out tasks, make judgments, and adjust to new information without direct programming from humans. Natural language processing, picture recognition, autonomous decision-making, and problem-solving are just a few of the many skills that go under the umbrella of AI. Making computers "smart" is simply one goal of this technology; another is to build systems that can process and comprehend enormous volumes of data, frequently at rates and scales that are far faster than those of humans.

AI has countless potential uses in a wide range of industries, including healthcare, banking, transportation, and entertainment. It is the impetus behind developments like self-driving cars, virtual personal assistants, and sophisticated medical diagnostics. It has the potential to transform industries, enhancing their effectiveness, efficiency, and responsiveness to the constantly changing needs of the modern world. AI does, however, also bring up significant ethical, privacy, and employment-related issues. Understanding how AI is changing our lives and the society we live in requires exploring both AI's capabilities and implications as it continues to develop. The path of discovery into the exciting world of AI only begins with this introduction.

Machines can execute intelligent jobs, learn from data, and make wise decisions thanks to AI. We can analyze and analyze enormous amounts of IoT-generated data using AI and IoT to gain insightful knowledge and enable real-time decision-making. AI algorithms can be implemented at the data generation edge to decrease latency and boost responsiveness.

### 17.1.3 Edge Cloud

Edge cloud computing eliminates the concept thatnecessitate to transport huge volume of data to centralized cloud servers by processing and storing data nearer to the source or client devices. IoT devices may process data in realtime by utilizing edge computing, leading to quicker reaction times, less network traffic, and more effectiveness. Additionally capable of supporting AI inference, edge cloud enables local AI model execution on edge devices.

A key innovation in contemporary computing and networking, edge cloud, denotes a fundamental change in how data is handled and distributed in the digital age. Essentially, the goal is to reduce latency and improve the performance of a variety of applications and services by moving the cloud's computing capacity closer to the locations where data is generated and needed. Cloud computing has historically utilized centralized data centers, which were frequently placed far from end users and data sources. Contrarily, edge cloud brings the capabilities of the cloud closer to the network's edge, enabling data to be processed and stored nearby where it is needed. Particularly in the area of IoT, autonomous systems, and real-time applications, this proximity has a significant impact.

Applications like autonomous vehicles making split-second choices, immersive augmented reality experiences, and precisely controlled industrial robots will all be made possible by edge cloud, according to the company. Additionally, it is essential for optimizing bandwidth utilization because it lessens the need for data transmission to far-off data centers. We will go into more detail about how it operates, how it affects various businesses, and the fascinating potential it has for computing and connection in the future. The development of this technology, which straddles the boundaries of cloud computing, networking, and the IoT, is changing how we interact with the digital world.

### 17.1.4 Blockchain

Blockchain is a decentralized ledger technology that guarantees security, immutability, and transparency in business dealings. Blockchain integration in IoT networks can improve security, privacy, and trust. It can offer decentralized governance over IoT networks, secure device authentication, and data integrity. Blockchain can also help with the development of new business models and enable secure, transparent transactions between IoT devices.

A blockchain runs on a network of computers, or nodes, thatcooperate to validate and store data, in contrast to typical centralized databases, where a single authority maintains control over the data. The term "blockchain" refers to a continuous chain of blocks formed by linking each new piece of data to the ones that came before it. Blockchain's capacity to guarantee data security and integrity without relying on a centralized authority is what makes it truly innovative. It makes entries unchangeable by utilizing sophisticated cryptographic methods; once information is stored on the blockchain, as stated by Yang Zen et al. (2021), it cannot be changed or removed.

As a result, there is an increased level of trust and openness, which has broad ramifications for many industries, including finance, supply chain management, healthcare, and voting systems. In this introduction, we will delve into the realm of blockchain technology and examine its foundational ideas, diverse uses, and opportunities and problems it poses. Understanding blockchain's complexities is crucial to navigating the constantly changing world of contemporary technology and business. Blockchain has the ability to fundamentally alter how we transact, manage identities, and secure data in the digital age.

## 17.2　THE FUSION

A powerful ecosystem where IoT devices gather data, 5G transmits it swiftly, AI analyses it, and blockchain protects its security and dependability is created by the blend of IoT, AI, edge cloud, and blockchain. This interaction has the prospective to lead to advances in a wide variety of sectors, together with manufacturing, transportation, and healthcare. The IoT, edge-fog-cloud computing, AI, and blockchain are just a few of the technologies that are convergent in several dimensions throughout the digital transformation, narrowing the line of distinction between the real world and digital world. Despite the fact that these technologies have emerged individually over time, they are now more interwoven than ever before, which is what is causing the creation of new business models according to Yasmin et al. (2021).

There has been a stableunion and blend of these technologies due to increased adaptation, adoption, and development. This is creating an exceptionalpatternswing that is anticipated to interrupt and restructure next-generation systems in erect domains so that the potential of the technologies arestreamlined in the best way to match one another. Although the convergence of the four technologies has the potential to address the primary flaws in the current systems, it is still in the early stages of adoption and is plagued by a number of problems, such as the lack of agreement on any bench marked models or best practices.

According to Sudharson et al. (2023), hyperautomation provides a multimodal structure for the strategic use of various automation technologies for software, either alone or in conjunction with AI and ML.

The industrial revolution advances by having AI as the brain where IoT devices are the data generators, 5G is the data carrier, and blockchain is the memory.

Figure 17.1 shows how the convergence of cloud, IoT, and blockchain are done. The fusion here is applied for areas like smart agriculture, smart city, smart healthcare, and many more can be implemented in the similar fashion.

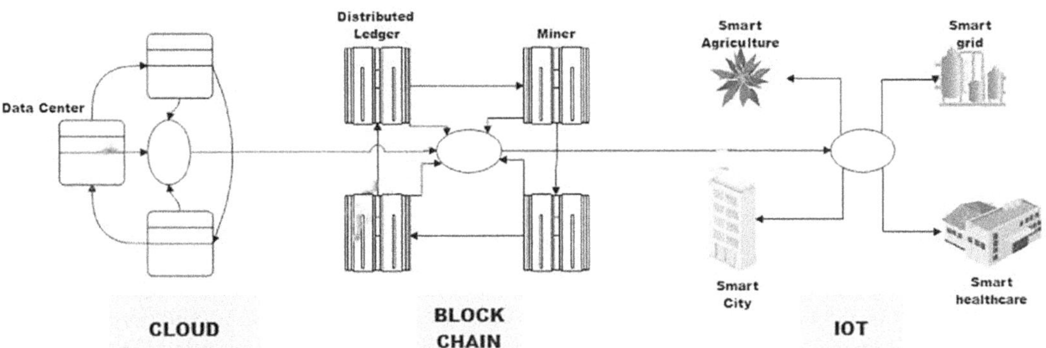


**FIGURE 17.1**　Fusion of cloud, IoT, and blockchain.

According to Firouzi et al. (2023), the IoT systems of the future generation are featured by the fusion of several technologies, bridging the distance between the real and digital worlds. These expertise ranges from edge-fog-cloud computing to AI and blockchain. Although these technologies were created independently over time, their synergy has advanced significantly. We are seeing a rapid convergence of these technologies, which will lead to a fundamental paradigm shift that will open up enormous advantages and opportunities for all vertical markets. However, there are still a number of obstacles preventing the complete merger of these technologies, such as a lack of concurrence on any suggested models or best practices. A comprehensive multidisciplinary layout addressing all aspects of the next generation of IoT systems via the fusion of edge, cloud, AI, and blockchain has been provided, while captivating the corresponding tasks into consideration. This includes solutions, architectures, protocols, services, and applications.

According to Goyal and Singh (2021), with the development of AI, the majority of services offered by businesses and organizations are now made digital. Workflow automation and robotic process automation (RPA) provide significant advantages over traditional business process automation. It increases a company process's accuracy, efficiency, productivity, and general customer satisfaction. There has been an analysis of the methods currently being used to automate the business process for customer relationship management. The discussion of several workflow automation solutions for enhancing the productivity and efficiency of current business operations has been given.

## 17.3 AI AS THE BRAIN FOR INDUSTRY AUTOMATION

According to Shah et al. (2023), the automobile sector will be greatly impacted by the introduction of AI and the development of related technologies. For instance, AI, which denotes the future of shipping and systems that will affect the concept of driving, is used in a technical innovation like autonomous driving. There will be an influx of new mobility-related firms, and those that already exist will need to change to accommodate them. The vehicle security domain uses a few security and AI techniques.

IoT device data is processed and analyzed by AI. Based on the patterns and information in the data, it derives insightful conclusions, predicts outcomes, and takes appropriate action. Depending on the requirements of the application, AI can function both centrally, in cloud-based setups, and at the edge, in devices themselves.

- Predictive Maintenance: Using data from sensors on industrial machines, AI can estimate equipment failure probabilities. This makes it possible for maintenance crews to make repairs before a breakdown happens, cutting downtime and boosting operational effectiveness.
- Quality Control: AI-powered cameras and sensors may check items being assembled for flaws and consistency issues, guaranteeing that only top-notch goods are released onto the market. Any departures from the norm can start automated processes to fix the problem.
- Process Optimization: AI systems are capable of analyzing intricate industrial processes and locating potential areas for improvement. Real-time parameter adjustments can be made to improve performance and reduce resource waste.
- Supply Chain Management: AI is capable of forecasting demand, maximizing inventory levels, and even foreseeing future supply chain interruptions, which supports producers in making decisions.
- Human-Robot Collaboration: AI can make it possible for humans and robots to work together in a secure and efficient manner. Robots with AI can undertake dangerous and monotonous duties while people concentrate on more intricate areas of production.
- Energy Management: AI may examine the patterns of energy use in a manufacturing facility and make recommendations on how to use less energy during off-peak hours or when specific equipment is not required.

- Flexibility and Customization: AI-driven automation can enable more tailored manufacturing runs. Without any downtime, machines may be swiftly modified to meet changing demands.
- Data analysis: AI can go through enormous amounts of data produced in an industrial context, revealing patterns and insights that manual analysis could miss.
- Safety Monitoring: AI may keep an eye out for any safety risks in the environment and send out notifications or initiate automated shutdowns if any irregularities are found.
- Decision Support: AI can help human operators and management on the production floor make wise decisions by analyzing real-time data.

Industrial automation that incorporates AI results in more precise processes, decreased waste, increased safety, and overall cost savings in addition to improved efficiency. It is an effective tool for modernizing production procedures.

## 17.4  IOT DEVICES AS DATA GENERATORS IN INDUSTRY AUTOMATION

IoT gadgets gather and send information from the real world. These gadgets can include sensors, cameras, wearables, cars, and other things. They give AI the raw data it needs to make decisions and gain insights. IoT devices can produce a wide range of data, from temperature readings to video streaming. Unquestionably, IoT devices are essential data generators for industrial automation. IoT gadgets help automate industries, as shown here:

- Sensors and Data Collection: IoT devices come with a variety of sensors that can track a number of variables, including temperature, pressure, humidity, vibration, and more. These sensors continuously gather information from machinery, tools, and the surrounding environment.
- Real-Time Monitoring: Industrial asset performance and condition can be tracked in real-time using IoT devices. This makes it possible to spot anomalies or operating circumstances that deviate from usual right away.
- Condition-Based maintenance: Condition-based maintenance techniques can be implemented using the data gathered by IoT sensors. Maintenance teams can reduce downtime and expenses by evaluating the data to forecast when equipment might break and carry out maintenance in advance.
- Remote Monitoring: Industrial equipment and operations can be monitored remotely using IoT devices. This is especially useful for large facilities or machinery that are situated in far-off locations.
- Data Driven Insights: By analyzing the data produced by IoT devices, patterns, trends, and correlations that might not be seen by manual observation can be found. Process optimization and increased productivity can be driven by these insights.
- Energy Efficiency: Real-time energy consumption monitoring is possible with IoT devices. The opportunities for cost and energy savings can then be found using this data.
- Inventory Management: IoT devices can give real-time data on stock levels in industries that use inventory, assisting in the optimization of inventory management and preventing shortages or excesses.
- Quality Control: IoT sensors can keep an eye on a product's quality at different production phases. Alerts and corrective measures may be triggered by deviations from quality requirements.
- Workflow Automation: Workflows can be automated using data from IoT devices. For instance, a specific activity may be initiated automatically if a given condition is met.
- Improving safety: IoT devices can keep an eye on working circumstances for any safety risks. Alerts can be sent to employees and supervisors in the event that hazardous situations are found.

- Customization: IoT devices have the ability to gather information on consumer preferences and usage trends, allowing manufacturers to provide more individualized products.

The data foundation required for intelligent decision-making, automation, and optimization in industrial settings is provided by IoT devices. Utilizing the power of IoT-generated data, businesses may increase productivity, cut costs, increase safety, and improve product quality.

## 17.5  5G AS THE DATA CARRIER IN INDUSTRY AUTOMATION

High-speed, low-latency, and high-capacity wireless communication are all made possible by 5G technology. It is necessary for sending the enormous amounts of data that IoT devices produce to AI systems for analysis. For applications that demand real-time answers, including autonomous vehicles and remote medical treatments, 5G's reduced latency is very important. Certainly, in the context of industrial automation, 5G technology acts as a potent data carrier. It has a number of benefits that play a crucial role in altering how industries run. Here are several ways that 5G is essential as a data carrier:

- High-Speed Data Transfer: When compared to earlier cellular network generations, 5G enables much faster data transfer rates. The massive amounts of data produced by IoT gadgets and sensors in industrial settings can now be transmitted in real time.
- Low Latency: One of the primary characteristics of 5G is its low latency, which entails a little amount of transmission delay. For applications like robotics and autonomous vehicles that need real-time responses, this is essential.
- Enormous Device Connectivity: 5G has the capacity to accommodate a huge number of connected devices at once. This functionality ensures easy connectivity and data exchange in an industrial setting with many IoT devices.
- Availability and Reliability: Businesses depend on ongoing operations. Because of 5G's reliability, there is less chance of downtime even in situations with high demand for data transfer.
- Network Slicing: The 5G standard supports network slicing, which enables the network to be split into virtual segments to meet different needs. This can guarantee that essential applications in industrial automation receive the required network resources.
- Support for Edge Computing: 5G can function flawlessly with edge computing, which moves data processing closer to the data source. This improves efficiency by reducing the need to send all data to centralized servers.
- Remote Control and Monitoring: 5G offers remote control and process monitoring thanks to its low latency and excellent dependability. This is especially helpful in circumstances when actual presence could be difficult.
- Augmented Reality (AR) and Virtual Reality (VR): Due to 5G's increased bandwidth and low delays, AR and VR may be used for tasks like remote maintenance, training, and design, which increases accuracy and productivity.
- Effective Resource Allocation: 5G's capacity to allocate network resources effectively means that data-intensive apps and other services can coexist peacefully on the same network.
- Dynamic Network Adaptation: Businesses can scale operations up or down as needed without sacrificing data transmission thanks to the network's capacity to react dynamically to changing demands.
- Enhanced Automation: By enabling real-time communication between machines and systems, 5G technology paves the way for sophisticated automation processes that boost efficiency and minimize human involvement.

Industrial automation is transformed by 5G's speed, low latency, large device connectivity, and reliability. It allows for seamless data interchange, instantaneous decision-making, and the adoption of cutting-edge technology that can revolutionize markets and boost productivity.

## 17.6  BLOCKCHAIN AS THE MEMORY IN INDUSTRY AUTOMATION

Blockchain offers a safe and tamper-resistant means to store and share data across the network, much how memory preserves the past information. It makes sure that data transfers are transparent and of high integrity. Blockchain's decentralized structure makes it perfect for keeping track of data transfers, safe financial transactions, and interactions between IoT devices. In the context of industry automation, the following section explains how blockchain technology might act as a safe and transparent memory:

- Data Integrity and Immutability: The ability to produce an unchangeable, tamper-proof record of transactions is the key characteristic of blockchain technology. This can be used in industrial automation to store important data like records of equipment maintenance, inspections for quality control, and supply chain movements. Data integrity and auditability are guaranteed after it has been recorded on the blockchain since it cannot be modified after the fact.
- Transparency of the Supply Chain: Using blockchain, the whole supply chain trip for both raw materials and finished goods can be transparently and tracably recorded. This openness assists in confirming the legitimacy and place of origin of components, lowering the possibility that fake or inferior materials would enter the manufacturing process.
- Smart Contracts for Automation: These contracts automatically carry out their conditions since they are written in code. These contracts can automate different industrial operations, such as triggering activities when specific circumstances are satisfied. For instance, when inventory levels reach a specific level, a smart contract may automatically place new orders for supplies.
- Decentralized Data Storage: Because traditional data storage systems are centralized, they are susceptible to cyberattacks and single points of failure. Data is dispersed throughout a network of nodes thanks to blockchain's decentralized structure, which increases its resistance to attacks and guarantees data availability.
- Authentication and Authorization: Blockchain can be utilized in industrial environments to create secure identity management for workers and equipment. As a result, crucial hardware and data are shielded from illegal access.
- Simplifying Interactions: By offering a shared, reliable source of data, blockchain can simplify interactions when many entities work together inside an industrial ecosystem. Shared records of orders, bills, and shipments can be a part of this.
- Data Monetization and Sharing: In certain circumstances, sectors may be able to monetize their data or even safely share it with partners. Controlled data sharing can be made easier by blockchain's cryptographic security, which also protects data ownership and authenticity.
- Regulatory Compliance: There are stringent restrictions in many businesses. Blockchain can assist in automating compliance by ensuring that documents are precise, open, and unchangeable.
- Data Privacy: Sensitive data is frequently used in industrial automation. Blockchain can offer a method for sharing important data while preserving privacy thanks to encrypted and permissioned access.
- Long-Term Data Storage: Some data, such as historical records and long-term performance measures, must be safely kept for a long time. The immutability and durability of blockchain can be useful in this situation.

Transparency, data security, and automation are improved when blockchain is used as a memory in industry automation. It makes certain that important data is safely kept and readily available while preserving its integrity over time. However, it's crucial to carefully consider if blockchain is appropriate for particular use cases and to balance its advantages with its computational and energy requirements, according to Yang et al. (2020).

Figure 17.2 shows how the blockchain technology has been used as memory units for storage. These can be applied to elements such as open shared ledger, consensus, shared contract, cryptography, etc.

## 17.7  FUSION OF AI AND BLOCKCHAIN

Abdulrahman et al. (2022) have spoken about the fusion of AI and blockchain that is implemented in aerospace engineering. The aforementioned technologies can assist in resolving a number of issues that the aerospace industry is now facing. This study uses an exploratory examination of the literature to assess blockchain and AI's possible applications in management and engineering of the aerospace industry. This study demonstrates how blockchain technology might be useful for managing records, particularly when it comes to maintenance, repair, and overhaul of airplanes. Additionally, AI offers important capabilities in navigation systems, flight path optimization, and predictive defect identification. The majority of these capabilities, however, still need to be experimentally validated and compliant with legal standards.

A blockchain-based system that enables data proprietors, cloud providers, and AI designers to work together on the preparation of machine learning models in a trustless AI market has been proposed by Baranwal Somy et al. (2019). Data is a crucial component of obtaining company insights

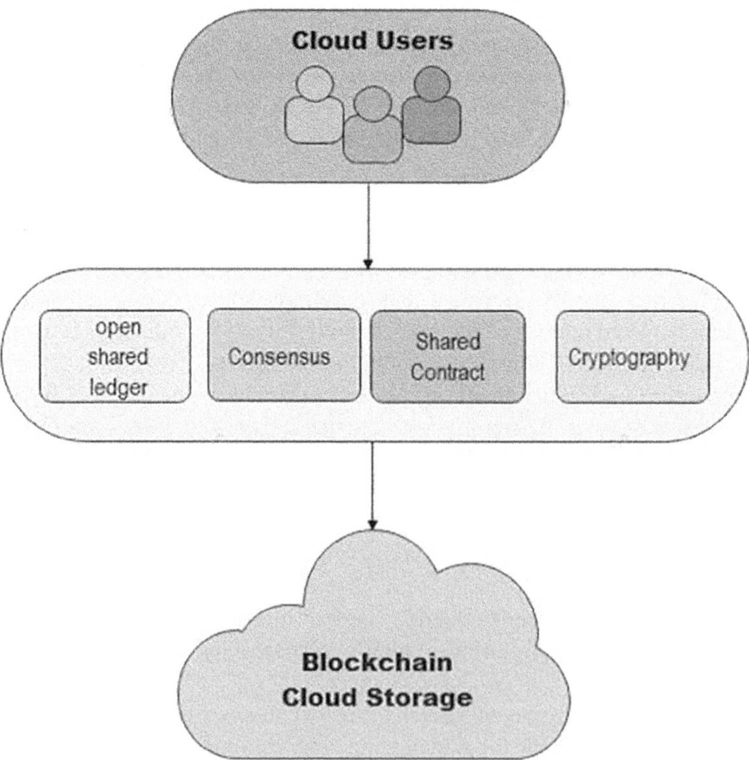


**FIGURE 17.2**  Use of blockchain as memory.

and is a highly treasured digital asset. The technology gives data owners the ability to maintain control and privacy over their information while yet enabling AI developers to use it for training. Similar to this, cloud computing companies' computational resources are available to AI developers without compromising proprietorship or secrecy of their trained models. In order for the blockchain system to provide provableconfirmation of wrongdoing and quarrel resolution, the system protocols are built up to motivate all three entities—data proprietors, cloud suppliers, and AI inventorstostraightforwardly record their activities on the dispersed ledger. The technology, which is built on the Hyperledger Fabric, can offer a workable substitute for centralized AI systems that cannot ensure the privacy of data or models. Its throughput and latency under a number of network structures, where peers on the blockchain may be dispersed across various datacenters and locations, are demonstrated experimentally through performance findings that are presented.

Figure 17.3 shows how the blockchain and AI has converged. The application areas where this fusion is used are shown in the figure. It involves components such as data storage, healthcare, financial services, supply chain, security, and authenticity verification.

The idea of utilizing a blockchain managed by AI to take use of the numerous features and benefits of blockchain services was put forth by Bouachir et al. (2022). The function of blockchain in the metaverse, its difficulties, the use of AI in developing intelligent blockchain features, and the effects of these on the metaverse ecosystem are discussed.

A paradigm for secure data exchange with blockchain assistance has been presented by Manogaran et al. (2022). The management of incoming and outgoing security in the collection and distribution of data falls under the purview of this paradigm. Recurrent learning is used to first categorize the inbound acquisition in order to find harmful data dissemination sequences. End-to-end authentication using blockchain data on reputation and sequence differentiation is used as an outbound security mechanism. The categorization and integrity confirmation in the business

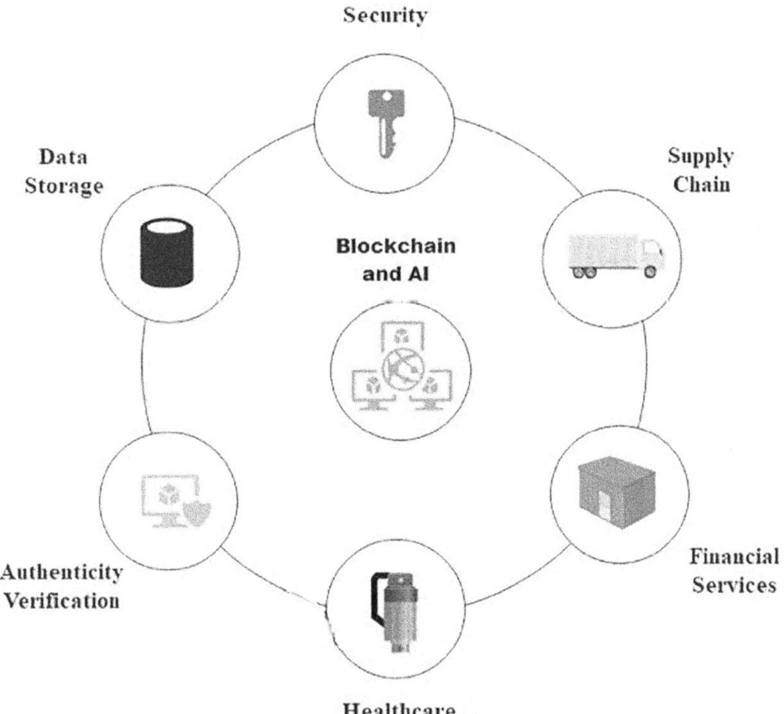


**FIGURE 17.3**   Fusion of blockchain and AI.

and processing workstations are how the blockchainmodelcontrols the data collection and distributioncases. In the smart industry, the functionality of the blockchain is divided for data collection and monitoring, while the non-mining blockchain terminal in the processing environment handles integrity and sequence verification for this purpose. By limiting false alarm progression, failure rate, and response time, the integrated security measures can maximize response rate.

In order to manage the parking system in automation service while minimizing potential problems, Rajagopal et al. (2022) have presented a thorough literature evaluation that is competitive in nature. Solutions for enhancing blockchain security by implementing AI in the development of various blockchain transportation systems are presented. The objective of this work is to investigate how blockchain technology and artificial intelligence will affect the automated industry. To add value and authenticity to the study, a secondary data collection approach has been used to obtain pertinent data and information on the research issue. Analogous to this, the resources engaged quantitative techniques to make the data easier to infer. The Industrial Revolution is described, along with some of its advantages. This focuses on the unresolved problems with workplace automation that can be resolved by blockchain and artificial intelligence.

Although AI and blockchain are primarily investigated independently, Rehman (2022) contend that blockchain and AI are complementary. For instance, a blockchain can help AI by managing and exchanging data. As AI systems depend largely on a lot of high-class training data, a blockchain may be utilized as a new stand to store and trade data. Regardless of the blockchain's vast prospective for exchange of data, this possible use case has not yet been thoroughly examined.

## 17.8  FUSION OF AI AND EDGE CLOUD

The combination of edge cloud and AI is a revolutionary confluence of cutting-edge technology that will have a significant impact on many different businesses. In order to accomplish this integration, AI capabilities must be implemented at the network's edge, which is where data is generated, processed, and consumed. This data is usually stored on local servers or decentralized devices. It greatly improves the effectiveness and responsiveness of AI-powered applications by doing this. This fusion has many important benefits. First off, by processing data locally, it lowers latency and produces faster response times—which are essential for applications like industrial automation and driverless cars. It also reduces the load on central data centers, saving electricity and network traffic.

Because of its ability to facilitate real-time decision-making, this convergence is extremely useful in situations where prompt data responses are necessary, like disaster relief or healthcare monitoring. Furthermore, in resource-constrained areas where uninterrupted Internet connectivity is not guaranteed, edge cloud computing can support AI-driven analytics. By making AI more approachable, effective, and flexible for a larger range of applications, the combination of edge cloud and AI has the potential to completely change a number of sectors, including manufacturing, IoT, healthcare, and transportation. In the end, this will change how we live and work. This technology has enormous potential for a more intelligent, responsive, and connected future as it develops.

Edge AI, according to Surianarayanan et al. (2023), is a paradigm of the future for developing and managing a large number of profitable real-time applications and services for both corporations and individuals. Edge computing and artificial intelligence are two incredibly prominent fields that are combined to create edge AI.

## 17.9  CONVERGENCE OF IOT AND EDGE CLOUD

The IoT and edge cloud convergence is a dynamic and revolutionary trend that is changing the data processing, analytics, and connectivity landscape. While edge cloud refers to decentralized computing resources and storage that are situated closer to the data source, IoT refers to the huge network of interconnected devices and sensors that gather and transmit data. There are a number of noteworthy results when these two technologies come together:

- High bandwidth efficiency
- Privacy and security
- Scalability
- Edge analytics
- Real-time processing
- Low latency
- Reliability

Real-time decision-making, reduced latency, and faster data processing are all made possible by locating computing resources to the edge. Applications such as augmented reality, industrial automation, and driverless cars depend on this. By minimizing the need to send all data to centralized data centers, edge cloud saves money on operating expenses and network traffic. IoT deployments that are remote or have limited resources might benefit greatly from the fact that only pertinent or processed data is transmitted to the cloud. Storing and processing data at the edge enhances data security and privacy by reducing exposure to potential breaches during data transmission. This is particularly crucial for delicate applications like smart homes and healthcare. Edge cloud allows for more scalable and flexible IoT deployments. Since more edge nodes can be added as needed, it is simpler to adjust for shifting needs. IoT devices may do advanced analytics locally using edge cloud power, gaining insightful knowledge from data without substantially depending on centralized cloud servers. By ensuring continuous operation even in the event of sporadic network connectivity or cloud disruptions, edge cloud strengthens and reliably IoT systems.

IoT and edge cloud convergence is fostering innovation in a range of industries, including manufacturing, smart cities, agriculture, and healthcare. This is because it enables enterprises to fully utilize IoT data while tackling critical issues like scalability, security, and latency. It signifies a fundamental change in the way we gather, analyze, and use data, which will eventually result in more adaptable and productive Internet of Things ecosystems.

According to Firouzi et al. (2023), the broad use of cloud computing in the past lowered the need for local edge storage and made it possible for edge devices to offload computing duties. However, when the network's edge produces an increasing amount of data, it is most appropriate to examine data there. For application that are sensitive to latency and that consume high bandwidth, numerous solutions, such as Cloudlet, have been introduced.

## 17.10 CONVERGENCE OF IOT AND AI

A system where the IoT logic is modeled to the requirements of industrial automation and reaps the benefits in the proper way has been developed by Nirmala et al. (2022). The proposed logic, which also makes use of AI, is referred to as the artificial-intelligence-assisted network paradigm (AIANP). The suggested AIANP greatly helps the automation industry regulate and observe the industrialized location without any safety issues or delays by introducing AI logic into its procedure. This is done by connecting Internet-enabled services to the industry to properly control the machinery. The research describes a variety of IoT-based automated devices, however due to their common flaws and weaknesses, it is necessary to come up with a novel approach to solving the difficulties with usual automation technologies. The suggested AIANP prototype provides users with a strong industrial automation competence, enabling them to appropriately control and track the sector.

The confluence of AI with IoT is a potent and profound synergy that is completely changing industries and applications. The term "convergence" describes how AI technologies are being incorporated into IoT ecosystems to enable more sophisticated and independent decision-making using the data produced by IoT devices. Some salient features of this convergence are as follows:

- Data-driven insights
- Predictive maintenance

- Enhanced automation
- Personalization
- Security and anomaly detection
- Scalability
- Energy efficiency

The IoT generates enormous amounts of data. AI systems are able to evaluate this data and derive valuable insights, forecast patterns, and spot abnormalities, allowing businesses to make data-driven decisions instantly. By analyzing IoT data, AI algorithms may identify when devices or equipment are likely to break, enabling proactive maintenance that minimizes downtime and improves asset management. AI integration can make processes more adaptive and automated in IoT systems. Without human input, devices are able to react to changing circumstances and make decisions. For example, in a smart city, traffic can be managed by devices, and temperature can be adjusted in smart homes.

AI can spot odd trends in IoT data, which aids in the detection and handling of security risks or unforeseen occurrences like cyberattacks or environmental shifts. AI and IoT together offer a scalable framework that can manage the growing number of connected devices and the necessary complexity of data processing. AI can optimize how resources are used in IoT systems, resulting in more environmentally and energy-friendly technologies.

Numerous industries, including healthcare, manufacturing, agriculture, transportation, and smart cities, are utilizing the confluence of IoT and AI. It's completely changing how companies and individuals use IoT data, allowing for improved automation, personalization, and decision-making while also tackling issues with complexity and data overload. At the vanguard of the fourth industrial revolution, this convergence has enormous future potential.

## 17.11  CONCLUSION

IoT, AI, edge cloud, and blockchain together form a dynamic confluence that is altering the technology environment and spurring innovation across numerous industries. This fusion has the potential to build a strong ecosystem that combines real-time data processing, intelligent decision-making, improved security, and decentralized trust to open up new possibilities and tackle difficult problems. The possibilities are essentially endless as these technologies develop and achieve more seamless integration. This merger has transformative potential, from enhancing manufacturing, healthcare, and logistics efficiency to enabling new paradigms in finance and supply chain management. Nevertheless, in order to ensure that the advantages of this fusion are achieved while minimizing potential hazards and ethical problems, it is essential to acknowledge the continued need for standards, interoperability, privacy safeguards, and regulatory modifications. As we advance in this exciting period of technology convergence, finding a balance between innovation and responsible use is crucial. A more connected, secure, and intelligent digital future is embodied by the combination of IoT, AI, edge cloud, and blockchain. To fully realize its promise and create a more effective and reliable digital world, it asks for cooperation, innovation, and responsible management.

## REFERENCES

Abdulrahman, Y., Parezanovic, V., & Svetinovic, D. (2022). AI-blockchain systems in aerospace engineering and management: Review and challenges. *2022 30th Telecommunications Forum (TELFOR)*. https://doi.org/10.1109/telfor56187.2022.9983700

Baranwal Somy, N., Kannan, K., Arya, V., Hans, S., Singh, A., Lohia, P., & Mehta, S. (2019). Ownership preserving AI market places using blockchain. *2019 IEEE International Conference on Blockchain (Blockchain)*. https://doi.org/10.1109/blockchain.2019.00029

Bouachir, O., Aloqaily, M., Karray, F., & Elsaddik, A. (2022). AI-based blockchain for the metaverse: Approaches and challenges. *2022 Fourth International Conference on Blockchain Computing and Applications (BCCA)*. https://doi.org/10.1109/bcca55292.2022.9922509

Firouzi, F., Jiang, S., Chakrabarty, K., Farahani, B., Daneshmand, M., Song, J., & Mankodiya, K. (2023). Fusion of IoT, AI, edge–fog–cloud, and blockchain: Challenges, solutions, and a case study in healthcare and medicine. *IEEE Internet of Things Journal*, 10(5), 3686–3705. https://doi.org/10.1109/jiot.2022.3191881

Goyal, N., & Singh, H. (2021). Process automation techniques in hospitality industry. *2021 9th International Conference on Reliability, Infocom Technologies and Optimization (Trends and Future Directions) (ICRITO)*. https://doi.org/10.1109/icrito51393.2021.9596303

Manogaran, G., Alazab, M., Shakeel, P. M., & Hsu, C.-H. (2022). Blockchain assisted secure data sharing model for internet of things based smart industries. *IEEE Transactions on Reliability*, 71(1), 348–358. https://doi.org/10.1109/tr.2020.3047833

Nirmala, P., Ramesh, S., Tamilselvi, M., Ramkumar, G., & Anitha, G. (2022). An artificial intelligence enabled smart industrial automation system based on internet of things assistance. *2022 International Conference on Advances in Computing, Communication and Applied Informatics (ACCAI)*. https://doi.org/10.1109/accai53970.2022.9752651

Rajagopal, B. R., Anjanadevi, B., Tahreem, M., Kumar, S., Debnath, M., & Tongkachok, K. (2022). Comparative analysis of blockchain technology and artificial intelligence and its impact on open issues of automation in workplace. *2022 2nd International Conference on Advance Computing and Innovative Technologies in Engineering (ICACITE)*. https://doi.org/10.1109/icacite53722.2022.9823792

Rehman, A. U. (2022). Application of Blockchain in restricting data access using AI. *2022 5th International Conference on Contemporary Computing and Informatics (IC3I)*. https://doi.org/10.1109/ic3i56241.2022.10072456

Shah, J. M., Natraj, N. A., Hallur, G. G., & Aslekar, A. (2023). Artificial intelligence (AI) in the automotive industry and the use of exoskeletons in the manufacturing sector of the automotive industry. *2023 International Conference on Sustainable Computing and Data Communication Systems (ICSCDS)*. https://doi.org/10.1109/icscds56580.2023.10105009

Sudharson, Bhuvaneshwaran, Tr, K., Kumar, S., Sushmita, & Lakshmi, J. (2023). A multimodal AI framework for hyper automation in industry 5.0. *2023 International Conference on Innovative Data Communication Technologies and Application (ICIDCA)*. https://doi.org/10.1109/icidca56705.2023.10099581

Surianarayanan, C., Raj, P., & Niranjan, S. K. (2023). The significance of edge AI towards real-time and intelligent enterprises. *2023 International Conference on Intelligent and Innovative Technologies in Computing, Electrical and Electronics (IITCEE)*. https://doi.org/10.1109/iitcee57236.2023.10090926

Yang, K., Liao, H.-M., Zhao, L.-H., Zheng, S.-Z., & Li, H.-W. (2020). Research on network security protection technology of energy industry based on blockchain. *2020 IEEE/CIC International Conference on Communications in China (ICCC Workshops)*. https://doi.org/10.1109/icccworkshops49972.2020.9209919

Yang Zen, T. H., Hong, C. B., Mohan, P. M., & Balachandran, V. (2021). ABC-verify: AI-blockchain integrated framework for tweet misinformation detection. *2021 IEEE International Conference on Service Operations and Logistics, and Informatics (SOLI)*. https://doi.org/10.1109/soli54607.2021.9672392

Yasmin, S., Sohan, M. F. A. A., Anwar, M. N. B., Hasan, M., & Farhad Hossain, G. M. (2021, January 5). SFC: A lightweight blockchain model for smart food industry. *2021 2nd International Conference on Robotics, Electrical and Signal Processing Techniques (ICREST)*. https://doi.org/10.1109/icrest51555.2021.9331215

# 18 Trustworthiness of Blockchain Technology in Healthcare 5.0 and Industry 5.0

*Kalaiselvi Thiruvenkadam and Veerakumar Pandi*

## 18.1 INTRODUCTION

Blockchain is one of the technological blooms that possess the potential to prosper in every possible discipline in the modern era. It is basically a decentralized system that is maintained by a network of computers. This technology can be employed in healthcare sector to handle patient health records in a secure, private, and complete manner. Blockchain reduces the difficulties in sharing medical data and maintain data privacy and integrity (Zhang & Ji, 2018).

Healthcare 5.0 is the most recent paradigm change in healthcare which can be called as smart healthcare. It adopts modern technologies to offer digital well-being, intelligent healthcare, and improved healthcare measures. The modern technologies such as smart sensors, nanotechnology, 5G, drones, blockchain, robotics, and cloud computing are used in Healthcare 5.0. Intelligent illness control, virtual care, and decision-making became possible because of the integration of these technologies (Saraswat et al., 2022).

Lack of data security is one of the problems faced by Healthcare 5.0. The data leakages in medical data should be controlled since it contains patients' sensitive data. It is also important to store patients' data digitally so that doctors can view patients' data and treatment history at anytime, anywhere with patients' permission. Blockchain technology is a solution to the data leakage problem in Healthcare 5.0. The adoption of this technology makes sure the medical data are securely stored and not tampered. Blockchain doesn't allow any modifications in data stored in the blocks. Hence, the medical data become tamper proof due to the adaptation of blockchain technology in Healthcare 5.0.

Similar to healthcare sector, the industry sector also evolved as Industry 5.0. This industrial revolution combines human and robot intelligence to enable critical thinking and labor-intensive tasks. Cobots are collaborative robots that can adapt to human brain changes and enhance efficiency in complex tasks. This revolution enables extraordinary levels of mass personalization in a variety of industries (Maddikunta et al., 2022).

Security and privacy are also a concern in Industry 5.0. Transparency and traceability of goods are always much needed in supply chain management. When there is transparency in supply chain, it establishes trust among manufacturers, distributors, retailers, and consumers, which enhances business relationship and results in smooth functioning of logistics. There is no centralized storage mechanism in blockchain network. The data are distributed among all the participants of the network. Hence, transparency along with security and privacy becomes possible in supply chain management due to blockchain. Blockchain can be employed for different operations in Industry 5.0, such as financial transactions, data security, goods management, quality control and supply chain.

Blockchain can contribute in Healthcare 5.0 and Industry 5.0 in various ways. The security challenges of blockchain have to be necessarily examined. The vulnerabilities of this technology



DOI: 10.1201/9781003442066-18

are exploited and solutions to those vulnerabilities are explored over time. To harness the growing power of blockchain technology, it is crucial to address its challenges and improve security.

The chapter's remaining sections are assembled in following ways. Related works are summarized in Section 2. Methodology of the proposed work is given in Section 3. Overview of Healthcare 5.0's evolution is given in Section 4. The evolution of Industry 5.0 is presented in Section 5. DLTs are discussed in Section 6. The blockchain basics are provided in Section 7. Section 8 lists the effects of blockchain in Healthcare 5.0, and Section 9 explains its impact on Industry 5.0. In Section 10, the security difficulties of blockchain technology are explored. The effect of quantum computing in strengthening blockchain will be read out in Section 11. The investigation comes to an end in Section 12.

## 18.2  RELATED WORKS

The most recent industrial and healthcare revolutions both greatly benefit from blockchain technology. The security and privacy features of blockchain technology make its employment easy in Healthcare 5.0 and Industry 5.0. Over the years, various research studies on the application of blockchain technology in both industry and healthcare have been carried out. There are numerous surveys conducted on the difficulties and restrictions of blockchain technology. As part of this work's literature review, a few of them are listed in the following.

Ahmad et al. highlighted blockchain technology's key features and some of its possible applications in telehealth and telemedicine (Ahmad et al., 2021). They discussed how blockchain can be handled to improve information security, privacy, and operational transparency. They also discussed different blockchain applications that doctors use for remote healthcare.

Hussien et al. performed a bibliometric analysis to determine the trends of blockchain technology in healthcare (Hussien et al., 2021). The study analyzed case studies of telecare medical information systems and e-health. They discussed the benefits of employing blockchain technology in healthcare-related industries.

Moosavi et al. performed a complete review using bibliometric and network analysis to determine how blockchain can improve supply chain management (Moosavi et al., 2021). They identified important papers, influential authors, and patterns of collaboration in the area of blockchain in supply chain management (SCM). The study identified key supply chain disciplines like supply chain management, finance, logistics, and security as areas where blockchain technology may be advantageous.

Verma et al. provided a comprehensive overview of blockchain-assisted applications. Their study proposed blockchain as a security enabler in Industry 5.0 (Verma et al., 2022). The article analyzed the main forces behind and prospective uses for blockchain in Industry 5.0. The goal was to assist researchers, academics, and business professionals in creating fresh blockchain-assisted solutions. They talked about how blockchain might be used in Industry 5.0 along with key enablers. They have provided a few essential definitions of Industry 5.0 that have been provided by professionals.

Khan et al. reviewed distributed ledger technology (DLT) in the context of the machine economy (Khan et al., 2022). They examined the technical features, difficulties, and advantages of DLTs. Additionally, they compared DLT models such the blockchain, directed acyclic graph, hashgraph, sidechain, and Holochain.

Odeh et al. discussed the problems involved in the utilization of blockchain technology healthcare along with its applications (Odeh et al., 2022). They looked at potential uses of blockchain technology to boost the efficiency of the healthcare industry. The concept of human-centric smart manufacturing system (HSM) was explained (Zhang et al., 2023). The authors discussed the significance and architecture of HSM. They explored the difficulties and constraints associated with the industry's adoption of HSM.

Kordestani et al. characterized the distinctive features of smart contracts on blockchain platforms in the pharmaceutical supply chain. They analyzed the working of smart contracts in the fight against fake medicines, and provided research areas for the future (Kordestani et al., 2023). Villarreal et al. carried out a survey on current blockchain frameworks addressing supply chain issues. (Villarreal et al., 2023). They examined the ways in which the reported blockchain frameworks address various supply chain difficulties. The article provided a summary of the characteristics of blockchain architecture for future supply chains. The study also examined supply chain applications for future blockchain frameworks, including difficulties and their full potential.

Ghosh et al. performed a literature on blockchain applications in the healthcare sector. They demonstrated how blockchain technology could be used in the healthcare industry. These highlighted challenges and identified future research areas by evaluating 144 papers (Ghosh et al., 2023). They analyzed several papers to highlight hot topics in blockchain-based healthcare systems. The authors explained blockchain technology and its features along with the current research themes of the technology.

Compared to surveys on alternatives to blockchain technology and comparisons of blockchain technology with its rival distributed ledger technologies, evaluation works on the applications and problems of blockchain are numerous and numerous in number. It is high time to look at the emerging DLTs that will soon compete with blockchain technology. The suggested study examines the security features and difficulties of the blockchain technology while contrasting it with alternative DLTs, such as Tangle, Hashgraph, Sidegraph and Holochain. In addition, quantum computing and its impact in strengthening blockchain technology is also investigated in this work.

Some of the most recent blockchain technology research studies in healthcare sector, industry, security issues, DLTs and quantum blockchain are mentioned in the Table 18.1.

**TABLE 18.1**

**Recent Surveys on Blockchain Technology**

| Author and Year | Healthcare | Industry | Security Issues | DLTs | Quantum Computing |
|---|---|---|---|---|---|
| (Bhushan et al., 2020) | ✗ | ✗ | ✓ | ✗ | ✗ |
| (Ahmad et al., 2021) | ✓ | ✗ | ✗ | ✗ | ✗ |
| (Hussien et al., 2021) | ✓ | ✗ | ✗ | ✗ | ✗ |
| (Verma et al., 2022) | ✗ | ✓(5.0) | ✗ | ✗ | ✗ |
| (Khan et al., 2022) | ✗ | ✓ | ✗ | ✓ | ✗ |
| (Odeh et al., 2022) | ✓ | ✗ | ✗ | ✗ | ✗ |
| (Nguyen, 2022) | ✗ | ✗ | ✗ | ✓ | ✗ |
| (Buser et al., 2023) | ✗ | ✗ | ✗ | ✗ | ✓ |
| (Swathi, 2022) | ✗ | ✗ | ✗ | ✗ | ✓ |
| (Guo & Yu., 2022) | ✗ | ✗ | ✓ | ✗ | ✓ |
| (Zhang et al., 2023) | ✗ | ✓(5.0) | ✗ | ✗ | ✗ |
| (Kordestani et al., 2023) | ✓ | ✗ | ✗ | ✗ | ✗ |
| (Villarreal et al., 2023) | ✓ | ✗ | ✗ | ✗ | ✗ |
| (Ghosh et al., 2023) | ✓ | ✗ | ✓ | ✗ | ✗ |
| (Kaur & Bansal, 2023) | ✓ | ✗ | ✗ | ✗ | ✗ |
| (Fiore et al., 2023) | ✓ | ✗ | ✗ | ✗ | ✗ |
| (Nair et al., 2023) | ✗ | ✓ | ✗ | ✗ | ✗ |
| (Jr & Khan, 2023) | ✗ | ✗ | ✗ | ✗ | ✓ |
| (Gomathi et al., 2023) | ✓(5.0) | ✓ (5.0) | ✗ | ✗ | ✗ |
| Proposed Study | ✓(5.0) | ✓ (5.0) | ✓ | ✓ | ✓ |

## 18.3  METHODOLOGY

The paper examined various research articles to summarize the contributions of blockchain technology to Healthcare 5.0 and Industry 5.0. The proposed study is a meta-analysis on blockchain technology to address the security challenges faced by blockchain and quantum computing solutions to improve blockchain security. Science Direct, Springer, and IEEE Explore are the major resources used for collecting articles. The search terms such as "blockchain," "blockchain and Industry 5.0," "blockchain and Healthcare 5.0," "blockchain security challenges," "distributed ledger technology," and "quantum computing for blockchain" are used for collecting the articles. The collected articles types are research, review, conference papers, and book chapters. A checklist is prepared to assess the quality of the papers. The checklist is used for inclusion of the papers based on relevance of paper's title to its contents, abstract, articles contribution to the research problems, alignment of conclusion to the abstract and journal index of the articles.

## 18.4  EVOLUTION OF HEALTHCARE 5.0

The healthcare sector has evolved over the years and grown as Healthcare 5.0 today. The growth can be attributed to the involvement of modern technologies such as artificial intelligence (AI), the Internet of Things (IoT), and robotics. The evolution of healthcare is shown in Figure 18.1. The figure shows the time period of each healthcare evolution.

The IT systems have emerged since the 1970s, when healthcare provision first became available (Tanwar et al., 2020). Healthcare 1.0 refers to this time period. Healthcare systems were not integrated with digital systems at that time due to lack of resources. Hence, paper prescriptions and reports were frequently used. This process increased the expenses and took more time. Chanchaichujit et al. explored the stages of the transformation of healthcare IT (Chanchaichujit

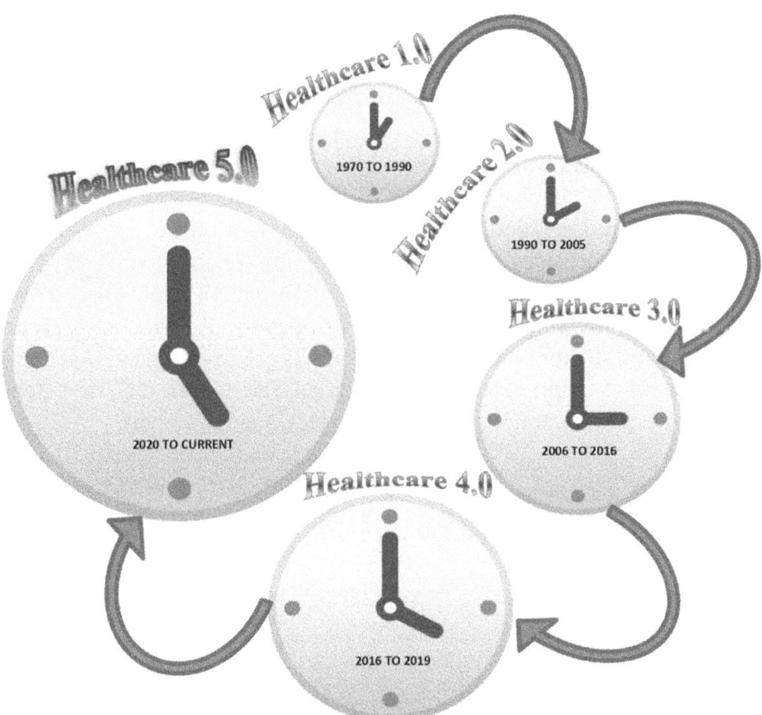


**FIGURE 18.1**  Healthcare evolution.

et al., 2019b). Healthcare 1.0 might arguably be defined as the years from 1970 to 1990. During the course of the following 15 years, most IT systems started networking. Administrative systems (AS) and laboratory information management system (LIMS) were important technologies in Healthcare 1.0 (Chanchaichujit et al., 2019a). Electronic health records (EHRs) were integrated with clinical imaging to give clinicians a better perspective. It was healthcare 2.0 in which electronic data interchange (EDI) and cloud computing were combined with HL7 messages for communication.

Healthcare 3.0 compiled all patient-related data into a single repository. Any authorized person may access the repository and amend it (Sharma et al., 2019). Healthcare 1.0 was centered on doctors and procedures. Healthcare 2.0 was dominated by technology. A key component of Healthcare 3.0 was the integration of technology and people (appinventiv.com). Technologies like electronic medical records (EMRs), big data, wearables, and optimization algorithms were used in Healthcare 3.0. Industry 4.0 and Healthcare 4.0 both took place at almost same time (Li & Carayon, 2021). The process of providing healthcare has evolved into a cyber-physical system. The modern technologies are utilized to produce connected and intelligent healthcare delivery. All the equipment and devices, homes and communities of the patients, were linked together in addition to the healthcare organizations and institutions. That was the rise of "Healthcare 4.0." Healthcare 4.0 made use of the technologies like IoT, blockchain, AI, and data analytics. The key technologies and target of healthcare versions are listed in Table 18.2.

The technologies used in Industry 5.0 are utilized by Healthcare 5.0. Healthcare 5.0 aspires to increase sustainability in the provision of healthcare, reduce costs, and enhance patient outcomes. Smart healthcare is referred to as Healthcare 5.0. It involves remotely controlling, managing, and handling various hospital system modules, ranging from outpatient visit department (OPD) to operations to pathology tests, etc., where all modules, including those for the super admin, admin, receptionist, doctor, accountant, pathologist, blood bank, radiologist, nurse, and patient are interconnected with one another and all modules are controlled by the main controller (Mohanta et al., 2019). Wazid et al. outlined the security needs for Healthcare 5.0 along with its possible uses. Applications including safe drug supply chain management, remote patient monitoring, disease detection and treatment, remote surgery, and hospital operations management can be used for a variety of healthcare services (Wazid et al., 2022). The security needs for Healthcare 5.0 are confidentiality, integrity, authentication, access control, non-repudiation, authorization, freshness, availability, forward secrecy, and backward secrecy.

The healthcare industry has evolved through five stages such as production, industrialisation, automation, digitalisation, and personalization. During the first phase, the sector concentrated on providing constant access to services and goods. The second phase of the industry's development focused on building an ecosystem of partners, including in-patient clinics and hospitals, to deliver improved services. In the third stage, automation was introduced to increase productivity. In the fourth stage, known as digitalization, new business models are investigated together with customer engagement. The fifth stage emphasizes personalization and marks the transition from patient-centered healthcare to customer-centric wellbeing services (medium.com).

**TABLE 18.2**

**Target and Technologies of Healthcare X.0**

| Healthcare | Target | Technologies |
|---|---|---|
| 1.0 | Doctor-centric approach | AS, LIMS |
| 2.0 | Technology-focused | EDI, cloud computing, HL7 |
| 3.0 | Integration of technology and people | EMR, big data, wearables, optimization algorithms |
| 4.0 | Interconnected and intelligent healthcare delivery | IoT, AI, blockchain, data analytics |
| 5.0 | Personalized patient-centric approach | Drones, explainable AI, fog computing, sensors, 5G, Internet of Medical Things |

## 18.5 EVOLUTION OF INDUSTRY 5.0

The First Industrial Revolution (1760–1840) is called Industry 1.0. It introduced machines and improved manual production and steam-powered engines. This industrial revolution transformed agriculture and the textile industry. The Second Industrial Revolution, Industry 2.0, occurred between 1870 and 1914 as a result of the introduction of railroads and telegraphs to various industries. This revolution was focused on mass manufacturing and spurred innovation in chemistry and related fields (Javaid & Haleem, 2019).

Industry 3.0 was seen with huge automation systems, digitalization, and networking of commercial and production processes. This was due to the advancements of electronics, computer and robotic technology (Li & Carayon, 2021). Industry 4.0 established a higher level of automation for operational productivity and efficiency (Akundi et al., 2022). It was a digital transformation of manufacturing and artificial practices, focused on cyber-physical systems, intelligent machines, automation, IoT integration, autonomous cars, AI, robots, nanotechnology, biotechnology, decentralized systems, and 3D printing (Silveira et al., 2019).

The next step in the evolution of manufacturing and production systems, known as Industry 5.0, integrates technology with human intelligence and skill (Gomathi et al., 2023). The Industry 4.0 was focused on mass manufacturing whereas Industry 5.0 shifts focus toward mass personalization. Mass customization (Wang, 2016) is the ability to generate products with a high level of customization while preserving efficiency and accessibility of mass manufacturing. Mass customization is a crucial element of Industry 5.0 as it provides companies the ability to make personalized goods to specific clients while yet enjoying the benefits of mass manufacturing techniques. The evolution of Industry X.0 is shown in Figure 18.2 with its timeline of and key focus.

Industry 5.0 extends benefits to society as a whole as well as to workers and employees. The adoption of resource-use technologies are promoted by the development of this sector (Joglekar et al., 2023). It supports human decision-making and profits from empowering technology that assists in the transformation of numerous areas. Digital twins, edge computing, big data analytics, the Internet of Everything (IoE), 6G, cobots, and blockchain are just a few examples of the technologies that aid organizations to become more efficient and deliver personalized products. The fifth industrial generation integrates human technicians into manufacturing revolution to enhance process efficiency (Leng et al., 2022b). It focuses on collaboration between autonomous machines and humans. This enables the workforce to understand and work alongside robots. This collaboration of machines and humans lead to efficient manufacturing processes, increased value, and reduced costs.

## 18.6 DISTRIBUTED LEDGER TECHNOLOGY

Distributed ledger technology (DLT) is becoming an innovative method of storing and updating data within and between organizations in recent years (Gorbunova et al., 2022). DLT is a decentralized network of computers where the ledger of transactions is distributed among all the participants of the network. Consensus protocols govern the administration of the decentralized network of DLTs (Bouras et al., 2020).

There are some emerging distributed ledger technologies such as blockchain, hashgraph, Tangle, sidechain, and Holochain. Blockchain is the first introduced distributed ledger technology. After the evolution of blockchain, other DLTs were developed over the years. The evolution and adoption of those technologies can also be seen as a challenge to future of blockchain. Bitcoin (Nakamoto, 2008) is the first created cryptocurrency whose mechanism is purely based on blockchain technology. Although blockchain concept was introduced earlier to bitcoin's arrival, the technology became very familiar after the introduction of bitcoin. Blockchain was initially used for financial transactions. Later the advancements in blockchain saw that the technology can be applied in various fields where it can offer secure data transfer, privacy, and transparency.

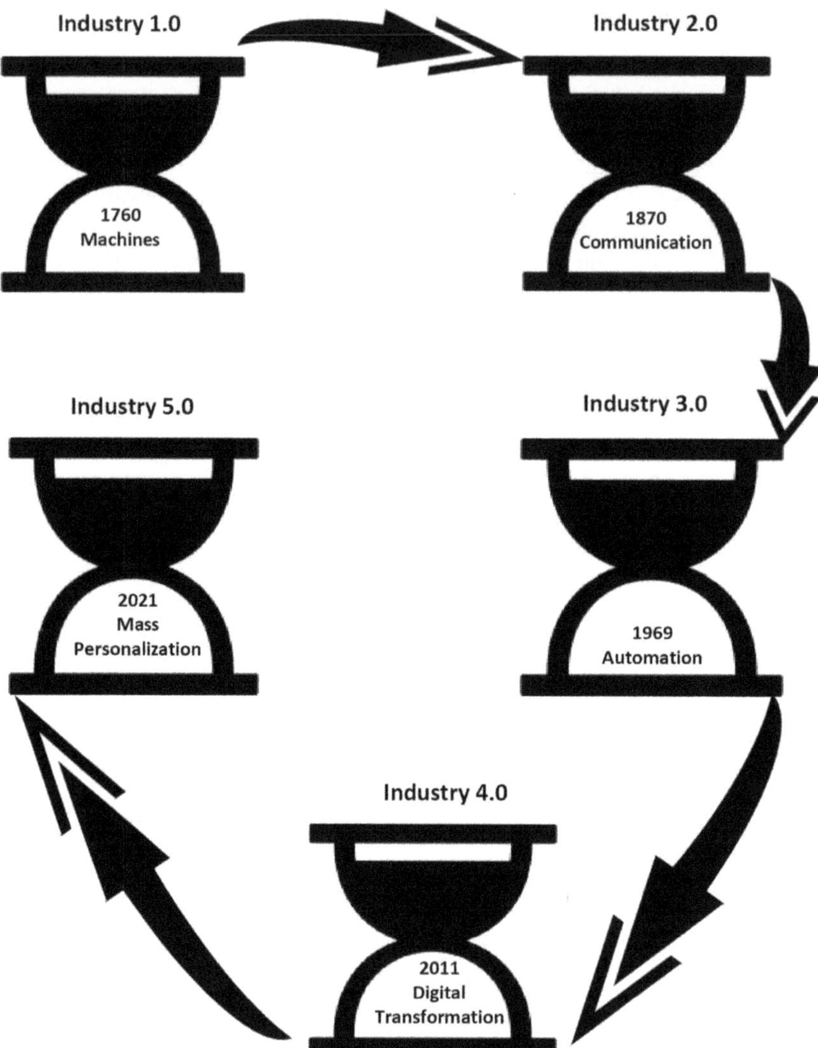


**FIGURE 18.2**   Industry evolution.

Hashgraph is developed to fix byzantine failures using gossip protocol. It is very fast in terms of transactions per second (TPS). Hashgraph is not widely adopted like blockchain. Tangle is made for IoT with high scalability and low energy consumption (Zhang et al., 2022). In Tangle, the directed acyclic graph (DAG) replaces the blocks when it comes to storage of transactions. Holochain is an agent-centric distributed generalized computing system. It is a network of agents where the agents maintain a unique source chain of their transactions (Harris-braun et al., 2018). The challenges involved in blockchain such as storage overhead and high energy consumption can be mitigated by Holochain. The 51% attack in blockchain is made impossible in Holochain (Kıyak et al., 2022).

The DLTs were discussed and compared based on various criteria (Akhtar, 2019). The architecture of Tangle and hashgraph is a DAG-based architecture. Blockchain architecture is linked-list-based architecture whereas sidechain is a multiple linked list architecture. Their comparison analysis showed that sidechain provide high privacy and hashgraph has low latency with high throughput.

A comparative analysis was performed for Blockchains based on different consensus mechanisms such as PoW, PoS, PPoS, and other DLTs (Arslan et al., 2021). Tempo is a recent distributed technology that performs far better than other DLTs in terms of throughput. The throughput of blockchain is very low than other technologies. The study reveals that energy consumption of blockchain is very high than its competing technologies. Energy consumption of tempo is considered very low and its storage usage is low as well. The comparison of DLTs is shown in Table 18.3. The table shows the comparison of DLTs such as blockchain, Tangle, sidechain, hashgraph, and Holochain based on criteria such as scalability, energy consumption, interoperability, throughput, etc. (Ahmad et al., 2021; Soltani et al., 2022; Akhtar, 2019; Arslan et al., 2021).

Although other DLTs have advantages, blockchain has many implementations whereas the rest are still in experimental level. The other technologies have better scalability than blockchain. The advantage of blockchain is that it is well established whereas its competitors are new to the market.

## 18.7  BLOCKCHAIN BASICS

Blockchain is a decentralized ledger that securely records every transaction (Dabbagh et al., 2019). A transaction is the exchange of money or any other kind of value between two parties. The transactions are hashed into a set of records called blocks, which is a growing list (Ranka et al., 2018). The blocks are connected to one another using cryptography. It is used to hold user-created transactions that include input fields like a timestamp and a public key. A transaction cannot be changed since doing so would result in a change to the transaction hash, which would prevent blocks from being linked properly. Hash is a 64-character long hexadecimal value. A common hashing technique generates a unique hash value for each transaction. Once generated, a hash cannot be reversed to reveal the specifics of a transaction. The cumulative hash value of all legitimate transactions makes up the merkle root hash. This is determined by pairing the transaction hash values and creating a new hash for the pair. This bottom-up pairing strategy continues until a single hash is obtained for the n number of transactions.

**TABLE 18.3**

**Comparison of Distributed Ledger Technologies**

| Criterion | Blockchain | Tangle | Hashgraph | Sidechain | Holochain |
|---|---|---|---|---|---|
| Scalability | Low | High | High | Medium | Theoretically unlimited |
| Interoperability | Medium | Low | Low | Low | Low |
| Energy consumption | High | Low | Low | High | Low |
| Smart contract | Yes | No | No | Yes | Yes |
| Application | Financial, smart contracts | Managing the IoT network and its payments | Event-based applications | Multi-blockchain structure | DApp-driven network |
| Architecture | Linked list blocks | Direct acyclic graph | Direct acyclic graph | Multiple linked lists | Distributed hash table |
| Copyright | Open source | Open source | Patented | Open source | Open source |
| Consensus | POW (SHA-256) | POW (hashcard) | Virtual voting | POW (Ethash) | Not required |
| Fee | Yes | No | No | Yes | Yes |
| Throughput | 5 to 20 TPS | 500–800 TPS | 100,000 TPS | Limited by main chain | Theoretically unlimited |
| Security | High | High | High | High | High |
| Platform | Bitcoin, Ethereum, Hyperledger Fabric | IOTA | Hedera | Monax | Holochain |

The main characteristics of blockchain include immutability, security, consensus, and decentralization. Blockchain is immutable because it is extremely difficult to change stored data. Due to distributed structure of the network wherein each node has a copy of the digital ledger, it is unlikely to add a transaction without the support of the majority of nodes. Once a transaction is recorded in the block, it cannot be changed again.

A bitcoin transaction is initiated in bitcoin network when client A wants to send some bitcoins to client B. The mining nodes approval is solicited to conduct the transaction. To begin the mining process, the transaction is broadcast to all network nodes. The transactions in the block will be assembled by the mining nodes and verified. The block and its verification will then be broadcast via a consensus procedure. If other nodes certify for the validity of each transaction in the block, it can be included to the ledger. This bitcoin transfer will be incomplete and regarded as illegitimate until other nodes accept the "block" containing the transaction (Zhang et al., 2019).

Blockchain network security is strengthened by the use of hashing algorithms, smart contracts, asymmetric-key cryptography, digital signatures, and consensus mechanisms. The key component of many cryptographic techniques is hash function. Using hash is an essential feature of blockchain technology (Fu et al., 2020). The hash function yields unique output for any size of input. Cryptography is used at every level of the blockchain, including the data layer, network layer, consensus layer, etc. In asymmetric encryption algorithm, the encryption key and the decryption key are distinct and are referred to as a public key and a private key, respectively. A random number algorithm is required to generate the private key, and an irreversible technique is used to calculate the public key (Zhai et al., 2019).

A signature algorithm and a verification algorithm are combined to produce the digital signature system. A digital signature controlled by a signature key. A verification method is utilized for validating the message's digital signature. Usually, the verification key controls the verification algorithm.

Blockchain technology uses consensus algorithms for quick and fair decision-making. A group of nodes uses the consensus method to approve block of transactions and validation. The blockchain network has no central decision-making body. However, it has a number of nodes that form a decentralized network and share control. Ismail and Materwala demonstrated the various computationally expensive consensus algorithms utilized in the blockchain literature. The merits and disadvantages of each consensus process were also discussed by the authors (Ismail & Materwala, 2019).

Self-executing contracts known as smart contracts are used in the blockchain platform to execute transactions automatically. The terms and agreements contained in the smart contract are moulded in the form of code. The smart contracts appreciate trust in the network. If the requirements and conditions are met, smart contracts will automatically execute transactions in a trustless environment. Smart contracts carry out the conditions of agreements between parties in the absence human. These agreements could take the form of arbitrary computer programs with conditional expressions (Sherman et al., 2019).

Once a transaction has been verified, its hash value is added to a block. Block data and block header are both components of a block. The metadata, which is another name for the information stored in block header, relates to the block itself. Hash values of each transaction are stored in block data whereas block header contains the Merkle tree root hash, the hash value of the previous block, the time stamp, and the nonce value. The block structure is shown in the Figure 18.3.

## 18.8 IMPACT OF BLOCKCHAIN IN HEALTHCARE 5.0

Blockchain is known for its secure data storage, data transfer and immutability of stored records. These security features draw attention of healthcare industry toward blockchain technology. Various blockchain-based applications, frameworks and prototypes are designed which are making great impact in medical industry. Few of them are summarized below.

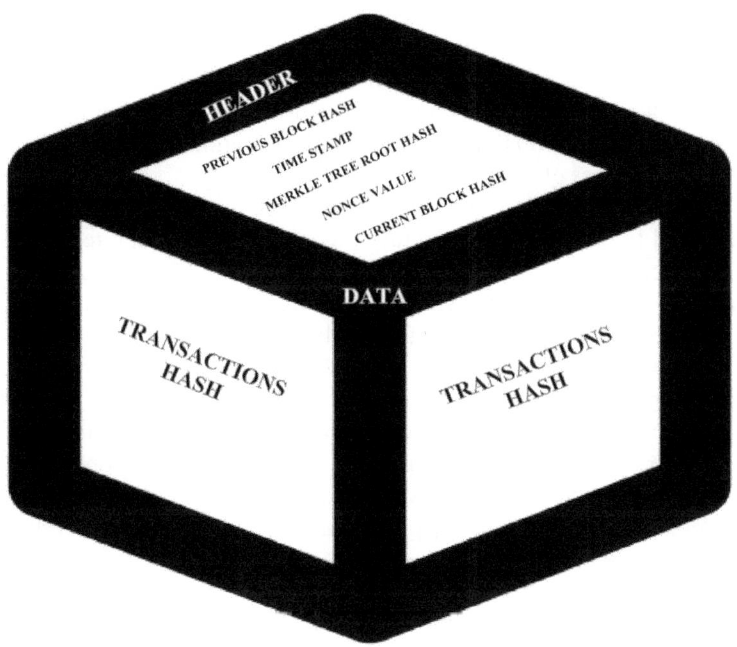


**FIGURE 18.3**  Block structure.

EHRs were introduced to store health data digitally instead of physical records to make them safer and more accessible. A blockchain prototype was designed to provide a proof of concept system for a secure and interoperable EHR system (Ekblaw et al., 2016). EHR contains patients' sensitive data which requires high level of secrecy as any patient will not want his health information to be exposed. Blockchain technology can be employed to provide a shared distributed view of health data such as genetic, diet, lifestyle, environmental and health data with guaranteed security and privacy protection (Linn & Koo, 2016). The health data will be stored in a distributed manner which means there is no central point of storage. Storing data at multiple points makes sure that data can be recovered even if it is deleted or tampered at one node.

Smart contract and IPFS were developed for storing and sharing neuroimaging data (Batchu et al., 2021). Image files were stored in IPFS whereas their hash values were being stored in smart contracts. IPFS was used for off-chain data storage for efficient insertion and retrieval. The proposed system prevents central point of failure and averts malicious corruption. Early detection of diseases helps in quick diagnosis. A blockchain-enabled framework could be used for an earlier detection of the diabetes disease (Chen et al., 2021). Patients' health information was collected from wearable devices and stored using InterPlanetary File System (IPFS). An EHR sharing framework combines system-based decease prediction, blockchain, and IPFS. Machine learning classification algorithms are executed on the data stored in IPFS. The results of the classification algorithms are then stored in the blockchain securely. The aim is to offer a secure system for storing, processing, and sharing patient health information. A smartphone-based DNA diagnostic system for malaria detection system uses deep learning for decision-making and blockchain for secure transactions of diagnostic outcomes (Guo et al., 2021). The accuracy of the approach was 97.83%. Blockchain performance was evaluated by considering the parameters such as send rate, average latency, and throughput.

Patient records, drug tracking, and device tracking are some opportunities for blockchain in healthcare sector. A vaccine tracking and monitoring system was developed using blockchain to trace the vaccines stored in health clinic. The entire history of the vaccine such that the day it was received in the clinic to the day it was consumed can be made available easily (Biswas et al., 2023). It is very crucial to maintain the integrity of the health data while maintaining patient records as any data tampering may cause a problem in treatment and. diagnosis. The immutability and tamper-proof qualities of the blockchain prevents a malicious user from changing the location history of a device or deleting it from record (Bell et al., 2018). The originality in drug tracking and device tracking ensures the timeliness of drugs and devices.

Computation and communication cost were a concern in healthcare data management. A blockchain-based novel EHR storage architecture was proposed to integrate the outsourced EHRs into immutable transactions on the blockchain (Ramesh et al., 2023). Communication and computation overheads are reduced since the EHRs are being stored on different IPFS nodes. For the management of healthcare data, a lightweight blockchain architecture was suggested to minimize processing and communication costs (Ismail et al., 2019). The proposed architecture attributes a lower network traffic and more rapid ledger update than the bitcoin network. The problems existed with traditional healthcare management systems such as single point of failure, data privacy, centralized data ownership, and system vulnerability are addressed in this proposed architecture. The suggested system group members in the network into clusters and allows one cluster to keep one entire copy of the ledger instead of one copy per participant. In this way the overheads of computation and communication are mitigated.

While storing a patient's personal health data on a server, the patient may want to own the control over his data. He may want his health data shared to doctors or hospitals with his permission only. A blockchain-network-based medical data management system allows patients to retain ownership over their own records while allowing hospitals to have easy access (Chen et al., 2019). The actual records are stored in a cloud platform and only the hash of these records kept in the network securely. Multi-signature contracts are introduced to handle the data ownership problem. This gives patient the ownership of their data but not to tamper the data without permission from hospitals. Blockchain can be integrated with AI to increase the availability of data needed for training and development, which might aid in personalized cardiovascular medicine. Blockchain offers secure integration of data from healthcare platforms and improves training and outcomes of AI (Krittanawong et al., 2020).

A web portal named Dwarna was proposed to connect different stakeholders of malta biobank (Mamo et al., 2020). Blockchain injects transparency and accountability into Dwarna's structure such that it safeguards research partners from data breaches. Blockchain stores research partners consent and increases reliability in bio banking process by providing more control to research partners. To solve the concerns of data privacy, authentication, and immutability, a patient-centric paradigm for a blockchain-enabled healthcare system was presented (Singh et al., 2021). A simple access control system using the hyperledger blockchain was developed and used in the healthcare industry. The issues related with confidentiality, access control, data integrity, level of authorization, authentication, and privacy of record are addressed by a new attribute-based and signature-based data encryption-decryption methods. An extended lightweight blockchain-based system enables multiple healthcare organizations to collaborate. A framework was developed to prevent data breaches and fraud in healthcare claims (Settipalli et al., 2023).

Maintaining the originality and secrecy of data is one important task in medical data management. Binance Smart Chain–based novel-scalable blockchain framework could be utilized for medical records management which provides secure access control for medical records (Monga & Singh, 2022). The system was the first of its kind to be deployed in Binance smart contract. The study shows that Binance smart contract is a better platform for blockchain compared to Ethereum network. The study concludes that the proposed system performs better than the state-of-the-art methods when it comes to medical record management. A medical data management system was developed to prevent the system from anonymous data access and protect sensitive patients' records (Tiwari et al., 2023). The system addresses potential security breaches in electronic healthcare systems. Kumar et al. proposed a novel scalable blockchain architecture to increase data integrity and secure data transmission by leveraging zero knowledge proof (ZKP) mechanism (Kumar et al., 2023). The off-chain storage, IPFS was put into service to address difficulties with data storage costs. The Ethereum smart contract was utilized to address data security issues.

The non-fungible token (NFT) was used as the mechanism to record and transmit the consent of the data subjects to use their data for research purposes (Cunningham et al., 2022). Only a legitimate consumer could make use of those consents and access the medical records. A blockchain-based system was proposed for storing and sharing pharmacokinetics (PGx) data (Albalwy et al., 2022). The system was implemented on a private Ethereum blockchain and achieved a large scale PGx data sharing. The essence of blockchain was to achieve data trust between unrelated parties. The trust was ensured by encryption and consensus algorithms (Wang, 2022). Blockchain technology supports emergency management of public health emergencies. Public health emergency decision-making and management system makes use of blockchain technology to realize the transparency and check of information in the whole process of emergency material transportation.

Summary of the mentioned works shows that blockchain is mainly used for secure storage of health data and its transfer purposes in the healthcare sector. The technology makes sure the patient's data are not tampered, not stolen, and not viewed by anyone other than patients and physicists. Application areas of blockchain in healthcare are shown in Figure 18.4.

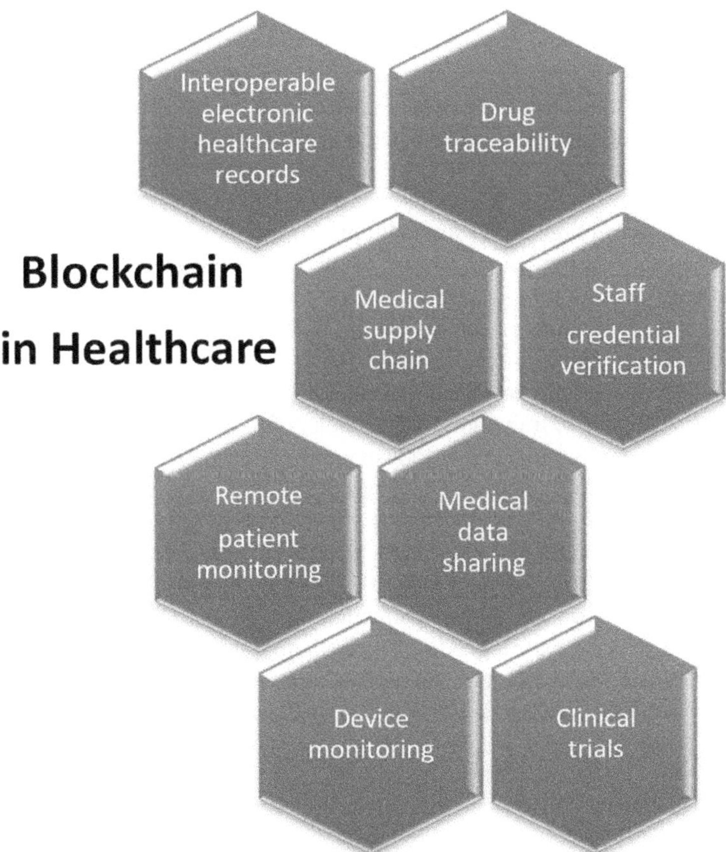


**FIGURE 18.4** Blockchain applications in healthcare.

## 18.9  IMPACT OF BLOCKCHAIN IN INDUSTRY 5.0

Blockchain is making an impact in the supply chain of the goods and products. The blockchain technology plays a role in SCM such that it keeps the reality in goods availability and location transparent to the stakeholders involved in the SCM. Industry 5.0 has emerged as a novel improvement to sustainable supply chains (SSCs) (Wang et al., 2023). AI and blockchain technology are utilized to monitor and manage manufacturing processes continuously. Multiple stakeholders are engaged in SSCs whose concerns are of more value in the adoption of blockchain technology.

Applications of blockchain technology and their benefit to SCM were investigated (Wang et al., 2022). A comprehensive framework of use case clusters was developed to analyze 53 applications of blockchain in SCM. Traditional blockchain uses Merkle trees to store data. The proof size was so large that it added more pressure to communication, causing end-to-end communication delays (Blossey et al., 2019). This in turn affected the stability and security of the system. The proposed security storage mechanism replaced the Merkle tree with the incremental aggregator subvector commitment to reduce the proof size.

Blockchain technology was used to design a data storage mechanism for Industry 5.0 (Liu et al., 2023). A sharded, two-layer Merkle tree was implemented to tackle low blockchain throughput. A special random low density parity check (LDPC) code was used to mitigate data availability attacks. The scalability issues were handled with the help of erasure code technology. Rupa et al. proposed an Industry 5.0–based blockchain application for medical record management. The system was developed on Remix Ethereum platform to ensure fraud prevention in medical certificates distribution (Rupa et al., 2021).

The issues with present single-chain agriculture supply chain systems are storage and scalability optimization, interoperability, security and privacy issues and privacy of personal data. The use of blockchain technology could enhance supply chain management. Bhat et al. developed a supply chain management system Agri-SCM-BIoT using blockchain and IoT to address these issues. The proposed system utilizes multiple blockchains that maintain their own ledger and have their terms and policies. The IoT gateways act as blockchain member nodes (Bhat et al., 2022). The key features of the blockchain such as confidentiality and data privacy challenges, light-weight consensus algorithms, deterministic smart contracts, fast information retrieval and flexible verification algorithms makes it suitable for SCM (Shakhbulatov et al., 2020).

Blockchain can provide security to industrial data management system against cyberattacks. An AI-induced constructive resilience model (AI-CRM) was introduced to strengthen cybersecurity in Industry 5.0. The study shows that proposed model reduces session drops by 10.88% and failure by 8.28% under the varying service transitions (Abuhasel, 2023). Blockchain combined with intrusion detection system can be applied to protect Industry 5.0 from cyberattack. Fraudulent transactions can be detected by blockchain technology (Ferrag et al., 2023). Some privacy protection can be adopted along with blockchain for effective privacy preservation.

Blockchain smart contract based system could boost timeliness and production control for a flexible individualized manufacturing (Leng et al., 2023). Three levels of smart contracts such as bottom level, middle level, and top level were implemented for better security and scalability. Industrial Internet of Things (IIoT) is crucial in production and supply chain. Traditional IIoT framework is a centralized system which is costly and vulnerable to attacks. A decentralized IIoT with secure blockchain middleware was developed (Leng et al., 2022a). The IIoT architecture has four layers such as perception layer, network layer, middleware layer, and application layer. The middleware layer stored and processed the data into which the blockchain was integrated to counterattack the security issues. Blockchain-based framework was proposed to address security and privacy issues associated with drone-assisted smart environments in beyond fifth generation (B5G) network. The framework was designed by leveraging blockchain and federated learning which allowed no space for single point failures and eliminated the need of central server (Alsamhi et al., 2023). Development of distributed trace-and-track systems could eliminate the risk of single-point failure.

The blockchain technology can be utilized for a better traceability and transparency in the food supply chain (Guruswamy et al., 2022).

A blockchain-based trust mechanism proof of authority was proposed to enhance data security and privacy (Sasikumar et al., 2023). Blockchain was combined with a digital twin for IIoT. One issue with Industry 5.0 is that the protocols used in its technology are centralized system based protocols which might go extinct in future where the need will be decentralized a system for a better and efficient control access (Oliveira et al., 2023). The issues present in Industry 5.0 are such as centralization, privacy preservation, latency, and security. A scheme named FusionFedBlock was developed to address these issues by integrating blockchain technology with federated learning (Singh et al., 2023).

Blockchain technology was integrated into banking systems for smarter processes. The core processes of the banks would become more transparent and secure with good efficiency (Patki & Sople, 2020). Decentralized and permissionless nature of blockchain technology brought a major change in finance sector (Guo & Liang, 2016). Some of the big international financial institutions have established their blockchain laboratories and working on its better adaption to the financial sector. More than 40 leading financial institutions of the world were brought together by R3 blockchain consortium to strengthen the exchange and cooperation. The finance sector has a strong desire to improve the backend efficiency of the blockchain and reduce the operational costs.

Technology and finance enterprises shift their attention toward developing blockchain prototypes. Blockchain technology eliminated the third party acting as a trust agent and allows a direct transaction between any two parties (Holotiuk et al., 2017). Blockchain can improve the time-consuming cross-border international transactions by making them quick and cheap. Dorfleitner and Braun introduced a blockchain-based fair payment (BCPay) framework for outsourcing services in cloud computing. It eliminated the need of a third party for fairness realization of the transaction (Dorfleitner & Braun, 2019). The BCPay was said to be cost-effective in terms of computational cost. This section explored the potentials of blockchain technology in Industry 5.0. In future, it is expected to make more contributions in different areas of industry. Application areas of blockchain in industry are shown in Figure 18.5.

## 18.10  SECURITY CHALLENGES

Despite security mechanisms such as asymmetric encryption, hashing techniques, and digital signatures consensus mechanisms, blockchain is still susceptible to attacks. As this technology is widely adopted, the attackers around the world are always trying and finding a new way to expose the vulnerability in blockchain. Besides attacks, blockchain itself has some challenges and issues such as scalability, energy consumption, and storage. The blockchain challenges, potential attacks, and solutions are presented in this section.

Blockchain immutability feature provides security, but it makes the modification of data impossible even if there is really a need to alter or delete data (Onik et al., 2019). To compromise this, two possible ways are out there. One is to create a new block by consensus from maximum number of nodes. The second way is to create a new chain. Both of these methods are said to be costly and infeasible. The fork problems that exist in blockchain technology and their types were discussed (Lin & Liao, 2017). The two types of fork are hard fork and soft fork, both of which happens when there is a modification is needed in a chain.

Meiklejohn presented ten obstacles to the adaption of DLT along with potential solutions. The obstacles are associated with the usability of distributed ledgers, governance of the system and rules making, meaningful comparisons, key management, agility, interoperability, scalability, cost-effectiveness, privacy and scalability (Meiklejohn, 2018).

Block withholding (BWH) attack is a threat to blockchain. The attack occurs when one of the miners of a mining pool solves the PoW problem and decides not to disclose it to the pool and causes

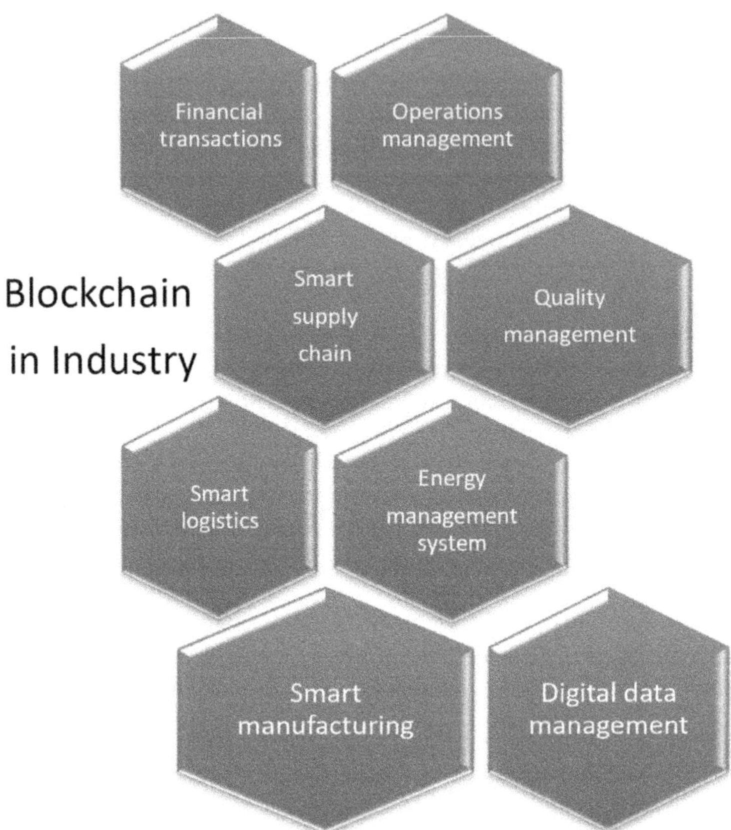


**FIGURE 18.5**  Blockchain applications in industry.

loss to the pool (Bag et al., 2017). The authors proposed a scheme to counter BWH attack using cryptography, which can be implemented on bitcoin protocol with minor modifications.

Black bird attack (BBA) is considered as a crucial threat to blockchain technology. The BBA tampers the fairness of the blockchain networks. BBA is possible if a particular miner gains the 51% hash rate generating speed. BBA is hard to detect and is efficient way to fetch the significant information from individuals. The authors proposed a case study which shows the reality of BBA is possible in blockchain systems. BBA mechanism makes the blockchain network vulnerable to double-spending attack (Xing & Chen, 2021). BBA is hard to implement in today's conventional blockchain network since doing so will require high computational power. In near future, BBA will become easy to implement in the post- quantum computing era as quantum computers are expected to be 100 million times faster than conventional computers. The authors designed a block access restriction (BAR) mechanism to counter black bird embedded double spending attacks (Xing & Chen, 2022).

Scalability is one of the issues in blockchain. It has low transaction throughput and high confirmation latency. Also its energy consumption is very high (Papadis & Tassiulas, 2020). Low throughput of bitcoin cannot satisfy the large-scale trading scenarios. The authors have confessed possible solutions to tackle the scalability problem (Zhou et al., 2020). The ever-growing size of blockchain makes it hard for casual users of the network to store an entire copy of network in their local systems (Henry et al., 2018). These users go after thin clients to compromise the storage issue. Thin clients run in simplified payment verification (SPV) mode. The blockchain queries are forwarded to semi-trusted intermediaries who make the thin clients vulnerable to privacy attacks and the network users may become susceptible to de-anonymization. Recent advancements in primitive information retrieval (PIR) protocols may help to maintain privacy in path-based transactions.

The summary of challenges involved in blockchain such as block size, high volume, transactions, and number of nodes and protocols were discussed, and two solutions—storage optimization and redesigning blockchain—to handle these challenges were offered (Mazlan et al., 2020). Dasgupta et al. confessed potential vulnerabilities to blockchain. Vulnerabilities in blockchain associated with cryptographic operations are cryptographic key vulnerability and hashing operation vulnerability. Identity vulnerability is associated with attacks such as replay attack, impersonation attack, and sybil attack. Replay attack happens when an attacker gains the access and steals the hash key for reusing. In impersonation attack, the access can be gained by imitating legitimate users of the network. Sybil attack isolates the target node from the network and use that node to perform attacks. The authors also discussed possible solutions to tackle these attacks in their paper (Dasgupta et al., 2019).

The low-level blockchain security risks involve 51% vulnerability, criminal activity, private key security, transaction privacy leakage, double spending, criminal smart contracts, under-priced operations, smart contract's vulnerabilities, and under-optimized smart contracts (Li et al., 2020). Smart pool is a mining pool system designed to improve efficiency and security of blockchain systems (Luu et al., 2017). High-level security risks associated with blockchain are network attacks, endpoint security, intentional misuse, code vulnerabilities, data protection, and human negligence (Guo & Yu, 2022). The authors listed various vulnerability analysis tools developed for smart contracts which can be used for detecting vulnerabilities.

The crypto wallets are kind of digital wallets that are used to store the private keys, the preservation of which is very crucial in order to secure the account. There are chances where the wallets are susceptible attacks. If an attacker is able to get the private key of an account by performing an attack on wallet, then he could own that account (Moubarak et al., 2018). Cryptocurrency exchange platforms have the provision to lock the funds that are found to be hacked from a wallet (Wright, 2020). Locking the hacked funds will make the attacker unable to move funds. Banking sector has its benefits from blockchain adoption, but the technology affects the bank at some cases. Regulatory policies that affect blockchain causes inconvenience its adoption. Blockchain implementation and execution is costly. Internet connectivity problem in India, particularly rural areas is also a barrier for blockchain implementation in India (Verma et al., 2023).

The challenges faced by blockchain in this classical computing era are discussed in this section. Researchers have presented various solutions for existing security challenges. It is always a good idea to prepare for future. Scientists are eying on security threats to blockchain systems that could be caused by quantum computers in future. Significant research works are implemented to use quantum computing solutions to strengthen blockchain systems.

## 18.11  THE QUANTUM IMPACT IN STRENGTHENING OF BLOCKCHAIN TECHNOLOGY

As quantum computers are in near future, it is necessary to address challenges that blockchain may face from quantum computers. Despite challenges explored in previous section, the security of blockchain which is maintained by consensus mechanism, cryptography and hashing techniques is robust in conventional computers. Quantum computers possess huge computational power that can easily solve cryptography puzzles of blockchain hence the security of the network will become doubtful. Research studies look at how quantum computing affects blockchain security and offer ways to integrate quantum computing with blockchain to increase security. In this section, we review academic papers that integrate blockchain with quantum computing.

For decades, digital computers have made it simpler for us to process information. However, quantum computers have the potential to revolutionize computing (www.mckinsey.com). Quantum computers make use of qubits, or quantum bits, which operate very differently from traditional bits. A qubit can concurrently represent one and zero, whereas conventional bits can only represent one or the opposite; this is true until the state is measured (scienceexchange.caltech.edu).

Steane gave a complete introduction to quantum computing and quantum information theory. There was discussion of fundamental quantum information concepts including qubits, data compression, quantum gates, and teleportation (Steane, 1998). Quantum computers are built on the core idea of quantum information (Gyongyosi & Imre, 2019). The use of quantum effects afforded by quantum mechanics allows for the representation of information in these computers as quantum states. Quantum algorithms utilize quantum computational complexity, with proposed methods showing significant speedups over classical algorithms due to the effects of quantum mechanics. Exponential parallelism is made possible in quantum systems by the exponential growth of the computing space with system size (Rieffel & Polak, 2000). This parallelism may result in quantum algorithms that are exponentially quicker than those that are conceivable with classical computing.

Blockchains use cryptographic algorithms to maintain data integrity (Alhadhrami et al., 2017). The security and integrity of the whole network is supposed to be compromised if quantum computers come into practice. Quantum computers possess high processing speed since they prefer qubits to binary bits. This may make it easy for an attacker to re-compute the hash values of the blocks.

The key issues faced by blockchains were discussed (Brotsis et al., 2022). The authors addressed best post-quantum cryptosystems to those issues. Theoretical backing for recent breakthroughs in post-quantum cryptography (PQC) was also offered in the study. Transactions are authenticated using the Elliptic Curve Digital Signature Algorithm (ECDSA). The authors confessed that blockchain's ECDSA was insufficient to counteract the quantum threat. It was demonstrated that the Shor algorithm favoured quantum over classical computing. The system's security can be jeopardized if an attacker uses this algorithm to extract the victim's private key from the system's public key. Quantum computing has more potential than the conventional computing due to quantum-mechanical processes. PQC refers to cryptographic solutions that can offer security against quantum computing. Post-quantum cryptography research focuses on using asymmetric algorithms to replace Rivest Shamir Adleman (RSA), Elliptic-Curve Diffie-Hellman (ECDH), ECDSA, and post-quantum secure hash functions for digital signature schemes.

Quantum computing has the potential to combine with blockchain technology and enable quantum blockchain. Its potential in medical records processing, thermal imaging, and patient monitoring were discussed (Kaushik & Kumar, 2023). Quantum blockchain is a decentralized, encrypted, and distributed system based on quantum information theory and quantum computing. A Web 3.0 framework powered by a quantum blockchain provided information-theoretic protection for decentralized transmission of data and payment operations (Xu et al., 2023). The future-proof security for data transmission and transaction information was discussed. In order to boost revenue and liquidity in Web 3.0, a use case for quantum NFTs was put up, and it was suggested that an optimal quantum deep learning auction be used for NFT trading. For secure communication, quantum blockchain employs quantum secure direct communication (QSDC) and quantum key distribution (QKD). QKD can offer provable security for one-time-pad (OTP) communication. Quantum blockchain combines the efficiency of quantum computers and quantum algorithms with the security of quantum networks.

Quantum-resistant blockchain systems were designed to handle quantum computing attacks (Zhang et al., 2021). The authors suggested replacing original signatures with digital signatures. The signature size and high public key might impact the performance of the system. The performance could be improved by putting hash data on the blockchain and the entire information on an IPFS. The quantum-based blockchain was used to design a sealed-bid auction system (Abulkasim et al., 2021). The sealed-bid auction system utilized blockchain to store transactions. The system was enabled by quantum computing and communication. This provided improved security and preserved anonymity.

Blockchain technology can be incorporated into the healthcare industry to improve stakeholder security and privacy. Blockchain technology could provide transparency and accountability and make sure that every transaction made in the system can be identified specifically. The traditional encryption technique is fortified by quantum security to defend quantum assaults. Block creation uses a quantum blind signature to protect against quantum threats. The healthcare ecosystem benefits from the integration of blockchain and quantum security because it increases efficiency, preserves stakeholder confidentiality and privacy, and guards against hostile activity (Bhavin et al., 2021).

An effective protocol was put forth for creating doubly hypergraph states-based quantum NFTs on a blockchain, where entanglement takes the place of traditional cryptographic hash functions (Pandey et al., 2022). The protocol tried to solve the issues with the present traditional NFTs' high costs and lack of security. By mounting a quantum state that represents the NFT on a blockchain rather than handing it physically to the owner, it proposed a novel method. The proposed protocol provided trustworthy and affordable NFTs.

These are recent studies that highlight how blockchain technology is impacted by quantum computing. More studies have been undertaken with the emphasis on quantum algorithms and blockchain. It is safe to say that blockchain and quantum computing could work together to make blockchain more secure.

## 18.12   CONCLUSION

The proposed work discussed blockchain technology and other DLTs briefly. The evolution healthcare and industry toward the fifth generation and the benefits of blockchain adaptation are explored. The findings reveal that application of blockchain technology in both healthcare and industry is mainly for security. The proposed study explored the trustworthiness of blockchain technology by discussing present blockchain security challenges and suggested existing solutions. The security threats that might harm blockchain systems in post-quantum computing are also discussed, and quantum solutions are presented. Since blockchain is getting involved in various fields for data storage, data transfer, and financial transactions, the security of blockchain systems should always be first priority. Hence, the proposed study focused on blockchain security. In future, with the arrival of quantum computers, many more threats are supposed to harm blockchain. The study suggests working on quantum computing based blockchain systems is one good research direction to harness blockchain technology for the betterment of future healthcare and industry.

## APPENDIX

### List of Abbreviations

1. AI—artificial intelligence
2. AI-CRM—AI-induced constructive resilience model
3. AS—administrative systems
4. B5G—beyond fifth generation
5. BBA—black bird attack
6. BCPay—Blockchain-Based Fair Payment
7. BWH—block withholding
8. DAG—directed acyclic graph
9. DBFT—Delegated Byzantine Fault Tolerance
10. DLT—distributed ledger technology
11. Dpos—delegated proof of stake
12. Dpow—delayed proof of work
13. ECDH—Elliptic-Curve Diffie-Hellman
14. ECDSA—Elliptic Curve Digital Signature Algorithm

15. EDI—electronic data interchange
16. EHRs—electronic health record
17. EMR—electronic medical record
18. FBA—Federated Byzantine Agreement
19. HSM—human-centric smart manufacturing system
20. IIoT—Industrial Internet of Things
21. IoE—Internet of Everything
22. IoT—Internet of Things
23. IPFS—InterPlanetary File System
24. LDPC—random low-density parity check
25. LIMS—laboratory information management system
26. OPD—outpatient visit department
27. OTP—one-time pad
28. PBFT—Practical Byzantine Fault Tolerance
29. Pgx—pharmacogenetic
30. PoB—proof of burn
31. PoS—proof of stake
32. PoSpace—proof of space
33. PoSV—proof of stake velocity
34. PoW—proof of work
35. PQC—post-quantum cryptography
36. QKD—quantum key distribution
37. QSDC—quantum secure direct communication
38. RSA—Rivest Shamir Adleman
39. SCM—supply chain management
40. SPV—simplified payment verification
41. SSCs—sustainable supply chains
42. TPS—transactions per second
43. ZKP—zero knowledge proof

## REFERENCES

Abuhasel, K. (2023, August). A Linear Probabilistic Resilience Model for Securing Critical Infrastructure in Industry 5.0. *IEEE Access*, 80863–80873. https://doi.org/10.1109/ACCESS.2023.3300650

Abulkasim, H., Mashatan, A., & Ghose, S. (2021). Quantum-Based Privacy-Preserving Sealed-Bid Auction on the Blockchain. *Optik*, 242(April), 167039. https://doi.org/10.1016/j.ijleo.2021.167039

Ahmad, R. W., Salah, K., Jayaraman, R., Yaqoob, I., Ellahham, S., & Omar, M. (2021). The Role of Blockchain Technology in Telehealth and Telemedicine. *International Journal of Medical Informatics*, 148(November 2020), 104399. https://doi.org/10.1016/j.ijmedinf.2021.104399

Akhtar, Z. (2019). From Blockchain to Hashgraph: Distributed Ledger Technologies in the Wild. *Proceedings—2019 International Conference on Electrical, Electronics and Computer Engineering, UPCON 2019*, 1–6. https://doi.org/10.1109/UPCON47278.2019.8980029

Akundi, A., Euresti, D., Luna, S., Ankobiah, W., Lopes, A., & Edinbarough, I. (2022). State of Industry 5.0—Analysis and Identification of Current Research Trends. *Applied System Innovation*, 5(1), 1–14. https://doi.org/10.3390/asi5010027

Albalwy, F., McDermott, J. H., Newman, W. G., Brass, A., & Davies, A. (2022). A Blockchain-Based Framework to Support Pharmacogenetic Data Sharing. *Pharmacogenomics Journal*, 22(5–6), 264–275. https://doi.org/10.1038/s41397-022-00285-5

Alhadhrami, Z., Alghfeli, S., Alghfeli, M., Abedlla, J. A., & Shuaib, K. (2017). Introducing Blockchains for Healthcare. *2017 International Conference on Electrical and Computing Technologies and Applications, ICECTA 2017*, 2018-January, 1–4. https://doi.org/10.1109/ICECTA.2017.8252043

Alsamhi, S. H., Rajput, N. S., Curry, E., Hawbani, A., Kumar, S., Hassan, U. U., & Scholar, G. (2023). *DataSpace in the Sky: A Novel Decentralized Framework to Dataspace in the Sky: A Novel Decentralized Framework to Secure Drones Data Sharing in B5G for.* https://doi.org/10.20944/preprints202305.0529.v1

Arslan, C., Sipahioğlu, S., Şafak, E., Gözütok, M., & Köprülü, T. (2021). Comparative Analysis and Modern Applications of PoW, PoS, PPoS Blockchain Consensus Mechanisms and New Distributed Ledger Technologies. *Advances in Science, Technology and Engineering Systems Journal, 6*(5), 279–290. https://doi.org/10.25046/aj060531

Bag, S., Ruj, S., & Sakurai, K. (2017). Bitcoin Block Withholding Attack: Analysis and Mitigation. *IEEE Transactions on Information Forensics and Security, 12*(8), 1967–1978. https://doi.org/10.1109/TIFS.2016.2623588

Batchu, S., Henry, O. S., & Hakim, A. A. (2021). A Novel Decentralized Model for Storing and Sharing Neuroimaging Data Using Ethereum Blockchain and the Interplanetary File System. *International Journal of Information Technology (Singapore), 13*(6), 2145–2151. https://doi.org/10.1007/s41870-021-00746-3

Bell, L., Buchanan, W. J., Cameron, J., & Lo, O. (2018). Applications of Blockchain Within Healthcare. *Blockchain in Healthcare Today, 1*, 1–7. https://doi.org/10.30953/bhty.v1.8

Bhat, S. A., Huang, N. F., Sofi, I. B., & Sultan, M. (2022). Agriculture-Food Supply Chain Management Based on Blockchain and IoT: A Narrative on Enterprise Blockchain Interoperability. *Agriculture (Switzerland), 12*(1). https://doi.org/10.3390/agriculture12010040

Bhavin, M., Tanwar, S., Sharma, N., Tyagi, S., & Kumar, N. (2021). Blockchain and Quantum Blind Signature-Based Hybrid Scheme for Healthcare 5.0 Applications. *Journal of Information Security and Applications, 56*(December 2020), 102673. https://doi.org/10.1016/j.jisa.2020.102673

Bhushan, B., Sinha, P., Sagayam, K. M., & Andrew, J. (2020). Untangling Blockchain Technology: A Survey on State of the Art, Security Threats, Privacy Services, Applications and Future Research Directions. *Computers and Electrical Engineering, October*, 106897. https://doi.org/10.1016/j.compeleceng.2020.106897

Biswas, K., Muthukkumarasamy, V., Bai, G., & Chowdhury, M. J. M. (2023). A Reliable Vaccine Tracking and Monitoring System for Health Clinics Using Blockchain. *Scientific Reports, 13*(1), 1–14. https://doi.org/10.1038/s41598-022-26029-w

Blossey, G., Eisenhardt, J., & Hahn, G. J. (2019). Blockchain Technology in Supply Chain Management: An Application Perspective. *Proceedings of the Annual Hawaii International Conference on System Sciences, 2019-January*, 6885–6893. https://doi.org/10.24251/hicss.2019.824

Bouras, M. A., Lu, Q., Zhang, F., Wan, Y., Zhang, T., & Ning, H. (2020). Distributed Ledger Technology for Ehealth Identity Privacy: State of the Art and Future Perspective. *Sensors (Switzerland), 20*(2), 1–20. https://doi.org/10.3390/s20020483

Brotsis, S., Kolokotronis, N., & Limniotis, K. (2022). Towards Post-Quantum Blockchain Platforms. *Security Technologies and Methods for Advanced Cyber Threat Intelligence, Detection and Mitigation*, 106–130. https://doi.org/10.1561/9781680838350.ch7

Buser, M., Dowsley, R., Esgin, M., Gritti, C., Kasra Kermanshahi, S., Kuchta, V., . . . Yu, J. (2023). A Survey on Exotic Signatures for Post-Quantum Blockchain: Challenges and Research Directions. *ACM Computing Surveys, 55*(12), 1–32.

Chanchaichujit, J., Tan, A., Meng, F., & Eaimkhong, S. (2019a). An Introduction to Healthcare 4.0. In *Healthcare 4.0* (pp. 1–15). Springer: Singapore. https://doi.org/10.1007/978-981-13-8114-0_1

Chanchaichujit, J., Tan, A., Meng, F., & Eaimkhong, S. (2019b). Healthcare 4.0. In *Healthcare 4.0*. https://doi.org/10.1007/978-981-13-8114-0

Chen, H. S., Jarrell, J. T., Carpenter, K. A., Cohen, D. S., & Huang, X. (2019). Blockchain in Healthcare: A Patient-Centered Model. *Biomedical Journal of Scientific & Technical Research, 10*(3), 1–10.

Chen, M., Malook, T., Rehman, A. U., Muhammad, Y., Alshehri, M. D., Akbar, A., Bilal, M., & Khan, M. A. (2021). Blockchain-Enabled Healthcare System for Detection of Diabetes. *Journal of Information Security and Applications, 58*(February), 102771. https://doi.org/10.1016/j.jisa.2021.102771

Cunningham, J., Davies, N., Devaney, S., Holm, S., Harding, M., Neumann, V., & Ainsworth, J. (2022). Non-Fungible Tokens as a Mechanism for Representing Patient Consent. *Studies in Health Technology and Informatics, 294*, 382–386. https://doi.org/10.3233/SHTI220479

Dabbagh, M., Sookhak, M., & Safa, N. S. (2019). The Evolution of Blockchain: A Bibliometric Study. *IEEE Access, 7*, 19212–19221. https://doi.org/10.1109/ACCESS.2019.2895646

Dasgupta, D., Shrein, J. M., & Gupta, K. D. (2019). A Survey of Blockchain from Security Perspective. *Journal of Banking and Financial Technology, 3*(1), 1–17. https://doi.org/10.1007/s42786-018-00002-6

Dorfleitner, G., & Braun, D. (2019). *Fintech, Digitalization and Blockchain: Possible Applications for Green Finance*. https://doi.org/10.1007/978-3-030-22510-0_9

Ekblaw, A., Azaria, A., Halamka, J. D., & Lippman, A. (2016, August). A case study for blockchain in healthcare: "MedRec" prototype for electronic health records and medical research data. In *Proceedings of IEEE Open & Big Data Conference* (Vol. 13, p. 13).

Ferrag, M. A., Maglaras, L., & Benbouzid, M. (2023). Blockchain and Artificial Intelligence as Enablers of Cyber Security in the Era of IoT and IIoT Applications. *Journal of Sensor and Actuator Networks, 12*(3), 40. https://doi.org/10.3390/jsan12030040

Fiore, M., Capodici, A., Rucci, P., Bianconi, A., Longo, G., Ricci, M., . . . Golinelli, D. (2023). Blockchain for the Healthcare Supply Chain: A Systematic Literature Review. *Applied Sciences, 13*(2), 686.

Fu, J., Qiao, S., Huang, Y., Si, X., Li, B., & Yuan, C. (2020). A Study on the Optimization of Blockchain Hashing Algorithm Based on PRCA. *Security and Communication Networks, 2020.* https://doi.org/10.1155/2020/8876317

Ghosh, P. K., Chakraborty, A., Hasan, M., Rashid, K., & Siddique, A. H. (2023). Blockchain Application in Healthcare Systems: A Review. *Systems, 11*(1). https://doi.org/10.3390/systems11010038

Gomathi, L., Mishra, A. K., & Tyagi, A. K. (2023, April). Industry 5.0 for Healthcare 5.0: Opportunities, Challenges and Future Research Possibilities. In *2023 7th International Conference on Trends in Electronics and Informatics (ICOEI)* (pp. 204–213). IEEE.

Gorbunova, M., Masek, P., Komarov, M., & Ometov, A. (2022). Distributed Ledger Technology: State-of-the-Art and Current Challenges. *Computer Science and Information Systems, 19*(1), 65–85. https://doi.org/10.2298/CSIS210215037G

Guo, H., & Yu, X. (2022). A Survey on Blockchain Technology and Its Security. *Blockchain: Research and Applications, 3*(2), 100067. https://doi.org/10.1016/j.bcra.2022.100067

Guo, X., Khalid, M. A., Domingos, I., Michala, A. L., Adriko, M., Rowel, C., Ajambo, D., Garrett, A., Kar, S., Yan, X., Reboud, J., Tukahebwa, E. M., & Cooper, J. M. (2021). Smartphone-based DNA Diagnostics for Malaria Detection Using Deep Learning for Local Decision Support and Blockchain Technology for Security. *Nature Electronics, 4*(8), 615–624. https://doi.org/10.1038/s41928-021-00612-x

Guo, Y., & Liang, C. (2016). Blockchain Application and Outlook in the Banking Industry. *Financial Innovation, 2*(1). https://doi.org/10.1186/s40854-016-0034-9

Guruswamy, S., Pojić, M., Subramanian, J., Mastilović, J., Sarang, S., Subbanagounder, A., Stojanović, G., & Jeoti, V. (2022). Toward Better Food Security Using Concepts from Industry 5.0. *Sensors, 22*(21), 1–24. https://doi.org/10.3390/s22218377

Gyongyosi, L., & Imre, S. (2019). A Survey on Quantum Computing Technology. *Computer Science Review, 31*, 51–71. https://doi.org/10.1016/j.cosrev.2018.11.002

Harris-braun, E., Luck, N., & Brock, A. (2018). Holochain White Paper. *Alpha 1*, 1–14. https://github.com/holochain/holochain-proto/blob/whitepaper/holochain.pdf

Henry, R., Herzberg, A., & Kate, A. (2018). Blockchain Access Privacy: Challenges and Directions. *IEEE Security & Privacy, 16*(4), 38–45.

Holotiuk, F., Pisani, F., & Moormann, J. (2017). The Impact of Blockchain Technology on Business Models in the Payments Industry. *WI 2017 Proceedings, September 2019*, 912–926.

Hussien, H. M., Yasin, S. M., Udzir, N. I., Ninggal, M. I. H., & Salman, S. (2021). Blockchain Technology in the Healthcare Industry: Trends and Opportunities. *Journal of Industrial Information Integration, 22*(November 2020), 100217. https://doi.org/10.1016/j.jii.2021.100217

Ismail, L., & Materwala, H. (2019). A Review of Blockchain Architecture and Consensus Protocols: Use Cases, Challenges, and Solutions. *Symmetry, 11*(10). https://doi.org/10.3390/sym11101198

Ismail, L., Materwala, H., & Zeadally, S. (2019). Lightweight Blockchain for Healthcare. *IEEE Access, 7*, 149935–149951. https://doi.org/10.1109/ACCESS.2019.2947613

Javaid, M., & Haleem, A. (2019). Industry 4.0 Applications in Medical Field: A Brief Review. *Current Medicine Research and Practice, 9*(3), 102–109. https://doi.org/10.1016/j.cmrp.2019.04.001

Joglekar, S., Kandam, S., & Dharmadhikari, S. (2023). Industry 5.0: Analysis, Applications and Prognosis. *The Online Journal of Distance Education and E-Learning, 11*(1), 257–264.

Jr, J. G., & Khan, S. (2023). *Fortifying the Blockchain: A Systematic Review and Classification of Post-Quantum Consensus Solutions for Enhanced Security and Resilience, 11*(June). https://doi.org/10.1109/ACCESS.2023.3296559

Kaur, A., & Bansal, S. (2023). *Blockchain in Healthcare: A Systematic Review and Future Perspectives* (Issue January). https://doi.org/10.1201/9781003373261-9

Kaushik, K., & Kumar, A. (2023). Demystifying Quantum Blockchain for Healthcare. *Security and Privacy, 6*(3). https://doi.org/10.1002/spy2.284

Khan, M. D., Schaefer, D., & Milisavljevic-Syed, J. (2022). A Review of Distributed Ledger Technologies in the Machine Economy: Challenges and Opportunities in Industry and Research. *Procedia CIRP, 107*(2021), 1168–1173. https://doi.org/10.1016/j.procir.2022.05.126

Kıyak, Y. S., Poor, A., Budakoğlu, I. İ., & Coşkun, Ö. (2022). Holochain: A Novel Technology Without Scalability Bottlenecks of Blockchain for Secure Data Exchange in Health Professions Education. *Discover Education, 1*(1). https://doi.org/10.1007/s44217-022-00013-y

Kordestani, A., Oghazi, P., & Mostaghel, R. (2023). Smart Contract Diffusion in the Pharmaceutical Blockchain: The Battle of Counterfeit Drugs. *Journal of Business Research, 158*(July 2022), 113646. https://doi.org/10.1016/j.jbusres.2023.113646

Krittanawong, C., Rogers, A. J., Aydar, M., Choi, E., Johnson, K. W., Wang, Z., & Narayan, S. M. (2020). Integrating Blockchain Technology with Artificial Intelligence for Cardiovascular Medicine. *Nature Reviews Cardiology, 17*(1), 1–3.

Kumar, P., Kumar, R., Gupta, G. P., Tripathi, R., Jolfaei, A., & Najmul Islam, A. K. M. (2023). A Blockchain-Orchestrated Deep Learning Approach for Secure Data Transmission in IoT-Enabled Healthcare System. *Journal of Parallel and Distributed Computing, 172*, 69–83. https://doi.org/10.1016/j.jpdc.2022.10.002

Leng, J., Chen, Z., Huang, Z., Zhu, X., Su, H., Lin, Z., & Zhang, D. (2022a). Secure Blockchain Middleware for Decentralized IIOT Towards Industry 5.0: A Review of Architecture, Enablers, Challenges, and Directions. *Machines, 10*(10), 858.

Leng, J., Sha, W., Lin, Z., Jing, J., Liu, Q., & Chen, X. (2023). Blockchained Smart Contract Pyramid-Driven Multi-Agent Autonomous Process Control for Resilient Individualised Manufacturing Towards Industry 5.0. *International Journal of Production Research, 61*(13), 4302–4321. https://doi.org/10.1080/002075 43.2022.2089929

Leng, J., Sha, W., Wang, B., Zheng, P., Zhuang, C., Liu, Q., Wuest, T., Mourtzis, D., & Wang, L. (2022b). Industry 5.0: Prospect and Retrospect. *Journal of Manufacturing Systems, 65*(August), 279–295. https://doi.org/10.1016/j.jmsy.2022.09.017

Li, J., & Carayon, P. (2021). Health Care 4.0: A Vision for Smart and Connected Health Care. *IISE Transactions on Healthcare Systems Engineering, 11*(3), 171–180. https://doi.org/10.1080/24725579.2021.1884627

Li, X., Jiang, P., Chen, T., Luo, X., & Wen, Q. (2020). A Survey on the Security of Blockchain Systems. *Future Generation Computer Systems, 107*, 841–853. https://doi.org/10.1016/j.future.2017.08.020

Lin, I. C., & Liao, T. C. (2017). A Survey of Blockchain Security Issues and Challenges. *International Journal of Network Security, 19*(5), 653–659. https://doi.org/10.6633/IJNS.201709.19(5).01

Linn, L. A., & Koo, M. B. (2016, September). Blockchain for health data and its potential use in health it and health care related research. In *ONC/NIST Use of Blockchain for Healthcare and Research Workshop* (pp. 1–10). Gaithersburg, Maryland, United States: ONC/NIST.

Liu, R., Yu, X., Yuan, Y., & Ren, Y. (2023). BTDSI: A Blockchain-Based Trusted Data Storage Mechanism for Industry 5.0. *Journal of King Saud University—Computer and Information Sciences, 35*(8), 101674. https://doi.org/10.1016/j.jksuci.2023.101674

Luu, L., Velner, Y., Teutsch, J., & Saxena, P. (2017). {SmartPool}: Practical decentralized pooled mining. In *26th USENIX Security Symposium (USENIX Security 17)* (pp. 1409–1426).

Maddikunta, P. K. R., Pham, Q. V., Prabadevi, B., Deepa, N., Dev, K., Gadekallu, T. R., . . . & Liyanage, M. (2022). Industry 5.0: A Survey on Enabling Technologies and Potential Applications. *Journal of Industrial Information Integration, 26*, 100257.

Mamo, N., Martin, G. M., Desira, M., Ellul, B., & Ebejer, J. P. (2020). Dwarna: A Blockchain Solution for Dynamic Consent in Biobanking. *European Journal of Human Genetics, 28*(5), 609–626. https://doi. org/10.1038/s41431-019-0560-9

Mazlan, A. A., Daud, S. M., Sam, S. M., Abas, H., Rasid, S. Z. A., & Yusof, M. F. (2020). Scalability Challenges in Healthcare Blockchain System-A Systematic Review. *IEEE Access, 8*, 23663–23673. https://doi.org/10.1109/ACCESS.2020.2969230

Meiklejohn, S. (2018). Top Ten Obstacles Along Distributed Ledgers Path to Adoption. *IEEE Security and Privacy, 16*(4), 13–19. https://doi.org/10.1109/MSP.2018.3111235

Mohanta, B., Das, P., & Patnaik, S. (2019). Healthcare 5.0: A Paradigm Shift in Digital Healthcare System Using Artificial Intelligence, IOT and 5G Communication. *Proceedings—2019 International Conference on Applied Machine Learning, ICAML 2019* (pp. 191–196). https://doi.org/10.1109/ICAML48257.2019.00044

Monga, S., & Singh, D. (2022). MRBSChain a Novel Scalable Medical Records Binance Smart Chain Framework Enabling a Paradigm Shift in Medical Records Management. *Scientific Reports, 12*(1), 1–12. https://doi.org/10.1038/s41598-022-22569-3

Moosavi, J., Naeni, L. M., Fathollahi-Fard, A. M., & Fiore, U. (2021). Blockchain in Supply Chain Management: A Review, Bibliometric, and Network Analysis. *Environmental Science and Pollution Research*. https:// doi.org/10.1007/s11356-021-13094-3

Moubarak, J., Filiol, E., & Chamoun, M. (2018). On Blockchain Security and Relevant Attacks. *2018 IEEE Middle East and North Africa Communications Conference, MENACOMM 2018*, 1–6. https://doi.org/10.1109/MENACOMM.2018.8371010

Nair, M. R., Rajan, N. B., & Satheesh, J. K. (2023). From Assistive Technology to the Backbone: The Impact of Blockchain in Manufacturing. *Evolutionary Intelligence, 0123456789.* https://doi.org/10.1007/s12065-023-00872-w

Nakamoto, S. (2008). Bitcoin: A peer-to-peer electronic cash system. *Satoshi Nakamoto.* https://www.poritz.net/jonathan/past_classes/winter16/CCatRU/BitcoinOriginalPaper.pdf

Nguyen, L. D. (2022). Analysis of Distributed Ledger Technologies for Industrial Manufacturing. *Scientific Reports.* https://doi.org/10.1038/s41598-022-22612-3

Odeh, A., Keshta, I., & Al-Haija, Q. A. (2022). Analysis of Blockchain in the Healthcare Sector: Application and Issues. *Symmetry, 14*(9). https://doi.org/10.3390/sym14091760

Oliveira, M., Chauhan, S., Pereira, F., Felgueiras, C., & Carvalho, D. (2023). *Blockchain Protocols & Edge Computing Targeting Average cost of IoT sensor. June.* https://doi.org/10.20944/preprints202306.1159.v1

Onik, M. M. H., Aich, S., Yang, J., Kim, C. S., & Kim, H. C. (2019). Blockchain in Healthcare: Challenges and Solutions. In *Big Data Analytics for Intelligent Healthcare Management*. Elsevier Inc. https://doi.org/10.1016/B978-0-12-818146-1.00008-8

Pandey, S. S., Dash, T., Panigrahi, P. K., & Farouk, A. (2022). *Efficient Quantum Non-Fungible Tokens for Blockchain*, 1–8. http://arxiv.org/abs/2209.02449

Papadis, N., & Tassiulas, L. (2020). Blockchain-based Payment Channel Networks: Challenges and Recent Advances. *IEEE Access, 8.* https://doi.org/10.1109/ACCESS.2020.3046020

Patki, A., & Sople, V. (2020). Indian Banking Sector: Blockchain Implementation, Challenges and Way Forward. *Journal of Banking and Financial Technology, 4*(1), 65–73. https://doi.org/10.1007/s42786-020-00019-w

Ramesh, D., Mishra, R., Atrey, P. K., Edla, D. R., Misra, S., & Qi, L. (2023). Blockchain Based Efficient Tamper-Proof EHR Storage for Decentralized Cloud-Assisted Storage. *Alexandria Engineering Journal, 68*, 205–226. https://doi.org/10.1016/j.aej.2023.01.012

Ranka, Y., Bagrecha, J., Gandhi, K., Sarvaria, B., & Chawan, P. M. (2018). A Survey on File Storage & Retrieval using Blockchain Technology. *International Research Journal of Engineering and Technology, 5*(10), 4.

Rieffel, E., & Polak, W. (2000). An Introduction to Quantum Computing for Non-Physicists. *ACM Computing Surveys (CSUR), 32*(3), 300–335.

Role of mHealth Apps in Healthcare Evolution from 1.0 to 3.0. https://appinventiv.com/blog/role-of-mhealth-apps-in-healthcare-evolution-from-1-0-3-0/ last accessed on 3rd September 2023.

Rupa, C., Midhunchakkaravarthy, D., Hasan, M. K., Alhumyani, H., & Saeed, R. A. (2021). Industry 5.0: Ethereum Blockchain Technology Based DApp Smart Contract. *Mathematical Biosciences and Engineering, 18*(5), 7010–7027. https://doi.org/10.3934/MBE.2021349

Saraswat, D., Bhattacharya, P., Verma, A., Prasad, V. K., Tanwar, S., Sharma, G., Bokoro, P. N., & Sharma, R. (2022). Explainable AI for Healthcare 5.0: Opportunities and Challenges. *IEEE Access, 10*(July), 84486–84517. https://doi.org/10.1109/ACCESS.2022.3197671

Sasikumar, A., Vairavasundaram, S., Kotecha, K., Indragandhi, V., Ravi, L., Selvachandran, G., & Abraham, A. (2023). Blockchain-Based Trust Mechanism for Digital Twin Empowered Industrial Internet of Things. *Future Generation Computer Systems, 141*, 16–27. https://doi.org/10.1016/j.future.2022.11.002

Settipalli, L., Gangadharan, G. R., & Bellamkonda, S. (2023). An Extended Lightweight Blockchain Based Collaborative Healthcare System for Fraud Prevention. *Cluster Computing, 4.* https://doi.org/10.1007/s10586-023-03973-4

Shakhbulatov, D., Medina, J., Dong, Z., & Rojas-Cessa, R. (2020). How Blockchain Enhances Supply Chain Management: A Survey. *IEEE Open Journal of the Computer Society, 1*(November), 230–249. https://doi.org/10.1109/OJCS.2020.3025313

Sharma, D., Singh Aujla, G., & Bajaj, R. (2019). Evolution from Ancient Medication to Human-Centered Healthcare 4.0: A Review on Health Care Recommender Systems. *International Journal of Communication Systems, May*, 1–40. https://doi.org/10.1002/dac.4058

Sherman, A. T., Javani, F., Zhang, H., & Golaszewski, E. (2019). On the Origins and Variations of Blockchain Technologies. *IEEE Security and Privacy, 17*(1), 72–77. https://doi.org/10.1109/MSEC.2019.2893730

Silveira, F., Rodeghiero Neto, I., Machado, F., da Silva, M., & Amaral, F. (2019). Analysis of Industry 4.0 Technologies Applied to the Health Sector: Systematic Literature Review: Personalentwicklung am Beispiel eines Tutorenprogramms. *Studies in Systems, Decision and Control*, 701–709.

Singh, A. P., Pradhan, N. R., Luhach, A. K., Agnihotri, S., Jhanjhi, N. Z., Verma, S., Kavita, Ghosh, U., & Roy, D. S. (2021). A Novel Patient-Centric Architectural Framework for Blockchain-Enabled Healthcare Applications. *IEEE Transactions on Industrial Informatics*, *17*(8), 5779–5789. https://doi.org/10.1109/TII.2020.3037889

Singh, S. K., Yang, L. T., & Park, J. H. (2023). FusionFedBlock: Fusion of Blockchain and Federated Learning to Preserve Privacy in Industry 5.0. *Information Fusion*, *90*(September 2022), 233–240. https://doi.org/10.1016/j.inffus.2022.09.027

Soltani, R., Zaman, M., Joshi, R., & Sampalli, S. (2022). Distributed Ledger Technologies and Their Applications: A Review. *Applied Sciences*, *12*(15), 7898.

Steane, A. (1998). Quantum Computing. *Reports on Progress in Physics*, *61*(2), 117–173. https://doi.org/10.1088/0034-4885/61/2/002

Swathi, P. (2022). A Survey on Quantum-safe Blockchain System. In *Proceedings of Annual Computer Security Applications Conference (ACSAC)* (Vol. 1, Issue 1). Association for Computing Machinery.

Tanwar, S., Parekh, K., & Evans, R. (2020). Blockchain-Based Electronic Healthcare Record System for Healthcare 4.0 Applications. *Journal of Information Security and Applications*, *50*. https://doi.org/10.1016/j.jisa.2019.102407

Tiwari, S., Dhanda, N., & Dev, H. (2023). A Real Time Secured Medical Management System Based on Blockchain and Internet of Things. *Measurement: Sensors*, *25*(September 2022), 100630. https://doi.org/10.1016/j.measen.2022.100630

Verma, A., Bhattacharya, P., Madhani, N., Trivedi, C., Bhushan, B., Tanwar, S., Sharma, G., Bokoro, P. N., & Sharma, R. (2022). Blockchain for Industry 5.0: Vision, Opportunities, Key Enablers, and Future Directions. *IEEE Access*, *10*(July), 69160–69199. https://doi.org/10.1109/ACCESS.2022.3186892

Verma, D., Kansra, P., & Kumar, P. (2023). Significance of Block Chain Technology and Industry 5.0 in Indian Banking Sector. *Opportunities and Challenges of Business 5.0 in Emerging Markets*, *January*, 263–269. https://doi.org/10.4018/978-1-6684-6403-8.ch014

Villarreal, E. R. D., Garcia-Alonso, J., Moguel, E., & Alegria, J. A. H. (2023). Blockchain for Healthcare Management Systems: A Survey on Interoperability and Security. *IEEE Access*, *11*(January), 5629–5652. https://doi.org/10.1109/ACCESS.2023.3236505

Wang, H. (2022). Public Health Emergency Decision-Making and Management System Sound Research Using Rough Set Attribute Reduction and Blockchain. *Scientific Reports*, *12*(1), 1–11. https://doi.org/10.1038/s41598-022-07493-w

Wang, J., Chen, J., Ren, Y., Sharma, P. K., Alfarraj, O., & Tolba, A. (2022). Data Security Storage Mechanism Based on Blockchain Industrial Internet of Things. *Computers and Industrial Engineering*, *164*(December 2021). https://doi.org/10.1016/j.cie.2021.107903

Wang, Y. (2016). CIRP Encyclopedia of Production Engineering. *CIRP Encyclopedia of Production Engineering, August 2017*. https://doi.org/10.1007/978-3-642-35950-7

Wang, Z. J., Chen, Z. S., Xiao, L., Su, Q., Govindan, K., & Skibniewski, M. J. (2023). Blockchain Adoption in Sustainable Supply Chains for Industry 5.0: A Multistakeholder Perspective. *Journal of Innovation & Knowledge*, *8*(4), 100425.

Wazid, M., Das, A. K., Mohd, N., & Park, Y. (2022). Healthcare 5.0 Security Framework: Applications, Issues and Future Research Directions. *IEEE Access*, *10*(December), 129429–129442. https://doi.org/10.1109/ACCESS.2022.3228505

What Is Quantum Computing. https://scienceexchange.caltech.edu/topics/quantum-science-explained/quantum-computing-computers last accessed on 3rd september 2023.

What Is Quantum Computing. https://www.mckinsey.com/featured-insights/mckinsey-explainers/what-is-quantum-computing last accessed on 3rd september 2023.

Wright, T. (2020). *Four-year Anniversary of Bitfinex Hack, and $12M of Stolen BTC Moved, Cointelegraph*. https://cointelegraph.com/news/four-year-anniversary-of-bitfinex-hack-and-12m-of-stolen-btc-moved last accessed on 14th October 2023.

Xing, Z., & Chen, Z. (2021). Black Bird Attack: A Vital Threat to Blockchain Technology. *Procedia Computer Science*, *199*, 556–563. https://doi.org/10.1016/j.procs.2022.01.068

Xing, Z., & Chen, Z. (2022). Using BAR Switch to Prevent Black Bird Embedded Double Spending Attack. *Procedia Computer Science*, *199*, 829–836.

Xu, M., Ren, X., Niyato, D., Kang, J., Qiu, C., Xiong, Z., Wang, X., & Leung, V. C. M. (2023). When Quantum Information Technologies Meet Blockchain in Web 3.0. *IEEE Network*, 1–8. https://doi.org/10.1109/MNET.134.2200578

Zhai, S., Yang, Y., Li, J., Qiu, C., & Zhao, J. (2019). Research on the Application of Cryptography on the Blockchain. *Journal of Physics: Conference Series, 1168*(3). https://doi.org/10.1088/1742-6596/1168/3/032077

Zhang, C., Wang, Z., Zhou, G., Chang, F., Ma, D., Jing, Y., Cheng, W., Ding, K., & Zhao, D. (2023). Towards New-Generation Human-Centric Smart Manufacturing in Industry 5.0: A Systematic Review. *Advanced Engineering Informatics, 57*(August), 102121. https://doi.org/10.1016/j.aei.2023.102121

Zhang, H., Zaman, M., Stacey, B., & Sampalli, S. (2022). A Novel Distributed Ledger Technology Structure for Wireless Sensor Networks Based on IOTA Tangle. *Electronics (Switzerland), 11*(15), 1–17. https://doi.org/10.3390/electronics11152403

Zhang, M., & Ji, Y. (2018). Blockchain for Healthcare Records: A Data Perspective. *PeerJ, 6*(May), 2–6.

Zhang, P., Wang, L., Wang, W., Fu, K., & Wang, J. (2021). A Blockchain System Based on Quantum-Resistant Digital Signature. *Security and Communication Networks, 2021*(2). https://doi.org/10.1155/2021/6671648

Zhang, R., Xue, R., & Liu, L. (2019). Security and Privacy on Blockchain. *ACM Computing Surveys, 52*(3). https://doi.org/10.1145/3316481

Zhou, Q., Huang, H., Zheng, Z., & Bian, J. (2020). Solutions to Scalability of Blockchain: A Survey. *IEEE Access, 8*, 16440–16455. https://doi.org/10.1109/aCCESS.2020.2967218

# 19 The Future of Trust
## *Exploring the Potential of Blockchain Technology*

*Divyajyothi MG, Rachappa Jopate, and Lenin J*

## 19.1  INTRODUCTION

Blockchain technology signifies a fundamental change in the way we think about and put into practice digital systems. Its immutability, transparency, and decentralized architecture present hitherto unheard-of possibilities for safe and effective transactions. Blockchain technology has enormous potential for innovation and disruption in a wide range of industries as it continues to gain traction. It allows users to deal directly with no middlemen by providing a strong and secure framework for logging and confirming data. Blockchain technology, with its decentralized structure, transparency, and immutability, has attracted a lot of interest and is changing the landscape of digital systems going forward. Blockchain is essentially a digital ledger that is distributed and decentralized, tracking transactions across multiple computers, or nodes. Blockchain operates on a peer-to-peer network, meaning that each user maintains a copy of the ledger, as opposed to traditional centralized systems that are controlled and verified by a single entity. By preventing a single party from controlling the entire system, this decentralized architecture improves transparency and does away with the need for middlemen. One of the key benefits of blockchain technology is transparency. Any transaction that has been added to the blockchain is visible to any user connected to the network. This transparency encourages trust and accountability since it allows all parties to independently check and audit transactions. As data maintained on the blockchain is immutable, once a transaction is recorded, it cannot be altered or tampered with. This immutability guarantees data integrity and offers a trustworthy, auditable record of transactions. Another key component of the platform is blockchain technology's ability to provide safe, effective peer-to-peer transactions without relying on a central authority. Participants can safely transfer value, swap assets, or directly share information with one another by using cryptographic protocols. By doing away with the need for middlemen like banks and clearinghouses, this lowers expenses, simplifies procedures, and boosts productivity. The most well-known use case for blockchain technology is cryptocurrency, but it has other uses as well. A number of industries, including finance, healthcare, supply chain management, and even governance, are investigating how blockchain technology might transform their business practices. Organizations may leverage the decentralized and transparent characteristics of blockchain to enhance security, reduce fraud, increase operational efficiency, and foster participant confidence.

The following sections will delve deeper into the underlying mechanisms and applications of blockchain, showcasing its transformative power in the modern digital landscape.

## 19.2  BLOCKCHAIN TECHNOLOGY APPLICATIONS

### 19.2.1  FINANCE SECTOR

The tokenization of assets, notably in the area of real estate, is one potential use of blockchain technology in the banking industry. To further appreciate how blockchain can transform the way real estate assets are purchased, sold, and managed, let's look at an example situation. In this scenario, a real estate developer aims to raise funds for a large-scale property development project. In the past, the developer would look to a select group of wealthy people or organizations for funding. But the developer chooses to tokenize the property and make fractional ownership available to more investors by utilizing blockchain technology. Using a blockchain platform, the developer first creates a digital version of the property. The underlying actual asset, in this example the real estate property, backs this representation, which is sometimes referred to as a security token. A small portion of the property's worth and ownership rights are represented by each security token. To guarantee regulatory compliance, the developer drafts a smart contract on the blockchain specifying the terms and circumstances of the investment. Regulations controlling profit distribution, investment caps, and eligibility restrictions are automatically enforced by the smart contract. It also gives investors the ability to trade their security tokens on secondary markets and describes the potential for liquidity. Investors who are interested in the project can now immediately purchase security tokens using the blockchain platform. The tokens provide a simple and international investment option and may be purchased with fiat money or cryptocurrencies. Because of the openness of the block chain, ownership records are kept safe and made available to all participants, which fosters a high degree of auditability and confidence. The developer updates the project's milestones and financial performance on a regular basis as the property development moves forward. Investors can monitor the project's progress, get financial reports, and, depending on the project's performance, receive dividends or capital appreciation through the blockchain platform. Moreover, investors can exchange their ownership holdings with other players in a decentralized secondary market thanks to the security tokens' liquidity. The opportunity for real estate fractional ownership is now available to a wider range of investors who may not have had the resources to invest in entire properties in the past. By using blockchain technology for asset tokenization, the financial industry can alter the financing, trading, and upkeep of real estate assets.

This paper (Wang & Nixon, 2021) offers a thorough analysis of the development of tokenization on the blockchain, which is crucial for managing various types of digital assets. For the purpose of tokenizing fungible, non-fungible, and semi-fungible assets, it examines general principles, useful schemes, and Ethereum standards. The study identifies challenges and suggests research directions to enhance the tokenization process on the blockchain, making it the first systematic exploration in this area. This research (Weerawarna et al., 2023; Varma, 2019) clarifies vlockchain technology in the finance sector from business, technological, and social perspectives. The study identifies gaps in knowledge, research, and implementation of blockchain in finance. It highlights the potential of blockchain in analyzing and managing financial data but also identifies concerns, such as big data, rules, and applications. The research suggests ways to bridge these gaps (Singh et al., 2023), including addressing technical factors, improving security and privacy, and promoting collaboration between academia, researchers, and financial institutions. It emphasizes the need for strategic planning and knowledge dissemination by governments to foster the exploration of blockchain in the finance industry. Thus, blockchain has the potential to transform traditional financial systems by eliminating intermediaries, improving transaction speed and security, and reducing costs, in areas such as cross-border payments, remittances, digital identity management, and decentralized finance (DeFi).

### 19.2.2 Healthcare

Blockchain technology in healthcare enables secure and decentralized storage of patient health records, tamper-proof audit trails for transactions and supply chain management, and decentralized networks for data sharing and collaboration in medical research, enhancing security, privacy, and interoperability. Health information sharing is a component of one of the earliest blockchain-based healthcare systems. This is challenging because it involves sensitive data that is categorized as personal information about the patient. This particular use case for blockchain technology has been covered (Patane et al., 2019; Xia et al., 2017). To increase the effectiveness, security, and privacy of electronic medical records (EMRs), MedRec is a blockchain-based solution. A decentralized, immutable record of patient data is created by the system using blockchain technology, assuring its integrity and lowering the possibility of illegal access or alteration. By facilitating secure data exchange and easy access to patient records across institutions, MedRec intends to improve interoperability across various healthcare providers. MedRec automates consent management and data governance through the use of smart contracts, providing patients more control over their personal health data. Additionally, the system includes data analytics tools to aid in population health management and research. The potential of MedRec in actual healthcare settings has been investigated in a number of studies (Ekblaw et al., 2016), which emphasize its advantages in terms of data security, privacy, and patient-centered treatment. The actual benefit of interoperability and cybersecurity can be unlocked through a blockchain-powered health information exchange (HIE). When it comes to population health management, this method has the ability to do away with the hassles and expenses associated with present third-party intermediaries. Better data integrity, cheaper transaction costs, decentralization, and the elimination of trust intermediaries are among the several claims made. In order to efficiently minimize unnecessary services and redundant testing while reducing costs and improving the efficacy of the continuum care cycle while adhering to all HIPAA rules and standards, patient care coordination via a blockchain HIE is necessary. Patientory (McFarlane et al., 2017) is a blockchain-based patient-centered protocol that is altering how healthcare stakeholders maintain electronic medical data and communicate with clinical care teams. Coral Health (Sharma et al., 2022) utilizes blockchain technology to create a comprehensive and secure health information exchange platform. It enables patients to control their health data and share it with trusted healthcare providers, researchers, and other stakeholders. A blockchain-based health data network called BurstIQ (Charles & Delgado, 2022) makes it possible to safely share, analyze, and profit from health data. It permits cooperation and data-driven innovation in healthcare while giving people ownership and control over their data. Medicalchain (C. Zhang et al., 2019) has developed a decentralized network for exchanging and storing electronic health records by utilizing blockchain technology. It ensures transparency and data integrity by allowing patients to provide medical professionals access to their records. A blockchain platform created especially for healthcare applications is offered by Gem. It permits safe exchange of health information, makes care coordination easier, and provides real-time analytics for population health management and research.

## 19.2.3  Supply Chain Management

Blockchain technology has garnered significant interest in the field of supply chain management because of its potential to enhance transparency, traceability, and security in supply chain operations (Dede et al., 2021). Numerous studies have looked into the application of blockchain technology to supply chain management (Bhalerao et al., 2019; Raj & B, 2021). A supply chain's worth of commodities may be tracked and verified by stakeholders thanks to blockchain technology, which creates an immutable and transparent record. Research has been done on the use of blockchain to enhance traceability in a number of industries, such as luxury goods, food, and pharmaceuticals (Song et al., 2019; Agrawal et al., 2021; Ayan et al., 2022). Further research is needed on the use of blockchain's smart contracts to automate and enhance supply chain processes (Alqarni et al., 2023; Prause, 2019). Smart contracts are self-executing programs that have predefined parameters and actions. Scholars have examined the potential of smart contracts to reduce errors, delays, and costs associated with supply chain operations by streamlining procedures such as order fulfillment, inventory control, and payment processing. The potential of blockchain to improve stakeholder engagement and supply chain visibility has also been researched (Difrancesco et al., 2022; Verny et al., 2020). Blockchain facilitates real-time information sharing by offering a transparent and decentralized platform, which enhances cooperation and confidence among supply chain participants. Research projects have looked into the integration of blockchain with other emerging technologies like the Internet of Things (IoT) and artificial intelligence (AI) in order to enable real-time data gathering, analysis, and decision-making in supply chain management (Som & Kayal, 2022; Bothra et al., 2023; Tyagi et al., 2023). Thus, blockchain can facilitate provenance tracking, increase supply chain transparency, reduce the prevalence of counterfeit items, and expedite processes like payment settlements and inventory management.

### 19.2.4 Intellectual Property Protection

Blockchain-based solutions have been proposed (Gürkaynak et al., 2018; Song et al., 2021) to address issues related to intellectual property rights and copyright infringement. Research has explored (Chen et al., 2020) how blockchain can create transparent and immutable records of intellectual property ownership, streamline licensing processes, and enable fair and transparent royalties' distribution. The use of blockchain technology for digital copyright protection is a cutting-edge technical strategy and security idea with a bright future that strives to defend the rights of copyright owners. This study (Luo, 2022) provides a thorough analysis of the situation of digital copyright protection today as well as the benefits and potential drawbacks of applying blockchain technology in three areas: transaction monitoring, transaction confirmation, and evidence preservation. Finally, a system design for blockchain technology is considered and suggested for the application of digital copyright protection. The study discovered that blockchain technology can be used to build a unified platform for digital copyright protection that completely and successfully records the entire process.

### 19.2.5 Voting and Governance

Blockchain can enhance the transparency, integrity, and security of voting systems. Research (Kshetri & Voas, 2018) has investigated blockchain-based voting platforms (Baudier et al., 2021; Curran, 2018; Mosley et al., 2022) that ensure tamper-proof voting records, enable remote and secure voting, and enhance voter trust in the electoral process (Verma & Sheel, 2022). As a result, blockchain technology has many advantages for voting and governance procedures. By offering a visible and immutable ledger where all transactions may be recorded, it assures transparency. The possibility of fraud or manipulation is eliminated because to this transparency. Through cryptographic techniques, it increases security and makes data very difficult for unwanted access or alteration (Febriyanto et al., 2020). Additionally, the immutable record spread across several nodes ensured by blockchain's decentralized structure further boosts system integrity. By eliminating intermediaries, blockchain streamlines processes, enhances efficiency, and reduces costs (Khan et al., 2020). Additionally, it enables broader participation by facilitating remote voting and eliminates geographical barriers. The tamper-resistant audit trail and smart contracts offered by blockchain add accountability and automation to governance procedures. Thus, blockchain's decentralized nature promotes a more democratic and inclusive approach to decision-making. While challenges exist, careful implementation can harness these benefits to revolutionize voting and governance systems.

## 19.3   IMPLEMENTATION OF BLOCKCHAIN

The deployment of blockchain technology involves a number of significant concerns and phases (Kwilinski, 2019; Suripeddi & Purandare, 2021). The particular use case for which blockchain technology might be useful must be identified first, and this is key. This calls for a thorough examination of a variety of marketplaces and industries, including voting processes, supply chain management, and decentralized apps (DApps). After the use case has been determined, selecting the optimal blockchain platform is essential (Muneeza et al., 2018; Tan et al., 2022). Scalability, consensus mechanisms, security features, and development tools are a few factors that must be taken into account to ensure the chosen platform (Rauta & Shah, 2021; Alu et al., n.d.) satisfies the requirements of the use case. Following platform selection, the blockchain network is designed (Kirpes et al., 2019; Tanrıverdi & Tekerek, 2019). This entails figuring out the members' roles and responsibilities as well as the consensus model and network structure. The creation of DApps and smart contracts (Shojaei et al., 2020) that are customized for the chosen platform (Khatoon, 2020) comes next, making sure that the logic and rules controlling interactions are properly written. The network infrastructure is then built up, with blockchain nodes configured and communication routes established between them. To assure functionality, security, and performance, the blockchain implementation is put through a rigorous testing process (Guo & Liang, 2016). To verify the system's behavior under various conditions, numerous tests and simulations are run. The blockchain network and related applications are deployed to the desired environment after testing is finished. It is crucial to establish governance structures that include decision-making procedures, consensus protocols, and participation guidelines. User-friendly interfaces and detailed instructions for dealing with the blockchain system promote user adoption. To guarantee efficient data flow and interoperability, integration with current systems or procedures can be required. To monitor the blockchain network, address performance or security concerns, and keep up with technological improvements, ongoing maintenance and upgrades are essential. The key to a successful implementation and adoption of blockchain technology is educating stakeholders about its advantages and capabilities. To traverse the complexity of implementation, cooperation with authorities in the legal, cybersecurity, and blockchain development fields may be required. A successful blockchain implementation that realizes the potential of this game-changing technology requires careful planning, diligent testing, and ongoing review (Roehrs et al., 2019).

### 19.3.1 Role of EdgeAI in Blockchain Technology

Edge AI's integration with blockchain technology has many benefits and significantly improves blockchain systems (Qiu et al., 2022; Cao, 2022). By implementing AI algorithms and models directly on edge devices, edge AI improves privacy and security (Hammoud et al., 2020) by keeping sensitive data closer to its source and lowering the likelihood of data breaches. It allows for real-time decision-making and enables blockchain networks to respond rapidly to urgent events by processing data locally. Edge AI also increases efficiency and scalability by minimizing resource usage and lightening the load on the blockchain network. The decrease in latency and bandwidth needs is one of the main advantages of edge AI in blockchain (Lu et al., 2020). Blockchain transactions are expedited and made more effective by processing data locally on edge devices, which reduces the need to send vast amounts of data to the cloud. Additionally, edge AI makes it possible for disconnected and offline operations, guaranteeing the continuation of crucial blockchain processes even when network access is poor or nonexistent (Ozdogan et al., 2022). Thanks to the integration of edge AI with blockchain technology, edge devices can now carry out intelligent computations, which boosts the effectiveness and performance of blockchain systems as a whole. It offers improved anonymity, real-time decision-making ability, scalability, effectiveness, lower latency, and offline operations. The incorporation of edge AI gives a possible route for unlocking the potential of blockchain applications as they continue to develop.

### 19.3.2 Role of Machine Learning Algorithms in Blockchain Technology

Blockchain technology is being improved, and its full potential is being unlocked, in large part because to machine learning algorithms. The blockchain ecosystem gains from using these algorithms in a variety of ways (Hirata et al., 2020). They allow for data analysis, which makes it possible to gain priceless insights from the enormous volume of data stored on the blockchain. Machine learning algorithms can help with decision-making and optimization procedures by spotting patterns and trends. Moreover, these algorithms contribute to fraud detection and prevention by leveraging historical data to identify suspicious transactions or fraudulent activities, bolstering the security and integrity of the blockchain network. Machine learning algorithms also enable predictive analytics, utilizing historical blockchain data to make forecasts and predictions that can be applied to market trends, supply chain optimization, and demand estimation. Additionally, machine learning algorithms can optimize smart contracts by adapting their behavior based on real-time data, improving efficiency and effectiveness. They also facilitate privacy preservation in blockchain systems by developing techniques like federated learning or differential privacy to protect sensitive data while still allowing valuable analysis. Furthermore, machine learning algorithms enhance network security by analyzing network traffic, identifying potential threats or attacks, and enabling proactive measures. Lastly, these algorithms aid in resource allocation within blockchain networks, optimizing the distribution of resources based on usage patterns and network demand, thereby improving scalability and performance. Although challenges such as data quality and model interpretability exist, the integration of machine learning and blockchain opens new avenues for innovation across industries (Wu et al., 2021).

### 19.3.3  ROLE OF IoT IN BLOCKCHAIN TECHNOLOGY

A wide range of opportunities are made possible by the combination of IoT devices and blockchain technology (Sharma et al., 2020a). Data security and integrity are two important functions of IoT in blockchain (Kumar & Mallick, 2018). Massive volumes of data being produced by IoT devices, and blockchain's immutable and tamper-proof ledger offers a safe platform for encoding and verifying transactions. Blockchain technology makes IoT data transparent, tamper-proof, and dependable. Another significant role of IoT in blockchain is establishing trust and authentication. With decentralized identity management systems powered by blockchain, IoT devices can securely authenticate themselves and communicate with other devices, fostering trust in the ecosystem. This enables seamless and secure interactions between devices, supporting autonomous decision-making and coordination. Supply chain and logistics also benefit from the combination of IoT and blockchain. Real-time data on variables like location, temperature, and handling conditions may be safely stored on the blockchain by integrating IoT devices into supply chain activities. By establishing an unchangeable audit trail, this improves the supply chain's transparency, effectiveness, and confidence. Blockchain and IoT integration improve automation and smart contracts. When paired with smart contracts built on the blockchain, IoT devices can perform transactions of their own accord based on predetermined criteria. For example, smart contracts can automatically trigger payment release once the IoT devices confirm successful delivery. Furthermore, IoT and blockchain enable individuals to retain ownership and control over their data. By securely recording data transactions on the blockchain, IoT devices empower individuals to monetize their data while maintaining control and privacy (Kim & Deka, 2020).

### 19.3.4  ROLE OF CLOUD SERVICES IN BLOCKCHAIN TECHNOLOGY

In order for blockchain technology to be implemented and run effectively, cloud services are essential (Gai et al., 2020). They provide the scalability, high availability, and infrastructure required to operate blockchain networks. Cloud services guarantee consistent performance even during periods of high usage since they have the capacity to dynamically scale resources based on demand. By using redundant servers and automated failover processes, the fault tolerance features offered by cloud services ensure the continuous operation of blockchain networks. Additionally, cloud services offer effective and affordable options for handling and storing the enormous amounts of data produced by blockchain networks (Sharma et al., 2020b). Businesses can use databases and cloud storage services to store and process blockchain data securely. Cloud-based analytics services give businesses access to insightful data that can be used to enhance decision-making and spur innovation. Cloud services make it easier to integrate blockchain networks with already-in-use business systems and apps. Organizations can easily connect their blockchain networks with legacy systems using cloud-based integration tools and services, facilitating effective data exchange and interoperability (Wang et al., 2019). Additionally, cloud services provide development tools and collaborative platforms that hasten the creation, testing, and deployment of blockchain applications. Organizations may streamline their blockchain development processes and promote team collaboration with the help of these tools, which offer programming environments, APIs, and pre-built templates. Using cloud services enables blockchain installation at a low cost, by only paying for the resources they actually use. Organizations can reduce costs and do away with the need to make sizable upfront capital expenditures in on-premises infrastructure. This is possible with the pay-as-you-go approach.

## 19.4 CHALLENGES TO BLOCKCHAIN ADOPTION

### 19.4.1 REGULATORY HURDLES

**Lack of Clarity:** Regulatory uncertainty regarding cryptocurrencies and blockchain technology inhibits adoption (Pandya et al., 2019). When regulations are unclear or subject to rapid change, investors and businesses may hesitate to enter the blockchain and cryptocurrency space. They fear potential legal consequences, fines, or the need to halt operations if they inadvertently violate evolving regulations (Al-Amri et al., 2019).

**Compliance Costs:** Compliance with evolving regulations is expensive and time-consuming for blockchain-based businesses. Adhering to constantly changing regulations can be expensive. Blockchain companies must allocate resources to ensure compliance, diverting funds and attention away from innovation and growth (Gaur, 2020).

### 19.4.2 SCALABILITY ISSUES

**Transaction Speed:** Blockchain's ability to handle large volumes of transactions is hampered by slow transaction processing times (Hashim et al., 2022). The quantity of transactions that can be confirmed and added to the blockchain in a given amount of time is constrained by slow transaction processing. When there is a spike in transaction demand, this constrained throughput becomes a bottleneck. To prioritize their transactions and have them processed quickly, users may choose to pay higher fees to miners. This fee competition drives up transaction costs, making blockchain less cost-effective for users.

**Network Congestion:** Scalability challenges result in network congestion and increased fees. Slow transaction processing times can inhibit micro-transactions (very small-value transactions) and high-frequency trading on blockchain networks. In these cases, fast confirmations are crucial, but slow speeds can hinder these activities.

### 19.4.3 INTEROPERABILITY CHALLENGES

**Blockchain Fragmentation:** Different blockchains often don't communicate effectively, limiting seamless data exchange. Most blockchains are designed as isolated networks with their own consensus mechanisms, rules, and data structures. They often operate independently of each other, making direct communication difficult (Worley & Skjellum, 2018).

**Smart Contract Compatibility:** Ensuring compatibility between various blockchain platforms and smart contracts is a complex task. Different blockchain platforms often use distinct programming languages for developing smart contracts. For example, Ethereum primarily uses Solidity, while other platforms might use languages like Rust, Vyper, or JavaScript. Developers need to learn and adapt to these varying languages

### 19.4.4 SECURITY CONCERNS

**51% Attacks:** The security of smaller blockchains is questioned since they are susceptible to 51% assaults (Abuidris et al., 2021; Khanum & Mustafa, 2023). A 51% assault, often referred to as a majority attack or a double-spend attack, happens when a single entity or collection of miners has more than 50% of the network's total hash rate. With this much power, they can alter the blockchain's transactions and possibly carry out harmful deeds like double spending money.

**Smart Contract Vulnerabilities:** Vulnerabilities in smart contracts can lead to significant losses (Krupp & Rossow, 2018). Smart contract vulnerabilities can indeed lead to significant losses, both in terms of financial assets and the reputation of blockchain projects. These vulnerabilities are often the result of coding errors, design flaws, or unexpected behaviors within the smart contract code. Here's how smart contract vulnerabilities can lead to losses.

### 19.4.5   LACK OF STANDARDIZATION

**Token Standards:** The absence of universal token standards makes it difficult for tokens to function across different platforms (Wang & Nixon, 2021). Tokens created on one blockchain may rely on specific smart contract functionality that is not available on another platform. This incompatibility prevents tokens from being directly ported or used across different blockchains.

**Data Standards:** Inconsistent data formats and structures hinder data sharing and integration. Inconsistent data formats require specialized parsers and data transformation procedures, adding complexity to data integration processes. Developers need to write custom code to extract, convert, and map data between systems.

### 19.4.6   USER EXPERIENCE

**Wallet Management:** Users find wallet management and private key security challenging (Liu et al., 2017). The various wallet options available to users include hardware wallets, software wallets, mobile wallets, and more. Each type has unique usage difficulties and security issues.

**Complexity:** The complexity of blockchain technology is a barrier for mainstream adoption (Prewett et al., 2020).

### 19.4.7   ENERGY CONSUMPTION

**Environmental Concerns:** Proof-of-work (PoW) consensus mechanisms contribute to high energy consumption, leading to sustainability concerns (Platt et al., 2021). PoW requires miners to solve complex mathematical puzzles through computational work. The competitive nature of mining encourages miners to use more and more computational power, leading to higher energy consumption (Sapra et al., 2023).

**Transition to PoS:** The shift to proof-of-stake (PoS) is a solution but faces resistance (Snider et al., 2018).

### 19.4.8   PRIVACY AND ANONYMITY

**Data Privacy:** It can be difficult to strike a compromise between openness and data privacy (Denker & Javaid, 2019; Liu et al., 2022). Striking a balance between transparency and privacy often involves obtaining informed consent from individuals regarding data usage. Ensuring that individuals fully understand the implications of data collection and use can be challenging.

**Regulatory Compliance:** Meeting privacy regulations like GDPR can be tricky on a public blockchain (W. Zhang et al., 2019).

### 19.4.9   COSTS AND RESOURCE CONSTRAINTS

**Initial Investment:** Implementing blockchain technology can be expensive, deterring some businesses (Tang et al., 2020).

**Skilled Workforce:** A shortage of blockchain talent can hinder adoption.

### 19.4.10 Resistance to Change

**Legacy Systems:** Organizations are often reluctant to transition from existing systems to blockchain (Atzori, 2015). Despite the enormous progress it has achieved, blockchain is still a relatively new and fast developing technology. Organizations may be hesitant to adopt a technology that is perceived as being in its early stages and subject to ongoing development and refinement.

**Cultural Shift:** Employees may resist the cultural changes associated with blockchain adoption (Choi et al., 2020). Blockchain is a relatively new and complex technology. Employees may feel overwhelmed by the need to learn and adapt to new tools, processes, and concepts, which can create resistance to change.

### 19.4.11 Tokenization Challenges

**Asset Tokenization:** Challenges in tokenizing real-world assets, like property or art, create barriers (Benedetti & Rodríguez-Garnica, 2023). Determining and ensuring the rightful ownership of real-world assets represented as tokens can be challenging. Custody solutions that securely hold and manage digital tokens linked to real assets are crucial but can be complex to implement.

**Legal Frameworks:** Legal and regulatory frameworks for tokenized assets are still evolving. Blockchain is inherently global, and digital assets can cross borders effortlessly. This presents challenges for regulators, as they need to consider how to regulate tokenized assets in a borderless digital environment, often with differing regulations in different jurisdictions.

### 19.4.12 Blockchain Education

**Lack of Understanding:** Blockchain technology adoption is hampered by a lack of knowledge and comprehension of it.

**Educational Resources:** Access to quality educational resources is essential for bridging this knowledge gap.

### 19.4.13 Network Security

**51% Attack Mitigation:** Developing effective strategies to mitigate 51% attacks is an ongoing challenge (Saad et al., 2020).

**Quantum Threat:** The potential future threat of quantum computing to blockchain security requires preemptive solutions (Denker & Javaid, 2019). The cryptographic techniques that now support the security of blockchain networks could be broken by quantum computers.

### 19.4.14 Cross-Border Challenges

**International Regulations:** Varying regulations across countries create complexities for cross-border blockchain applications (W. Zhang et al., 2019).

**Data Localization Laws:** Compliance with data localization laws can hinder global blockchain solutions.

### 19.4.15 Ethical Concerns

**Decentralization vs. Centralization:** Balancing the benefits of decentralization with the potential for abuse is a complex ethical dilemma (Tang et al., 2020).

**Social Impact:** Ethical considerations surrounding blockchain's impact on society and privacy must be addressed.

## 19.5  CONCLUSION

Blockchain has emerged as a disruptive force with the ability to redefine the fundamental foundations of how we establish, verify, and keep trust in the constantly changing landscape of technology and trust. We are at a critical point in "The Future of Trust: Exploring the Potential of Blockchain Technology," where the seeds of innovation have been sowed and the opportunities are endless, as we complete this chapter. Blockchain's promise lies not only in its ability to secure and decentralize data but also in its capacity to foster transparency, empower individuals, and democratize trust. It is a testament to human ingenuity and collaboration, transcending borders and industries to pioneer a new era of trust and accountability. As we look ahead, the future of trust through blockchain technology is poised to touch every facet of our lives. From supply chains and finance to healthcare, governance, and beyond, blockchain's potential is limited only by our imagination and dedication to harnessing its power for the betterment of society. However, let us not forget that this journey is not without its challenges and complexities. Regulatory frameworks must evolve to adapt to the digital age, security must remain paramount, and inclusivity should be at the heart of our endeavors.

## REFERENCES


Abuidris, Y., Kumar, R., Yang, T., & Onginjo, J. (2021). Secure large-scale E-voting system based on blockchain contract using a hybrid consensus model combined with sharding. *ETRI Journal*, 43(2), 357–370.

Agrawal, T. K., Kumar, V., Pal, R., Wang, L., & Chen, Y. (2021). Blockchain-based framework for supply chain traceability: A case example of textile and clothing industry. *Computers & Industrial Engineering*, 154, 107130. ISSN 0360-8352. https://doi.org/10.1016/j.cie.2021.107130

Al-Amri, R., Zakaria, N. H., Habbal, A., & Hassan, S. (2019). Cryptocurrency adoption: Current stage, opportunities, and open challenges. *International Journal of Advanced Computer Research*, 9(44), 293–307.

Alqarni, M. A., Alkatheiri, M. S., Chauhdary, S. H., & Saleem, S. (2023). Use of blockchain-based smart contracts in logistics and supply chains. *Electronics*, 12(6), 1340. MDPI AG. http://doi.org/10.3390/electronics12061340

Alu, E. S., Ahubele, B. O., & Nnodi, J. T. (n.d.). A proposed model for decentralized governance using blockchain technology.

Atzori, M. (2015). *Blockchain technology and decentralized governance: Is the state still necessary?* Available at SSRN 2709713.

Ayan, B., Güner, E., & Son-Turan, S. (2022). Blockchain technology and sustainability in supply chains and a closer look at different industries: A mixed method approach. *Logistics*, 6(4), 85. MDPI AG. http://doi.org/10.3390/logistics6040085

Baudier, P., Kondrateva, G., Ammi, C., & Seulliet, E. (2021). Peace engineering: The contribution of blockchain systems to the e-voting process. *Technological Forecasting and Social Change*, 162, 120397.

Benedetti, H., & Rodríguez-Garnica, G. (2023). Tokenized assets and securities. In *The Emerald Handbook on Cryptoassets: Investment Opportunities and Challenges* (pp. 107–121). Emerald Publishing Limited.

Bhalerao, S., Agarwal, S., Borkar, S., Anekar, S., Kulkarni, N., & Bhagwat, S. (2019). Supply chain management using blockchain. In *2019 International Conference on Intelligent Sustainable Systems (ICISS)* (pp. 456–459). Palladam, India. https://doi.org/10.1109/ISS1.2019.8908031

Bothra, P., Karmakar, R., Bhattacharya, S., & De, S. (2023). How can applications of blockchain and artificial intelligence improve performance of Internet of Things?—A survey. *Computer Networks*. https://doi.org/10.1016/j.comnet.2023.109634

Cao, L. (2022). Decentralized ai: Edge intelligence and smart blockchain, metaverse, web3, and desci. *IEEE Intelligent Systems*, 37(3), 6–19.

Charles, W. M., & Delgado, B. M. (2022). Health datasets as assets: Blockchain-based valuation and transaction methods. *Blockchain Healthc Today*, 5. https://doi.org/10.30953/bhty.v5.185

Chen, W., Zhou, K., Fang, W., Wang, K., Bi, F., & Assefa, B. (2020). Review on blockchain technology and its application to the simple analysis of intellectual property protection. *International Journal of Computational Science and Engineering*, 22(4), 437–444.

Choi, D., Chung, C. Y., Seyha, T., & Young, J. (2020). Factors affecting organizations' resistance to the adoption of blockchain technology in supply networks. *Sustainability*, 12(21), 8882.

Curran, K. (2018). E-voting on the blockchain. *The Journal of the British Blockchain Association*, 1(2).

Dede, S., Köseoğlu, M. C., & Yercan, H. F. (2021). Learning from early adopters of blockchain technology: A systematic review of supply chain case studies. *Technology Innovation Management Review*, 11(6).

Denker, K., & Javaid, A. Y. (2019). Quantum computing as a threat to modern cryptography techniques. In *Proceedings of the International Conference on Foundations of Computer Science (FCS)* (pp. 3–8). The Steering Committee of The World Congress in Computer Science, Computer Engineering and Applied Computing (WorldComp).

Difrancesco, R. M., Meena, P., & Kumar, G. (2022). How blockchain technology improves sustainable supply chain processes: A practical guide. *Operations Management Research*, 1–22. https://doi.org/10.1007/s12063-022-00343-y

Ekblaw, A., Azaria, A., & Halamka, J. D. (2016). A case study for blockchain in healthcare: "MedRec" prototype for electronic health records and medical research data. In *Proceedings of IEEE Open & Big Data Conference* (Vol. 13, p. 13).

Febriyanto, E., Rahayu, N., Pangaribuan, K., & Sunarya, P. A. (2020, October). Using blockchain data security management for e-voting systems. In *2020 8th International Conference on Cyber and IT Service Management (CITSM)* (pp. 1–4). IEEE.

Gai, K., Guo, J., Zhu, L., & Yu, S. (2020). Blockchain meets cloud computing: A survey. *IEEE Communications Surveys & Tutorials*, 22(3), 2009–2030.

Gaur, N. (2020). Blockchain challenges in adoption. *Managerial Finance*, 46(6), 849–858.

Guo, Y., & Liang, C. (2016). Blockchain application and outlook in the banking industry. *Financial Innovation*, 2, 1–12.

Gürkaynak, G., Yılmaz, I., Yeşilaltay, B., & Bengi, B. (2018). Intellectual property law and practice in the blockchain realm. *Computer Law & Security Review*, 34(4), 847–862.

Hammoud, A., Sami, H., Mourad, A., Otrok, H., Mizouni, R., & Bentahar, J. (2020). AI, blockchain, and vehicular edge computing for smart and secure IoV: Challenges and directions. *IEEE Internet of Things Magazine*, 3(2), 68–73.

Hashim, F., Shuaib, K., & Zaki, N. (2022). Sharding for scalable blockchain networks. *SN Computer Science*, 4(1), 2.

Hirata, E., Lambrou, M., & Watanabe, D. (2020). Blockchain technology in supply chain management: Insights from machine learning algorithms. *Maritime Business Review*, 6(2), 114–128.

Khan, S., Arshad, A., Mushtaq, G., Khalique, A., & Husein, T. (2020). Implementation of decentralized blockchain e-voting. *EAI Endorsed Transactions on Smart Cities*, 4(10).

Khanum, S., & Mustafa, K. (2023). A systematic literature review on sensitive data protection in blockchain applications. *Concurrency and Computation: Practice and Experience*, 35(1), e7422.

Khatoon, A. (2020). A blockchain-based smart contract system for healthcare management. *Electronics*, 9(1), 94.

Kim, S., & Deka, G. C. (Eds.). (2020). *Advanced Applications of Blockchain Technology*. Berlin and Heidelberg, Germany: Springer.

Kirpes, B., Mengelkamp, E., Schaal, G., & Weinhardt, C. (2019). Design of a microgrid local energy market on a blockchain-based information system. *IT-Information Technology*, 61(2–3), 87–99.

Krupp, J., & Rossow, C. (2018). teEther: Gnawing at ethereum to automatically exploit smart contracts. In *27th USENIX Security Symposium (USENIX Security 18)* (pp. 1317–1333).

Kshetri, N., & Voas, J. (2018). Blockchain-enabled e-voting. *IEEE Software*, 35(4), 95–99.

Kumar, N. M., & Mallick, P. K. (2018). Blockchain technology for security issues and challenges in IoT. *Procedia Computer Science*, 132, 1815–1823.

Kwilinski, A. (2019). Implementation of blockchain technology in accounting sphere. *Academy of Accounting and Financial Studies Journal*, 23, 1–6.

Liu, L., Li, X., Au, M. H., Fan, Z., & Meng, X. (2022, April). Metadata privacy preservation for blockchain-based healthcare systems. In *International Conference on Database Systems for Advanced Applications* (pp. 404–412). Cham: Springer International Publishing.

Liu, Y., Li, R., Liu, X., Wang, J., Zhang, L., Tang, C., & Kang, H. (2017, October). An efficient method to enhance Bitcoin wallet security. In *2017 11th IEEE International Conference on Anti-counterfeiting, Security, and Identification (ASID)* (pp. 26–29). IEEE.

Lu, Y., Huang, X., Zhang, K., Maharjan, S., & Zhang, Y. (2020). Low-latency federated learning and blockchain for edge association in digital twin empowered 6G networks. *IEEE Transactions on Industrial Informatics*, 17(7), 5098–5107.

Luo, L. (2022). Application of blockchain technology in intellectual property protection. *Mathematical Problems in Engineering*, 2022.

McFarlane, C. T., Beer, M., Brown, J., & Prendergast, N. (2017). *Patientory: A Healthcare Peer-to-Peer EMR Storage Network v 1. 1* (pp. 3, 19). Addison, TX: Entrust Inc.

Mosley, L., Pham, H., Guo, X., Bansal, Y., Hare, E., & Antony, N. (2022). Towards a systematic understanding of blockchain governance in proposal voting: A dash case study. *Blockchain: Research and Applications*, 3(3), 100085.

Muneeza, A., Arshad, N. A., & Arifin, A. T. (2018). The application of blockchain technology in crowdfunding: Towards financial inclusion via technology. *International Journal of Management and Applied Research*, 5(2), 82–98.

Ozdogan, M. O., Carkacioglu, L., & Canberk, B. (2022, May). Digital twin driven blockchain based reliable and efficient 6G edge network. In *2022 18th International Conference on Distributed Computing in Sensor Systems (DCOSS)* (pp. 342–348). IEEE.

Pandya, S., Mittapalli, M., Gulla, S. V. T., & Landau, O. (2019). Cryptocurrency: Adoption efforts and security challenges in different countries. *HOLISTICA–Journal of Business and Public Administration*, 10(2), 167–186.

Patane, R., Nadar, A., Dubey, V., & Nadar, C. (2019). Medical data access and permission management using blockchain. *JETIR Research Journal*, 6, 655–658.

Platt, M., Sedlmeir, J., Platt, D., Xu, J., Tasca, P., Vadgama, N., & Ibañez, J. I. (2021, December). The energy footprint of blockchain consensus mechanisms beyond proof-of-work. In *2021 IEEE 21st International Conference on Software Quality, Reliability and Security Companion (QRS-C)* (pp. 1135–1144). IEEE.

Prause, G. (2019). Smart contracts for smart supply chains. *IFAC-PapersOnLine*, 52(13), 2501–2506. ISSN 2405-8963. https://doi.org/10.1016/j.ifacol.2019.11.582

Prewett, K. W., Prescott, G. L., & Phillips, K. (2020). Blockchain adoption is inevitable—Barriers and risks remain. *Journal of Corporate Accounting & Finance*, 31(2), 21–28.

Qiu, X., Yao, D., Kang, X., & Abulizi, A. (2022). Blockchain and K-means algorithm for edge AI computing. *Computational Intelligence and Neuroscience*, 2022.

Raj, Y., & B, S. (2021). Study on supply chain management using blockchain technology. In *2021 6th International Conference on Inventive Computation Technologies (ICICT)* (pp. 1243–1247), Coimbatore, India. https://doi.org/10.1109/ICICT50816.2021.9358768

Rauta, N., & Shah, K. (2021). Implementation of ethereum blockchain in healthcare using IPFS. *Pulse*, 2(2).

Roehrs, A., da Costa, C. A., da Rosa Righi, R., da Silva, V. F., Goldim, J. R., & Schmidt, D. C. (2019). Analyzing the performance of a blockchain-based personal health record implementation. *Journal of Biomedical Informatics*, 92, 103140.

Saad, M., Spaulding, J., Njilla, L., Kamhoua, C., Shetty, S., Nyang, D., & Mohaisen, D. (2020). Exploring the attack surface of blockchain: A comprehensive survey. *IEEE Communications Surveys & Tutorials*, 22(3), 1977–2008.

Sapra, N., Shaikh, I., & Dash, A. (2023). Impact of proof of work (PoW)-Based blockchain applications on the environment: A systematic review and research agenda. *Journal of Risk and Financial Management*, 16(4), 218.

Sharma, P. K., Jindal, R., & Borah, M. D. (2020a). Blockchain technology for cloud storage: A systematic literature review. *ACM Computing Surveys (CSUR)*, 53(4), 1–32.

Sharma, P. K., Kumar, N., & Park, J. H. (2020b). Blockchain technology toward green IoT: Opportunities and challenges. *IEEE Network*, 34(4), 263–269.

Sharma, V., Gupta, A., Ul Hasan, N., Shabaz, M., & Isaac, O. (2022). Blockchain in secure healthcare systems: State of the art, limitations, and future directions. *Security and Communication Networks*, 2022, 1–15. https://doi.org/10.1155/2022/9697545

Shojaei, A., Flood, I., Moud, H. I., Hatami, M., & Zhang, X. (2020). An implementation of smart contracts by integrating BIM and blockchain. In *Proceedings of the Future Technologies Conference (FTC) 2019: Volume 2* (pp. 519–527). Springer International Publishing.

Singh, A., Shahare, P., Vikram, P., Srivastava, V., Manpreet, K., & Maan. (2023). Financial sector and blockchain technology: Challenges and applications. https://doi.org/10.47750/pnr.2023.14.02.201

Snider, M., Samani, K., & Jain, T. (2018). Delegated proof of stake: features & tradeoffs. *Multicoin Capital*, 19, 1–19.

Som, A., & Kayal, P. (2022). *AI, Blockchain, and IOT*. https://doi.org/10.1007/978-3-031-11545-5_8

Song, H., Zhu, N., Xue, R., He, J., Zhang, K., & Wang, J. (2021). Proof-of-contribution consensus mechanism for blockchain and its application in intellectual property protection. *Information Processing & Management*, 58(3), 102507.

Song, J. M., Sung, J., & Park, T. (2019). Applications of blockchain to improve supply chain traceability. *Procedia Computer Science*, 162, 119–122. https://doi.org/10.1016/j.procs.2019.11.266

Suripeddi, M. K. S., & Purandare, P. (2021, July). Blockchain and GDPR–a study on compatibility issues of the distributed ledger technology with GDPR data processing. In *Journal of Physics: Conference Series* (Vol. 1964, No. 4, p. 042005). IOP Publishing.

Tan, A., Gligor, D., & Ngah, A. (2022). Applying blockchain for halal food traceability. *International Journal of Logistics Research and Applications*, 25(6), 947–964.

Tang, Y., Xiong, J., Becerril-Arreola, R., & Iyer, L. (2020). Ethics of blockchain: A framework of technology, applications, impacts, and research directions. *Information Technology & People*, 33(2), 602–632.

Tanrıverdi, M., & Tekerek, A. (2019, November). Implementation of blockchain based distributed web attack detection application. In *2019 1st International Informatics and Software Engineering Conference (UBMYK)* (pp. 1–6). IEEE.

Tyagi, A. K., Dananjayan, S., Agarwal, D., & Thariq Ahmed, H. F. (2023). Blockchain—internet of things applications: Opportunities and challenges for industry 4.0 and society 5.0. *Sensors*, 23(2), 947. MDPI AG. http://doi.org/10.3390/s23020947

Varma, J. (2019). Blockchain in finance. *Vikalpa*, 44, 1–11. https://doi.org/10.1177/0256090919839897

Verma, S., & Sheel, A. (2022). Blockchain for government organizations: Past, present and future. *Journal of Global Operations and Strategic Sourcing*, 15(3), 406–430.

Verny, J., Oulmakki, O., Cabo, X., & Roussel, D. (2020). Blockchain & supply chain: Towards an innovative supply chain design. *Projectics / Proyéctica / Projectique*, 26, 115–130. https://doi.org/10.3917/proj.026.0115

Wang, G., & Nixon, M. (2021, December). SoK: Tokenization on blockchain. In *Proceedings of the 14th IEEE/ACM International Conference on Utility and Cloud Computing Companion* (pp. 1–9). https://doi.org/10.1145/3492323.3495577.

Wang, S., Wang, X., & Zhang, Y. (2019). A secure cloud storage framework with access control based on blockchain. *IEEE Access*, 7, 112713–112725.

Weerawarna, R., Miah, S. J., & Shao, X. (2023). Emerging advances of blockchain technology in finance: A content analysis. *Personal and Ubiquitous Computing*. https://doi.org/10.1007/s00779-023-01712-5

Worley, C., & Skjellum, A. (2018, July). Blockchain tradeoffs and challenges for current and emerging applications: Generalization, fragmentation, sidechains, and scalability. In *2018 IEEE International Conference on Internet of Things (iThings) and IEEE Green Computing and Communications (GreenCom) and IEEE Cyber, Physical and Social Computing (CPSCom) and IEEE Smart Data (SmartData)* (pp. 1582–1587). IEEE.

Wu, Y., Wang, Z., Ma, Y., & Leung, V. C. (2021). Deep reinforcement learning for blockchain in industrial IoT: A survey. *Computer Networks*, 191, 108004.

Xia, Q. I., Sifah, E. B., Asamoah, K. O., Gao, J., Du, X., & Guizani, M. (2017). MeDShare: Trust-less medical data sharing among cloud service providers via blockchain. *IEEE Access*, 5, 14757–14767.

Zhang, C., Xu, C., Xu, J., Tang, Y., & Choi, B. (2019). GEM^2-tree: A gas-efficient structure for authenticated range queries in blockchain. In *2019 IEEE 35th International Conference on Data Engineering (ICDE)* (pp. 842–853). Macao, China. https://doi.org/10.1109/ICDE.2019.00080

Zhang, W., Yuan, Y., Hu, Y., Nandakumar, K., Chopra, A., Sim, S., & De Caro, A. (2019). Blockchain-based distributed compliance in multinational corporations' cross-border intercompany transactions: A new model for distributed compliance across subsidiaries in different jurisdictions. In *Advances in Information and Communication Networks: Proceedings of the 2018 Future of Information and Communication Conference (FICC)*, Vol. 2 (pp. 304–320). Springer International Publishing.

# 20 Demystifying the Industry 5.0 Version

*Venkatesan Ramachandran, Feroze Ahamed Zahir Ahamed,
Thanga Helina Stalin, and Shirley Chellathurai Pon Anna Bai*

## 20.1 INTRODUCTION

The history of industry has been characterized by waves of transformation that have redefined the interaction between humans and machines and ushered in novel eras of technological progress. As we approach the dawn of the modern industrial era, Industry 5.0 presents itself as the most recent development in this continuous story, offering the convergence of cutting-edge technology to influence manufacturing and other sectors of the economy. It is critical to deconstruct the complexities of Industry 5.0 as businesses and societies throughout the globe negotiate this period of unparalleled transformation. Industry 5.0 emphasizes a cooperative relationship between humans and robots, building on the groundwork established by its predecessors. Industry 5.0 lays a strong emphasis on the integration of human capabilities, in contrast to other industrial revolutions that frequently concentrated on automation and efficiency improvements. The goal is to establish a symbiotic partnership where the advantages of both humans and machines are combined to produce previously unheard-of levels of sustainability, innovation, and production.

This chapter aims to provide a full exploration of Industry 5.0, with a focus on demystifying its essential components, core concepts, and multifarious influence. We explore the technology foundations that shape this new industrial paradigm, from the merging of cyber-physical systems to the function of artificial intelligence and the Internet of Things. To give a detailed knowledge of how Industry 5.0 is changing conventional manufacturing processes and global supply chains, real-world applications and implications are examined closely. We expand our research of Industry 5.0 to include its socioeconomic aspects in addition to its technical aspects.

This transformation is about more than just robots and algorithms; it's about people being empowered, skills being improved, and innovation being approached from a human perspective. We face possibilities and difficulties as we peel back the layers of Industry 5.0, realizing that an integrated approach that takes into account the intertwined domains of technology, society, and economics is vital. This exploration attempts to provide researchers, practitioners, and policymakers navigating the unknown seas of Industry 5.0 with a guiding light through an interdisciplinary perspective. Understanding the subtleties of this most recent industrial revolution is becoming important not only for maintaining a competitive edge but also for responsible and sustainable advancement as industries adopt it.

### 20.1.1 BACKGROUND AND CONTEXT

Each new industrial revolution has brought forth revolutionary changes in the ever-changing industrial landscape; the advent of Industry 5.0 is a turning point in this continuum. Gaining an understanding of Industry 5.0's history and setting is essential to deciphering its nuances and negotiating the challenges it poses to conventional production methods. The origins of Industry 5.0 can be found in the earlier industrial revolutions, which were all distinguished by unique technological developments. Industry 4.0 paved the way for the incorporation of digital technology into manufacturing



DOI: 10.1201/9781003442066-20

with its emphasis on automation, networking, and data exchange. Industry 5.0, on the other hand, goes beyond the constraints of simple automation to adopt a more comprehensive paradigm that emphasizes the cooperation between humans and robots.

Industry 5.0 represents a break from the conventional understanding of automation as a substitute for human labor as we exist at the intersection of technical innovation and industrial reinterpretation (Marinelli, 2023).

Rather, it imagines a time where machines and people coexist peacefully, with each utilizing their special talents to build a more productive and dynamic industrial environment. This change in viewpoint emphasizes the augmentation of human capabilities with cutting-edge technologies, creating a mutually beneficial connection that goes beyond the confines of traditional manufacturing. Recent breakthroughs in artificial intelligence, the Internet of Things, and cyber-physical systems additionally impact the backdrop of Industry 5.0. These technologies serve as Industry 5.0's cornerstone, enabling networked systems that speed up data interchange and decision-making in real time.

In light of this, understanding Industry 5.0 becomes not only an academic project but also a necessary practical step for global industry and governments. A thorough awareness of this emergent paradigm's history and context will help us navigate new territory as we explore its many facets, which range from human-machine collaboration to socioeconomic effects. We hope to understand the technical nuances of Industry 5.0 as well as its wider implications and potential problems for our industrial fabric through this investigation.

### 20.1.2 Significance of Industry 5.0

The enormous effect that Industry 5.0 is expected to make on manufacturing productivity and efficiency further emphasizes the significance. The Internet of Things, artificial intelligence, and cyber-physical systems all work together to provide previously unthinkable levels of interconnectivity and data sharing (Chakir et al., 2023). The seamless exchange of real-time information among human operators and machines facilitates unprecedented precision in simplifying operations and empowering decision-making processes. Furthermore, Industry 5.0 is a reaction to the changing demands of a linked and globalized society. Industry 5.0 is characterized by its capacity to quickly adjust to shifting market demands, modify products at scale, and develop adaptable manufacturing methods.

In a time when markets are becoming more unpredictable and variable, and consumer expectations are changing rapidly, this flexibility is essential. Industry 5.0 is not just important on the manufacturing floor. It penetrates supply networks, impacting inventory control, logistics, and other aspects of industrial ecosystems. This connectivity creates new opportunities for cooperation, creativity, and sustainability in addition to improving operational efficiency.

## 20.2 FOUNDATIONS OF INDUSTRY 5.0

### 20.2.1 Historical Evolution of Industrial Revolutions

The development of industry is replete with discrete revolutions that each signifies a radical shift in the way societies manufacture, market, and consume commodities. It is essential to examine the genealogy of industrial revolutions that cleared the way for this modern paradigm shift in order to comprehend the origins of Industry 5.0. The late 1700s saw the onset of the first industrial revolution, which was defined by mechanization and the use of steam power (Poompavai & Elakkiya, 2022). Mass industrialization began with the transition from rural economies, signaled by the invention of steam engines and mechanized textile manufacture. This historical period saw the emergence of urbanization and an entirely novel category of industrial workers in addition to revolutionizing manufacturing and societal systems.

The development of mass production, assembly lines, and electricity during the late 19th and beginning of the 20th centuries defined the second industrial revolution. Unprecedented economic growth was propelled by inventions like the internal combustion engine and the telegraph. Large-scale industrial enterprises emerged during this time, and urbanization expanded even more, changing the face of the world economy. The latter part of the 20th century saw the emergence of the third industrial revolution, also known as the Digital Revolution. Automation and the development of computerized systems became primarily driven by advances in computing, electronics, and telecommunications technology.

The spread of digital technologies has drastically changed how people work, communicate, and conduct business. The Fourth Industrial Revolution, often known as Industry 4.0, began to take shape in the early 21st century, building on the groundwork established by the Digital Revolution. The Internet of Things, data analytics, and smart technology integration into manufacturing processes were the defining features of this stage of development. An increasingly linked and effective industrial environment resulted from the centralization of automation, networking, and real-time data sharing. As we approach the dawn of the 21st century, Industry 5.0 appears as the most recent development in this historical story. Automation and connectivity were the main features of Industry 4.0, while Industry 5.0 boldly moves things further by emphasizing human-machine collaboration (Shanmuganathan & Elango, 2023). These industrial revolutions' paths show how technology has advanced as well as how human-machine interaction has changed, starting with the mechanization of tasks.

### 20.2.2   INDUSTRY 4.0 VS. INDUSTRY 5.0

The next phase of collaborative intelligence is being ushered in by the differences between Industry 4.0 with the newly formed model of Industry 5.0, which represent a major development in the approach to industrialization. Although they are both distinguished by cutting-edge technologies and digital integration, important distinctions show how one industrial revolution led to the next.

### 20.2.3   KEY PRINCIPLES AND CONCEPTS

Industry 5.0 presents a series of ideas and precepts that set it apart as a paradigm change in the manufacturing sector (Sundaravadivazhagan et al., 2021). These guiding concepts are a reflection of the fundamental ideas of Industry 5.0's ideology:

- *A Human-Centric Approach:*
  - *Principle:* Understanding that each human has distinct cognitive, creative, and emotional intelligence, Industry 5.0 centers manufacturing processes on the needs of its workforce.
  - *Idea:* The concept emphasizes the notion that, instead of taking the place of human labor, technology should improve human capacities and decision-making.
- *Intelligence that collaborates:*
  - *Principle:* An essential element of Industry 5.0 is human-machine collaboration. It highlights the benefits that result from the cooperation of mechanical accuracy and human cognitive capacities.
  - *Idea:* The goal of collaborative intelligence is to create a manufacturing environment where people and machines work together to enhance efficiency, creativity, and productivity.
- *Customization at Scale:*
  - *Principle:* Industry 5.0 makes it possible to produce highly personalized goods at scale in order to meet the unique needs of each client.
  - *Idea:* This idea is for a manufacturing system which can easily adjust to a range of client needs, providing customization and flexibility in production.
- *Flexibility and Agility:*
  - *Principle:* Industry 5.0 places a strong emphasis on the requirement for agile and adaptable production processes that can quickly adapt to changes in the market.

**TABLE 20.1**

**Industry 4.0 vs. Industry 5.0**

| Major key | Industry 4.0 | Industry 5.0 |
| --- | --- | --- |
| **Foundation and Focus** | The Fourth Industrial Revolution, or Industry 4.0, is distinguished by the digitization of production processes. It places a strong emphasis on leveraging data analytics, the Internet of Things (IoT), and smart technologies to build intelligent, networked systems. A major component that improves manufacturing accuracy and efficiency is automation. | Industry 5.0 presents a paradigm change by putting people back at the core of manufacturing, building on the digital foundation of Industry 4.0. Industry 5.0 emphasizes the value of human-machine collaboration rather than just automation, highlighting the complementary abilities of both species. |
| **Human-Machine Collaboration** | The primary role of humans in Industry 4.0 is to supervise and manage automated operations. Although people are still essential, the focus is on developing "smart factories," where robots can interact and make choices on their own, eliminating the need for continual human supervision. | In contrast, Industry 5.0 places a heightened emphasis on collaboration between humans and machines. It envisions a workplace where machines augment human capabilities, fostering a symbiotic relationship. Tasks that require creativity, problem-solving, and emotional intelligence are areas where human involvement becomes crucial. |
| **Role of Automation** | On the other hand, Industry 4.0 emphasizes human-machine collaboration even more. It shows a workplace in which humans and machines coexist in a symbiotic connection as machines enhance human capabilities. Human intervention becomes essential for tasks requiring creativity, problem-solving, and emotional intelligence. | Automation is still essential, but Industry 5.0 goes beyond repetitive jobs. Automation is viewed as a tool to supplement human abilities instead of substitutes them, creating a setting where people and machines work together to solve challenging problems. |
| **Flexibility and Customization** | Industry 4.0 highlights how data-driven insights can be used to increase the flexibility of manufacturing processes. Real-time modifications and flexible methods enable customization. | Industry 5.0 incorporates human judgment and creativity to further enhance personalization. Working together, humans and robots can produce highly customized items at scale and respond to changing market demands more quickly. |
| **Socioeconomic Impact** | Industry 4.0's socioeconomic effects can be seen in lower costs, more productivity, and the development of new business models. The optimization of industrial processes is the main objective of the transformation. | The socioeconomic impact of Industry 5.0 goes above operational effectiveness. In order to create a more diverse and people-centered industrial environment, there are consequences for employment roles, skill development, and social well-being from a focus on human-centric values and collaboration. |

- *Idea:* The idea is to design adaptable production systems that are simple to reorganize in response to changes in customer demands, product requirements, and new trends.
- *Integrative Technologies:*
  - *Principle:* Industry 5.0's core tenet is the adoption of cutting-edge technology, such as artificial intelligence, cyber-physical systems, and the Internet of Things.
  - *Idea:* The idea behind this notion is to create a seamless and integrated industrial ecosystem by means of a comprehensive technology integration that goes beyond specific applications.

- *Ethical and Responsible Innovation:*
  - *Principle:* Industry 5.0 addresses social concerns about job displacement, privacy, and environmental impact by emphasizing ethical issues and responsible innovation.
  - *Idea:* In order to ensure that the advantages of Industry 5.0 technologies are broad and inclusive, the idea emphasizes the necessity of making moral decisions at the development and application stages of the technology.
- *Empowerment and Skill Development:*
  - *Principle:* Industry 5.0 acknowledges the value of ongoing skill development for workers, enabling people to collaborate with cutting-edge technologies.
  - *Idea:* This idea entails developing educational and training initiatives that give people the tools they need to prosper in an Industry 5.0 setting while promoting a culture of lifelong learning.
- *Sustainability and the Circular Economy:*
  - *Principle:* Sustainability is a fundamental tenet of Industry 5.0, which advocates for the shift to a circular economy by reducing waste and maximizing resource utilization.
  - *Idea:* The idea is to create goods and procedures that put the environment's sustainability first, fostering an industrial ecosystem that is more socially and environmentally conscious. Together, these fundamental ideas and concepts serve as Industry 5.0's cornerstone, directing its application and development toward a future of cooperative, adaptive, and responsible manufacturing.

## 20.3 HUMAN-MACHINE COLLABORATION

### 20.3.1 THE ROLE OF HUMANS IN INDUSTRY 5.0

Industry 5.0 represents a shift from the traditional perspective of technology as a substitute for human labor, emphasizing the role of humans. Industry 5.0 ushers in a new era in which people are no longer just operators but vital partners who contribute their special cognitive abilities to forge a harmonious alliance with cutting-edge technologies (Khurshid et al., 2023). This change in the function of people includes multiple important aspects:

- *Innovative Approach to Problem Solving:* People are recognized in Industry 5.0 for their ability to solve problems and be creative. The focus lies in utilizing human creativity to tackle intricate problems that might be difficult for machines to handle independently. Industrial processes gain a degree of adaptability and creativity from the human touch in creative issue solving.
- *Critical Thinking and Decision-Making:* When making decisions that call for subtle judgment, human decision-making and critical thinking skills are crucial. Humans are expected to make strategic decisions in Industry 5.0, guided by their experiences, instincts, and moral principles. It is believed that making decisions with the needs of people in mind is essential to managing uncertainty and producing responsible results.
- *Emotional Intelligence:* Humans are unique in that they possess emotional intelligence. Industry 5.0 acknowledges the significance of emotions in the workplace and the role emotional intelligence plays in cooperation, communication, and employee well-being. Humans foster a happy and cooperative work atmosphere because of their emotional intelligence.
- *Handling Complicated Tasks:* Industry 5.0 sees people managing complicated jobs requiring a range of abilities, including creativity, emotional intelligence, and flexibility. Machines can perform repetitive, routine activities, but humans are better at things that require a more complex, context-aware approach.
- *Continuous Learning and Adaptation:* Because Industry 5.0 is dynamic, workers need to be flexible and agile. People are essential for lifelong learning, skill acquisition, and

technological adaptation. This dedication to lifelong learning guarantees that human labor will always be at the forefront of technology innovation.

- *Handling Complicated Tasks:* Industry 5.0 sees people managing complicated jobs requiring a range of abilities, including creativity, emotional intelligence, and flexibility. Machines can perform repetitive, routine activities, but humans are better at things that require a more complex, context-aware approach.
- *Continuous Learning and Adaptation:* Because Industry 5.0 is dynamic, workers need to be flexible and agile. People are essential for lifelong learning, skill acquisition, and technological adaptation. This dedication to lifelong learning guarantees that human labor will always be at the forefront of technology innovation.

## 20.3.2  Synergies between Humans and Machines

At the time of my most recent knowledge update in January 2022, the term "Industry 5.0" was not well-known or established (Tortorella et al., 2023). I can, however, share some knowledge about the possible benefits of human-machine cooperation within the framework of Industry 4.0 and related developments in the manufacturing and industry. For the most recent information, please consult more recent sources if the idea of Industry 5.0 has undergone any changes since then. Industry 4.0 refers to how industries are changing as a result of the integration of cutting-edge technologies like automation, big data analytics, the Internet of Things, and artificial intelligence. An increasingly cooperative and synergistic working environment is being created by the expanding interplay between humans and machines.

- *Augmented Intelligence:* Industry 4.0 places a strong emphasis on the idea of augmented intelligence, in which humans and robots work together to improve each other's capacities. Large volumes of data can be swiftly processed and analyzed by machines, giving humans insightful information that can be used to make decisions.
- *Collaborative Robots (Cobots):* These are made to collaborate with people to increase productivity and security. They can carry out laborious or physically taxing chores, freeing up human workers to concentrate on more intricate and mental aspects of their employment.
- *Data-Driven Decision-Making:* Data-driven decision-making is made possible by the mix of machine analytics and human expertise. Humans are able to decipher the insights that machines supply and use their ingenuity and experience to tackle challenging challenges.
- *Skill Enhancement and Training:* As a result of technology integration, there is a greater emphasis on retraining and upskilling workers. The latest technologies require human comprehension, operation, and maintenance, creating an ecosystem that is always learning.
- *Human-Machine Interfaces:* Wearable technology and user-friendly interfaces help improve human-machine communication. This lowers the learning curve for new technology by encouraging a more natural and intuitive connection.
- *Flexibility and Adaptability:* Human employees offer to the workplace their creativity, emotional intelligence, and flexibility. While people are able to adjust to changes and navigate uncertain situations, machines are capable of handling routine jobs.
- *Ethical and Social Considerations:* When it comes to tackling ethical and social issues around technology, humans are essential. This entails addressing the effects of automation on society, as well as guaranteeing equity, accountability, and transparency.

It is reasonable to assume that Industry 5.0 will highlight the cooperative and mutually beneficial connection that exists between humans and machines even more. The secret is striking the correct balance and utilizing human and machine talents to build an industrial ecosystem that is more inventive, efficient, and sustainable.

## 20.4  TECHNOLOGICAL UNDERPINNINGS

### 20.4.1  Cyber-Physical Systems

When the physical and digital realms combine, we get cyber-physical Systems (CPS). They are intelligent, networked systems that come from the seamless fusion of state-of-the-art computer, communication, and control technologies with physical processes. These technologies serve as a conduit between the virtual world of algorithms and the concrete; real-world objects that software algorithms impact (Zayat et al., 2023). Applications for CPS can be identified in many different areas, such as manufacturing, infrastructure, and healthcare. The core of cyber-physical systems is the intimate integration of computational algorithms and physical processes, made possible by embedded systems including the Internet of Things. These systems consist of intelligent, networked devices with the ability to perceive, monitor, and relate to their physical environment in real time.

CPS collects data from the physical world, analyzes it in real time, and reacts dynamically to changes through advanced sensors, actuators, and communication networks, resulting in a closed-loop feedback system. CPS has the potential to have a significant influence and transform the way we plan, oversee, and manage complex systems. For instance, CPS can automatically change parameters in manufacturing to enhance output quality and efficiency. CPS applications have the potential to improve health outcomes in the healthcare industry by enabling real-time, individualized patient monitoring. Additionally, CPS support improved public services, energy efficiency, and effective traffic control in smart cities. Critical factors in the design and implementation of CPS are security and resilience.

As these systems grow more and more ingrained in our daily lives, it is critical to protect against cyberattacks and guarantee the dependability of the interconnected parts. Furthermore, the correct application of CPS technology depends heavily on ethical issues pertaining to data protection, responsibility, and transparency (Demir & Cicibaş, 2019). The development of CPS is evidence of how technology has the ability to fundamentally alter how humans engage with the physical environment. With further advancements in this field of study and creativity, CPS has the potential to boost productivity, enhance judgment, and build a more intelligent and connected environment. In order to fully realize the promise of CPS, a multidisciplinary approach combining domain-specific knowledge, data science, computer science, and engineering experience is needed to open up new avenues for innovation and societal improvement.

### 20.4.2  Artificial Intelligence in Industry 5.0

Artificial intelligence (AI) is at the cutting edge of Industry 5.0, which is an entirely novel phase of industrial revolution that is just around the corner. Redefining the connection between humans and machines with an emphasis on collaboration and synergy, Industry 5.0 aims to build upon the basis of Industry 4.0, which included advanced automation and digitization. This makes AI a key factor promoting innovation in a range of industrial domains (Al-Banna et al., 2023). Neural networks, machine learning algorithms, and sophisticated data analytics enable machines to learn from their interactions and adapt to new situations in addition to carrying out jobs precisely. When AI and Industry 5.0 come together, the result is a dynamic, intelligent manufacturing environment where human workers and machines work together harmoniously to improve the quality of output, efficiency, and productivity.

Industry 5.0 uses AI in ways that go beyond simple automation. AI-enabled smart factories can anticipate maintenance requirements, optimize manufacturing processes, and automatically modify workflows in accordance with real-time data. Greater flexibility in production is made possible by this degree of adaptability, which enables quick reactions to shifting market conditions and demand. The idea of "cognitive manufacturing," in which robots are endowed with the capacity for autonomous understanding, reasoning, and decision-making, is central to AI in Industry 5.0. AI systems are able to evaluate large, complicated datasets, spot trends, and offer insightful analysis to decision-makers because of this cognitive ability. In consequently, human workers work in tandem with AI systems to take use of their analytical prowess, fusing the advantages of AI processing capacity with human intuition.

AI not only increases operational effectiveness but also fosters the development of novel goods and services. By utilizing machine learning algorithms and predictive analytics, organizations can enhance their competitiveness by anticipating market trends, streamlining supply chains, and tailoring products to unique customer demands. Industry 5.0's adoption of AI, however, is not without its difficulties. These include moral dilemmas, privacy issues with data, and the requirement for AI systems that are visible and understandable. An intelligent assessment of the societal implications of new technologies is necessary to strike a balance between the advantages of automation and the human touch.

### 20.4.3 INTERNET OF THINGS INTEGRATION

The pervasiveness and application of the Internet of Things (IoT) in a wide range of industries mark a significant advancement toward a networked and intelligent society. IoT integration is the process of seamlessly connecting common things, sensors, and physical equipment to the Internet so they can trade, gather, and use data (Bahulikar et al., 2023). The coming together of the digital and physical spheres has the potential to revolutionize how we work, live, and engage with our surroundings. Smart houses in the IoT integration age are outfitted with networked gadgets that allow for monitoring energy consumption, security system, and appliance monitoring and control. Through the use of sensors built into wearable technology, real-time health data is gathered, enabling more individualized treatment.

Industries including manufacturing, agriculture, and transportation use IoT to improve decision-making, streamline operations, and increase efficiency outside of the consumer space. The capacity to build networks of devices that communicate with one other effortlessly is one of the main characteristics of IoT integration. The foundation of smart cities is their interconnection, wherein IoT sensors and devices are used to monitor traffic, control energy use, and improve public safety. These gadgets produce data that helps build intelligent urban ecosystems that adapt dynamically to the requirements of their resident. The Industrial Internet of Things (IIoT) makes it easier to maintain equipment in an industrial context by enabling real-time equipment monitoring, predictive maintenance, and process optimization.

Businesses may increase operational efficiency, decrease downtime, and make innovative, data-driven decisions by integrating IoT. IoT integration is becoming widely used, but there are drawbacks as well, such as worries about interoperability, security, and data privacy. Preserving the enormous volume of data produced by IoT devices is essential to preserving confidence in these networked systems. Standardized protocols and strong cybersecurity measures are also necessary to guarantee that various platforms and devices may communicate with each other without any problems. The evolution of IoT integration has led to a growing significance for edge computing development. By processing data closer to its point of origin, edge computing lowers latency and improves the responsiveness of IoT systems. The increasing needs for real-time analytics and decision-making are being met in large part by this move toward decentralized computing.

## 20.5 REAL-WORLD APPLICATIONS

### 20.5.1 CASE STUDIES IN MANUFACTURING

Of certainly, let's look at a few case studies that illustrate how technology has affected the manufacturing sector, especially with regard to Industry 4.0:

### 20.5.1.1   Siemens' Amberg Facility

- *Background:* Industry 4.0 ideas were introduced by the multinational technology giant Siemens at its Amberg Electronics Plant in Germany. Industrial automation uses Simatic controllers, which are produced at this site.
- *Implementation:* The Amberg facility integrated robotics, data analytics, and IoT sensors as part of a completely digitalized and networked approach. A digital thread linked every step of the production process, from design to delivery.
- *Findings:*
  - *Efficiency Gains:* A 99.99885% production accuracy rate was achieved after deployment.
  - *Flexibility:* The plant managed to achieve little downtime when switching between products.
  - *Reduced Lead Times:* There was a notable reduction in the lead times for production.
  - *Key Takeaway:* The Siemens factory in Amberg serves as an example of how a thorough adoption of Industry 4.0 principles may lead to appreciable improvements in precision, flexibility, and efficiency.

### 20.5.1.2   The Brilliant Factory Initiative by General Electric

- *Context:* General Electric (GE) started a project to convert its conventional manufacturing methods into "Brilliant Factories."
- *Implementation:*
  - *Digital Twin Technology:* To enable real-time monitoring and optimization, GE used digital twin technology to build virtual reproductions of actual industrial *systems.*
  - *Advanced Analytics:* By using advanced analytics, maintenance plans were optimized and equipment breakdowns were predicted.
  - *IoT Sensors:* Using IoT sensors to collect data from machinery and equipment in real time.
- *Findings:*
  - *Decreased Downtime:* Unplanned downtime was significantly decreased as a result of predictive maintenance.
  - *Enhanced Productivity:* Improvements in overall equipment effectiveness (OEE) were made possible by the application of data analytics.
  - *Cost Savings:* By preventing pointless repair tasks, the predictive maintenance approach reduced costs.
  - *Key Takeaway:* GE's Brilliant Factory effort shows how digital twin technology, advanced analytics, and the IoT can be combined to improve manufacturing processes' efficiency cut down on downtime, and save costs.

These case studies demonstrate how manufacturing can undergo revolutionary changes as a result of the incorporation of cutting-edge technology under the purview of Industry 4.0, resulting in enhanced efficacy, flexibility, and cost-effectiveness. Additionally, they stress the significance of adopting a comprehensive strategy that incorporates digital technology at every stage of the value chain. GE's Brilliant Factory effort shows how digital twin technology, advanced analytics, and the IoT can be combined to improve manufacturing processes' efficiency cut down on downtime, and save costs.

### 20.5.2   Impact on Productivity and Efficiency

A new era in manufacturing has been brought about by the integration of modern technologies, especially within the context of Industry 4.0, which has had a substantial impact on productivity and efficiency across a variety of industries (Gadekar et al., 2022). Traditional manufacturing methods have been redefined by this technological revolution, which has brought in a variety of intelligent technologies that cooperate to improve overall performance and expedite operations.

- *Enhanced Precision and Automation:* Increasing production on factory floors has been made possible by the use of robotics and automation. Robotic systems are becoming increasingly adept at doing labor-intensive and repetitive tasks that formerly required human interaction. The precision and consistency with which these machines function helps to minimize errors and faults, which in turn raise the caliber of products that are produced.
- *Real-Time Monitoring and Data Analytics:* Manufacturers now have access to a constant stream of data from different phases of the production cycle thanks to the development of real-time monitoring via the IoT and sensor technologies. With so much data available, decisions may be made quickly and in accordance with real performance indicators. With the use of sophisticated data analytics, useful insights are progressively extracted, workflows are optimized, bottlenecks are found, and upkeep needs are anticipated. This proactive strategy reduces downtime and improves overall productivity.
- *Predictive Maintenance:* Machine learning algorithms and IoT sensors have made it possible to incorporate predictive maintenance tactics, which have revolutionized sectors dependent on machinery. These systems can foresee equipment breakdowns before they happen and enable prompt interventions by studying data trends.
- *Customization and Flexibility:* Industry 4.0 technologies have made it easier for production processes to become more adaptive and flexible. In order to quickly adapt to changing market needs, smart factories may quickly modify production lines to meet different product specifications. Since it takes less time and money to switch between different goods or production lines, this degree of flexibility improves efficiency.
- *Optimized Supply Chain Management:* Industry 4.0 affects the whole supply chain, not just the manufacturing floor. Real-time supply chain visibility, from the procurement of raw materials to the delivery of the finished product, is made possible by interconnected digital technologies. Improved inventory control, demand forecasting, and communication between distributors, manufacturers, and suppliers are all made possible by this transparency. The end effect is a more reactive and efficient supply chain that have been optimized.
- *Empowering the Workforce:* Industry 4.0 performance depends heavily on the human workforce, even while technology serves a crucial role. With the use of digital tools, employees may concentrate on more difficult and worthwhile jobs. When people and machines work together, their individual abilities complement one another, creating a synergistic partnership that encourages creativity and problem-solving in the workplace.

### 20.5.3 Socioeconomic Impacts and Challenges

The assimilation of cutting-edge technologies, especially in the context of Industry 4.0 and beyond, has significant socioeconomic ramifications that influence how enterprises operate, how societies function, and how people engage with the quickly changing technological environment (Krstić et al., 2022). Even though these developments present previously unheard-of chances for creativity, effectiveness, and economic expansion, they also present important obstacles that must be carefully considered in order to guarantee a fair and equitable transition.

#### 20.5.3.1 Positive Socioeconomic Impacts
- *Economic Growth and Job Creation:* By boosting productivity and encouraging innovation, the implementation of Industry 4.0 technology has the potential to stimulate economic

growth. Businesses that invest in digitalization, automation, and modern manufacturing processes create new industries and job prospects.

- *Enhanced Productivity and Life Quality:* Technological developments lead to greater productivity across a range of industries, which lowers costs, makes better use of resources, and produces goods and services of higher caliber. Smart technologies can also improve people's quality of life in general by bringing about advances in urban planning, transportation, and healthcare.
- *Global Connectivity and Market Expansion:* Thanks to digital technologies, businesses can now reach a wider audience and consumers can now access a wider variety of goods and services. An increasingly interconnected global economy is a result of this interconnection, which encourages international cooperation and trade.
- *Opportunities for Education and Skill Development:* The need for digital skills is increasing in line with the development of technology. In order to prepare the workforce for employment of the future, this opens chances for skill development and education in cutting-edge disciplines like cybersecurity, data science, and artificial intelligence.

### 20.5.3.2  Challenges and Considerations

- *Employment Displacement and Skills Gap:* Automation and digitization of sectors may result in employment displacement, especially for routine and repetitive roles (Concepcion et al., 2022). Programs for reskilling and upskilling the workforce are desperately needed to close the skills gap and make sure people are prepared for the changing nature of the labor market.
- *Economic inequalities and Inequality:* There are worries about economic inequalities and inequality as a result of the uneven distribution of the advantages of technology breakthroughs. In order to meet this challenge, proactive steps must be taken to guarantee that everyone in society may benefit from Industry 4.0.
- *Data Security and Privacy Issues:*
  Concerns around cybersecurity and data privacy are brought up by our increasing reliance on data-driven technologies. Finding a balance between using data to drive innovation and safeguarding people's privacy is a difficult task that calls both strong legal frameworks and moral considerations.
- *Ethical and Social Implications:* As technology develops, moral issues take on greater significance. To guarantee that technology benefits humans in a morally and positively way, concerns about algorithmic bias, the responsible application of artificial intelligence, and the effects of automation on the well-being of society should be addressed.
- *Transitioning Workforce and Societal Resistance:* People and communities that are impacted by change may become resistant due to the quick speed of technology advancement. In order to ensure a seamless transition and increase public confidence in developing technology, inclusive methods, effective communication, and education are important.

### 20.5.4  Opportunities for Inclusive Growth

Making that the advantages of economic advancement are distributed fairly requires equitable expansion, which is broad-based economic development that helps all facets of society (Soltani et al., 2023). In the framework of Industry 4.0 and technology developments, there are various chances to promote equitable growth:

- *Digital Inclusion:*
  *Technology Access:* It is imperative to guarantee that digital technology, such as cellphones and the Internet are widely *accessible*. This entails closing the digital divide

by resolving infrastructural deficiencies and encouraging accessible, cost-effective use of digital resources.

- *Programs for Skill Development:*
  *Upskilling and Reskilling:* Putting in place comprehensive skill-development initiatives that address the changing demands of the labor market. To enable people to engage in the digital economy, this involves offering training in data analysis, digital literacy, and emerging technologies.
- *Innovation and Entrepreneurship:* Assistance for New Businesses building an ecosystem that encourages entrepreneurship, particularly in domains where technology is a driving force. This entails supporting startups and small enterprises with resources, finance, and mentorship in order to promote innovation and employment development.
- *Opportunities for Education and Training:*
  *STEM Education:* Giving priority to STEM education in order to prepare people for the abilities required in the digital age. STEM stands for science, technology, engineering, and mathematics. Promoting diversity in STEM disciplines can help create a workforce that is more inclusive.
- *Social Impact Projects:*
  Promoting and funding technology-driven projects that tackle social issues is known as "Tech for Good." This involves funding initiatives that have beneficial effects on communities in the fields of education, healthcare, long-term viability and the environment.
- *Flexibility and Remote Work:*
  *Possibilities for Remote Work:* Increasing the number of remote work options can give people in various geographic places access to jobs. This can be especially helpful for people who live in rural areas or places where employment prospects are scarce.
- *Inclusive Technology Design:*
  *Features of Accessibility:* Giving inclusive design first priority while creating new digital platforms and technologies. In order to ensure that a broad user base can utilize technology, accessibility features that accommodate those with varying abilities must be incorporated (Harn et al., 2023).
- *Community Engagement:*
  *Community-Led Development:* Involving local communities in the creation and execution of technological initiatives is known as community engagement or community-led development. This guarantees that initiatives take into account local requirements, are culturally sensitive, and enable communities to actively engage in technology breakthroughs.
- *Rules and Policies of the Government:*
  Adopting laws and policies that support inclusive development is known as inclusive policy-making. This could involve social safety nets to assist disadvantaged groups throughout economic downturns, laws prohibiting discrimination, and tax incentives for companies that promote inclusion.
- *Collaborative-Private Alliances:*
  *Collaborative Initiatives:* Promoting cooperation to solve societal issues between the public and private sectors. Through public-private partnerships, lasting solutions that serve a larger population can be created by utilizing the assets of both sectors.
- *Financial Inclusion:*
  *Access to finance:* Encouraging financial inclusion by giving people and companies, particularly those in underprivileged areas, access to finance. Fintech, or innovative financial technologies, and inclusive banking methods can help with this.
- *Workplace Inclusion and Diversity:*
  *Diverse Workforce:* Encouraging inclusivity and diversity in companies. Having a workforce that is varied in terms of demographics, experiences, and backgrounds fosters innovation and a more welcoming workplace atmosphere.

## 20.6  FUTURE TRENDS AND PREDICTIONS

### 20.6.1  Emerging Technologies in Industry 5.0

Industry 5.0 wasn't a commonly used word as of the final knowledge update in January 2022, and it's possible that the most recent advancements in the industry were not fully taken into account (Saharan & Pathak, 2023). However, given the way Industry 4.0 is developing and broader technological trends, a number of new technologies are probably going to have a big impact on the industrial environment. The following technologies might continue to influence industry futures and be applicable in a growing Industry 5.0 setting:

- *Artificial Intelligence (AI) and Machine Learning:* As these fields develop, machines will be able to analyze data, anticipate outcomes, and make better decisions thanks to the algorithms behind AI and machine learning. These technologies may be further incorporated into quality assurance, predictive maintenance, and production processes in Industry 5.0.
- *5G Technology:* The extensive deployment of 5G networks has the potential to completely transform industrial connection. For real-time data sharing, which speeds up decision-making and promotes the expansion of the Industrial Internet of Things (IIoT), high-speed, low-latency connectivity is essential.
- *Digital Twins:* Virtual copies of actual systems or procedures, or digital twins, are developing in sophistication. They make it possible to monitor, analyze, and optimize physical assets in real time. Digital twins could provide more thorough insights across the whole product lifecycle in Industry 5.0.
- *Edge Computing:* To cut down on latency and speed up reaction times, edge computing processes data nearer to the point of generation. This can facilitate real-time decision-making and increase the efficiency of data-intensive procedures in industrial settings.
- *Advanced Robotics:* Cobots, or collaborative robots, are one type of robotics that is developing to work more smoothly alongside people. Improved automation, increased manufacturing precision, and adaptable and flexible production lines are all possible with advanced robotics.
- *Virtual Reality (VR) and Augmented Reality (AR):* These technologies are used in design, maintenance, and training. These technologies could be useful in Industry 5.0 to provide virtual design simulations, remote support, and immersive training experiences.
- *Blockchain Technology:* Supply chains that are transparent and traceable can benefit from blockchain's decentralized and secure structure. Blockchain may be used in Industry 5.0 to improve cybersecurity, validate transactions, and guarantee data integrity.
- *Quantum Computing:* Although it is still in its infancy, this technology has the power to completely transform data processing and tackle challenging issues at a rate that traditional computers are unable to match. Quantum computing may have an effect on simulation and optimization jobs in Industry 5.0.
- *Biotechnology and Nanotechnology:* New materials, procedures, and sensors can result from developments in biotechnology and nanotechnology. These technologies could be used in manufacturing, materials science, and healthcare, resulting in more effective and sustainable industrial processes.
- *Human-Machine Collaboration Systems:* Industry 5.0 places a strong emphasis on cooperation between humans and machines and takes a human-centric perspective. In order to realize this collaborative vision, systems that improve ergonomics, interface design, and human-machine interaction will be essential.
- *Sustainable Technologies:* In Industry 5.0, sustainable technologies like eco-friendly materials, circular economy strategies, and renewable energy sources should become more popular. The emphasis on sustainability is in line with international initiatives to lessen the effect on the environment and build more robust industrial systems.

- *Cybersecurity Solutions:* Strong cybersecurity solutions are becoming more and more important as connectivity rises. Advanced cybersecurity measures will be necessary in Industry 5.0 to safeguard confidential information, thwart online attacks, and guarantee the dependability of networked systems.

## 20.6.2 ANTICIPATED TRANSFORMATIONS IN INDUSTRIAL PRACTICES

Predicted changes in manufacturing procedures include merging of advanced technology, emphasis on human-centric methods, and development of resilient and sustainable practices, especially as we progress into Industry 5.0 (Emanuilov & Yordanova, 2022). The following significant changes are anticipated to mold the industrial landscape:

- *Human-Centric Partnership:*
  *Collaboration Is Encouraged:* Industry 5.0 places a strong emphasis on a human-centric strategy that fosters cooperation between people and machines. Technology integration seeks to complement human qualities rather than to replace them, promoting a mutually beneficial partnership in which people provide their creativity, critical thinking, and emotional intelligence.
- *Intelligent and Adaptive Manufacturing:*
  *AI and ML Adoption:* AI- and ML-powered intelligent solutions will become standard equipment in manufacturing operations. Real-time data analysis, production workflow optimization, maintenance demand prediction, and overall operational efficiency enhancement are all features of these systems.
- *Customization and Flexibility:*
  *Growing Need for Personalization:* Industry 5.0 predicts a rise in the desire for individualized and customized goods. Manufacturing methods that are flexible and adaptive will allow for quick changes in product configurations in response to specific customer demands and market trends.
- *Detailed Digital Twins:*
  *Utilizing Digital Twins for Lifecycle Management:* Digital twins—virtual copies of actual resources or operations—will advance to encompass a product's whole lifecycle. Digital twins will offer real-time insights from design and production to operation and maintenance, facilitating proactive problem-solving and better-informed decision-making.
- *Edge and Decentralized Computing:*
  *The Emergence of Edge Computing:* As edge computing becomes more widely used, data processing and analysis will be possible closer to the location where the data is generated (Sassanelli et al., 2022). In industrial contexts, this change facilitates decentralized decision-making, lowers latency, and improves real-time capabilities.
- *Eco-Friendly and Sustainable Practices:*
  *The Fundamentals of the Circular Economy:* A greater focus on sustainability and circular economy principles will be seen in Industry 5.0. Sustainable procedures will be included into industries' operations, ranging from cost-effective production methods to materials recycling and reuse.
- *Digitalization of the Supply Chain: Building*
  *Robust and Flexible Supply Chains:* Supply chains will become more digitally integrated, improving responsiveness, visibility, and transparency. Through this digital revolution, firms will be able to optimize inventory management, create more robust supply networks, and respond swiftly to changes in demand.
- *Materials and Nanotechnology Innovations:*
  *Advanced Materials:* Materials innovation, especially nanotechnology-based materials, will help create stronger, lighter, and more environmentally friendly materials. The

design of products, production methods, and overall resource efficiency will all be impacted by these developments.
- *Applications of Augmented Reality (AR) and Virtual Reality (VR):*
  *AR and VR for Training and Maintenance:* AR and VR technologies will be widely used in remote help, maintenance, and training. These immersive technologies will help with maintenance jobs, enhance training programs, and promote group problem-solving.
- *Integration of Cybersecurity:*
  *Enhanced Measures of Cybersecurity:* Strong cybersecurity measures are going to be more and more important as connectivity grows. Advanced cybersecurity solutions will be integrated into Industry 5.0 to safeguard confidential information, guarantee the integrity of networked systems, and fend off online attacks.
- *A Motivated Workforce and Lifelong Learning:* Emphasis on ongoing education on Industry 5.0 recognizes the value of having a workforce that is knowledgeable and flexible. Initiatives for lifelong learning will be given top priority, enabling employees to grow their skill sets, stay current in a rapidly evolving technology environment, and actively engage in the cooperative human-machine environment.
- *Global Standards and Interoperability:*
  *Standardization:* Global standards and interoperability will be essential as Industry 5.0 develops. Standardized protocols and standards will guarantee interoperability in networked systems, encourage cross-industry collaboration, and enable smooth technology integration.

The changes that are expected to occur in industrial processes are part of a more comprehensive evolution that is being fueled by the confluence of sustainable, human-centered, and technical concepts. Adaptability, inventiveness, and a dedication to moral and responsible behavior will be crucial elements in constructing a future where technology benefits humanity universally as industries traverse this revolutionary path (Adel, 2022).

## 20.7  CONCLUSION

In general, Industry 5.0 is expected to bring about significant changes that will fundamentally alter the way that industries operate. An appealing outlook regarding the development of global industries is painted by this paradigm shift, which is being driven by the convergence of cutting-edge technology, a renewed emphasis on human-centric collaboration, and a dedication to sustainable approaches. The core of Industry 5.0 is a dynamic human-machine synergy that prioritizes cooperation over displacement. Artificial intelligence, real-time analytics, and intelligent systems are augmenting human talents and ushering in a new era of production where innovation, analytical thinking, and interpersonal skills are considered important elements of industrial processes. One recurring element is flexibility, which is best exemplified by clever and flexible manufacturing procedures that can quickly adjust to the unique needs of each customer and the constantly changing market environment.

Because they provide thorough insights at every stage of the product lifecycle, digital twins are essential for proactive asset management and well-informed decision-making. In addition to improving real-time performance, the shift to edge and decentralized computing supports eco-friendly methods and the concepts of the circular economy. In order to maintain a strong worldwide network, Industry 5.0 anticipates supply chains that are fast and flexible, supported by digitization, transparency, and flexibility.

Innovation is reshaping the fundamentals of product design and manufacturing, especially in materials science and nanotechnology. Sustainable materials support the general commitment to environmental consciousness and help create a future that is resource-efficient. The focus is on human empowerment, with lifelong learning programs making sure that workers are flexible and involved in a cooperative human-machine context.

In an era of increased connectedness, cybersecurity becomes an unavoidable priority, protecting sensitive data and networked systems. Industry 5.0 is built on global standards and interoperability, which enable smooth integration of technology and promote cross-industry cooperation. This group's perspective for the future emphasizes diversity, sustainability, and social responsibility rather than just technology innovation. The guiding principles of collaboration, innovation, and moral responsibility will direct industries through this transformative landscape and pave the way for an era where technology enhances human experience and contributes to a more sustainable, flexible, and accessible global industrial ecosystem. Industry 5.0 presents a fascinating picture of a world where people and industry coexist peacefully alongside the intelligent technology that drives progress, with a focus on human-centric values and advanced technology.

## REFERENCES


Adel, A. (2022). Future of industry 5.0 in society: Human-centric solutions, challenges and prospective research areas. *Journal of Cloud Computing*, 11, 40. https://doi.org/10.1186/s13677-022-00314-5

Al-Banna, A., Rana, Z. A., Yaqot, M., & Menezes, B. (2023). Interconnectedness between Supply Chain Resilience. *Industry 4.0, and Investment. Logistics*, 7(3), 50.

Bahulikar, S., Chattopadhyay, A., & Hudnurkar, M. (2023). Framework for integrating lean thinking with industry 4.0: Way ahead for entrepreneurs in Indian MSME's. *The Journal of Entrepreneurship*, 32(2), 271–306.

Chakir, O., Rehaimi, A., Sadqi, Y., Krichen, M., Gaba, G. S., & Gurtov, A. (2023). An empirical assessment of ensemble methods and traditional machine learning techniques for web-based attack detection in industry 5.0. *Journal of King Saud University-Computer and Information Sciences*, 35(3), 103–119.

Concepcion, R., Ramirez, T. J., Alejandrino, J., Janairo, A. G., Baun, J. J., Francisco, K., . . . & Izzo, L. G. (2022, December). A look at the near future: Industry 5.0 boosts the potential of sustainable space agriculture. In *2022 IEEE 14th International Conference on Humanoid, Nanotechnology, Information Technology, Communication and Control, Environment, and Management (HNICEM)* (pp. 1–6). IEEE.

Demir, K., & Cicibaş, H. (2019). *The Next Industrial Revolution: Industry 5.0 and Discussions on Industry 4.0* (pp. 247–260). Berlin, Germany: Peter Lang GmbH, Internationaler Verlag der Wissenschaften.

Emanuilov, I., & Yordanova, K. (2022). Business and human rights in Industry 4.0: A blueprint for collaborative human rights due diligence in the Factories of the Future. *Journal of Responsible Technology*, 10, 100028.

Gadekar, R., Sarkar, B., & Gadekar, A. (2022). Model development for assessing inhibitors impacting Industry 4.0 implementation in Indian manufacturing industries: An integrated ISM-Fuzzy MICMAC approach. *International Journal of System Assurance Engineering and Management*, 1–26

Harn, O. Y., Ching, N. T., Chiet, C. W., Suan, L. M., & Chian, Y. M. (2023). The relationship of industry 4.0 and business performance in Malaysian manufacturing firms: A PLS-SEM model. *International Journal of Business and Technology Management*, 5(1), 431–445.

Khurshid, K., Danish, A., Salim, M. U., Bayram, M., Ozbakkaloglu, T., & Mosaberpanah, M. A. (2023). An in-depth survey demystifying the Internet of Things (IoT) in the construction industry: Unfolding new dimensions. *Sustainability*, 15(2), 1275.

Krstić, M., Agnusdei, G. P., Miglietta, P. P., Tadić, S., & Roso, V. (2022). Applicability of industry 4.0 technologies in the reverse logistics: A circular economy approach based on Comprehensive Distance Based Ranking (COBRA) method. *Sustainability*, 14(9), 5632.

Marinelli, M. (2023). From industry 4.0 to construction 5.0: Exploring the path towards human–robot collaboration in construction. *Systems*, 11(3), 152.

Poompavai, N., & Elakkiya, E. (2022). Feed the globe utilizing IOT-driven precision agriculture. *Advances in Computational Sciences and Technology*, 15(1), 11–20.

Saharan, T., & Pathak, A. (2023). Government implications of infrastructural development and CSR in industry 4.0. In *Industry 4.0 and the Digital Transformation of International Business* (pp. 251–271). Singapore: Springer Nature Singapore.

Sassanelli, C., Arriga, T., Zanin, S., D'Adamo, I., & Terzi, S. (2022). Industry 4.0 driven result-oriented PSS: An assessment in the energy management. *International Journal of Energy Economics and Policy*, 12(4), 186–203

Shanmuganathan, B., & Elango, E. (2023). *Exploring Recent Advances of IOT in Ambient Intelligence (AMI) & USE Case.* Book—Applications of IOT in Science and Technology, Publisher: Innovation Online Training Academy (IOTA) Publishers, 159–167.

Soltani, S., Maxwell, D., & Rashidi, A. (2023). The state of industry 4.0 in the Australian construction industry: An examination of industry and academic point of view. *Buildings*, 13(9), 2324.

Sundaravadivazhagan, B., Subashini, B., & Ashik, M. (2021). A review on Internet of Things (IoT): Security challenges, issues and the countermeasures approaches. *Psychology and Education*, 58(2), 6544–6560.

Tortorella, G. L., Saurin, T. A., Hines, P., Antony, J., & Samson, D. (2023). Myths and facts of industry 4.0. *International Journal of Production Economics*, 255, 108660.

Zayat, W., Kilic, H. S., Yalcin, A. S., Zaim, S., & Delen, D. (2023). Application of MADM methods in Industry 4.0: A literature review. *Computers & Industrial Engineering*, 109075.

# 21 Edge AI for Connected Healthcare in Internet of Medical Things for Smart Cities

*Mohamed Sirajudeen Mohamed Hanifa, Karima Salim Hashil Alnaamani, Gnanasankaran Natarajan, and Elakkiya Elango*

## 21.1 INTRODUCTION

The combination of cutting-edge technologies has served as an engine for revolutionary break-throughs in the quickly changing field of healthcare. The merging of edge AI (artificial intelligence at the edge) with the Internet of Medical Things (IoMT), a phenomenon that has gained importance in the field of smart cities, is one example of a paradigm-shifting integrating them (Rathi et al., 2021). Urban environments are embracing technological connections more and more to tackle complex problems and the healthcare industry will gain a lot from edge AI and IoMT working together. Smart cities have arrived at the intersection of utilizing Internet of Things (IoT) improvements to improve the standard of life for their residents. They are distinguished by the integration of cutting-edge technologies and digital infrastructure. In this regard, the combination of edge AI and IoMT has great potential to transform the way healthcare is provided. Together, edge AI—which deals with locally analyzing information on devices during the edge of the network—and IoMT—which links medical systems and devices over the Internet—offer a framework that has the potential to address significant issues related to medical provisioning.

The objective of this chapter is to explore the complex relationship between edge AI and IoMT, with a particular emphasis on how they are used in linked healthcare throughout the context of smart cities. In addition to lowering latency and bandwidth usage, edge computing's close proximity to medical devices allows for the analysis of vital medical data in actual time. We will navigate via the domains of cutting-edge diagnostics, personalized treatment, and the creation of proactive healthcare systems as we investigate the possible effects of this integration. But there are difficulties through this convergence. To guarantee the smooth and responsible implementation of edge AI in connected healthcare, concerns like security, privacy, and interoperability must be thoroughly examined and addressed. This chapter will explore the complex world of edge AI for associated healthcare in the era of medical things inside the framework of smart cities as we set out on this journey, illuminating the opportunities, difficulties, and potentially revolutionary possibilities that lie ahead.

### 21.1.1 BACKGROUND

Technology breakthroughs are bringing about a significant shift in the healthcare industry, with the potential to change how patients receive and interact with care. The integration of edge AI via the IoMT is one of the key technological intersections at the cutting-edge of this shift in technology (Kelly et al., 2020). In the context of smart cities, where data-driven solutions and networked systems are becoming essential elements, edge AI and IoMT together have enormous potential to transform healthcare. The smooth and timely delivery of medical services is frequently hampered by issues with latency, bandwidth limitations, and centralized processing that plague traditional healthcare systems. Acknowledging these drawbacks, edge AI's rise delivers a paradigm change by facilitating localized data processing directly on devices, reducing latency issues, and maximizing bandwidth utilization. In addition, IoMT makes it easier for wearables, medical devices, and health monitoring systems to connect with each other online, forming a network that makes it possible to gather extensive and ongoing health data.

In the framework of smart cities, in which integrating technology is essential to solving urban problems, edge AI and IoMT combined become especially pertinent to healthcare delivery. In order to improve the standard of life for its citizens, smart cities use data and connectivity, and a key element of this goal is healthcare. Urban environments are dynamic, so healthcare solutions that are responsive, flexible, and able to deliver individualized care at scale are required. This investigation aims to investigate the complex interplay between edge AI and IoMT, particularly in the context of associated healthcare in smart cities (Rodrigues et al., 2023). This chapter aims to present insights into the manner in which this transformative technology in addition may transform the delivery of healthcare in the backdrop of rapidly changing urban landscapes through examining the fundamentals of edge AI and IoMT, examining their potential uses in healthcare, and tackling the difficulties connected with their integrating them. By navigating through the context of edge AI for connected healthcare in the IoMT for smart cities, we establish the groundwork for a thorough comprehension of the consequences, difficulties, and opportunities that come with this merging of technologies.

### 21.1.2 Significance of Edge AI and IoMT Integration in Healthcare

The convergence of edge AI and IoMT is a game-changer for healthcare, ushering in a period of more effective, responsive, and individualized care. Fundamental to this importance is the capacity to tackle enduring issues that have impeded the best possible provision of healthcare. First off, edge AI's proximity computing transforms the way healthcare data is processed. Edge AI dramatically lowers latency through allowing confined data analysis instantly on devices or at the edge of the network, guaranteeing that vital medical data can be handled in real time. This improves the general adaptability of healthcare systems and is especially important in situations of emergency or for applications requiring quick decisions.

Second, IoMT offers a networked ecosystem of sensors and medical devices connected by the Internet, facilitating the smooth exchange of health-related data. Because of their interconnectedness, patients can be continuously monitored, giving medical professionals a comprehensive understanding of each patient's health. IoMT enables thorough health monitoring outside of conventional healthcare settings, from wearable devices monitoring vital signs to smart medical equipment transferring real-time data. In the framework of smart cities, the interaction among edge AI and IoMT grows particularly significant. The combined use of these innovations improves the ability to expand of healthcare services in urban environments, where there is a high population density and medical facilities are frequently expanded. Because of edge AI's localized the process, centrally located servers are not overworked and computational tasks are successfully managed. Concurrently, IoMT facilitates the development of an interconnected healthcare network, enabling more efficient data exchange and better coordination between diverse medical systems and devices.

Additionally, the development of diagnosis and treatment customization is aided by the integration of edge AI and IoMT. Large-scale datasets produced by IoMT devices can be analyzed by machine learning algorithms at the edge, resulting in quicker and more precise diagnosis. Based on each person's specific health data, personalized treatment plans are subsequently rapidly created, encouraging a move away from general healthcare approaches and toward more specialized and successful interventions.

### 21.1.3 Contextualizing within Smart Cities

The growth of healthcare services gains further significance and relevance when edge AI and the IoMT are contextualized inside the smart cities framework. The strategic application of digital technologies and data-driven solutions to improve the effectiveness and standard of urban living define smart cities (Rathi et al., 2021). Here, the combination of edge AI and IoMT is a natural fit with the larger goals of smart city projects. Smart cities use technology to solve a range of urban issues, such as resource optimization, accessibility to healthcare, and the general health of citizens. By offering clever and adaptable solutions for healthcare delivery, the integration of edge AI and IoMT directly advances these goals.

- **Optimizing Resource Usage:** Making effective use of scarce resources is a problem that smart cities frequently encounter. Edge AI's localized processing powers minimize the need for centralized data processing, which aids in the optimization of computing resources. This guarantees that computational efforts are allocated effectively, keeping obstacles in using resources in addition to improving the rapidity of healthcare services.
- **Enhancing Urban Health Monitoring:** Continuous and remote health monitoring is made possible by the networked ecosystem of IoMT in smart cities. Individuals can create a comprehensive and current health profile by using real-time health data generated by wearables, smart medical equipment, and other IoMT devices. Proactive monitoring and early intervention are made possible by the seamless integration of this data into the larger urban health infrastructure.
- **Reactive Healthcare Systems:** Edge AI's real-time processing powers guarantee that healthcare systems in Smart Cities can react quickly to medical emergencies. The combined use of Edge AI and IoMT responds to the require for adaptable healthcare systems in dynamic urban environments, whether it is through the analysis of health data from a network of sensors throughout emergencies in public health or the provision of instantaneous diagnostic insights in smart ambulances.
- **Personalized Health Services:** Citizen-centric and personalized services are given priority in smart cities. Delivering extremely individualized healthcare services is made possible by Edge AI in conjunction with the extensive information produced by IoMT devices. In line with the larger philosophy of citizen well-being in Smart Cities, machine learning algorithms at the edge can evaluate individual health data to customize treatment plans, preventive measures, and lifestyle recommendations.

Essentially, the Smart City context's adoption of Edge AI and IoMT turns healthcare compared to a reactive service into a proactive, citizen-centric system. Smart Cities can address current healthcare issues and establish the groundwork for a more robust, adaptable, and flexible urban healthcare infrastructure by utilizing the advantages of these technologies.

### 21.1.4 Foundations of Edge AI and IoMT

Figure 21.1 illustrates the fundamentals of Edge AI and the IoMT, which are essential to comprehending the revolutionary effects of their integration in healthcare (Lim, 2023). Now let's explore the fundamental elements of Edge AI and IoMT:

#### 21.1.4.1 Foundations of Edge AI

- **Definition and Core Principles:** Edge AI involves the processing of data locally on devices, often at the periphery of the network, as opposed to relying solely on centralized cloud servers. This proximity computing minimizes latency and enhances real-time processing capabilities.

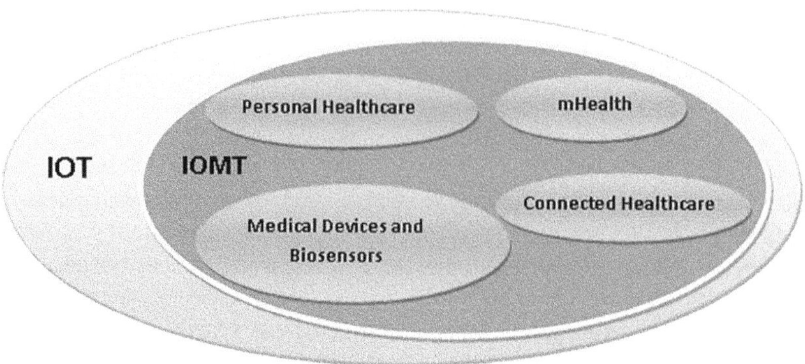


**FIGURE 21.1**   Integration of IOT and IOMT in healthcare.

- **Artificial Intelligence:** At its core, Edge AI leverages machine learning algorithms and AI models to analyze and derive insights from data at or near the data source. This enables devices to make intelligent decisions without heavy reliance on external servers.

- **Applications in Healthcare:**
  - **Real-time Diagnostics:** Edge AI facilitates real-time analysis of medical data, allowing for swift diagnostics and immediate decision-making.
  - **Local Data Processing:** The ability to process data locally on medical devices ensures timely responses and reduces the need for extensive data transfers.

### 21.1.4.2   Foundations of IoMT

- **Key Components and Architectural Framework:**
  - **Connected Devices:** The IoMT is a network of wearables, sensors, and other medical equipment that is networked together.
  - **Communication Protocols:** Data exchange between various medical devices is made possible by standardized communication protocols like HL7 and DICOM.
  - **Cloud Integration:** IoMT frequently uses cloud-based analytics and storage, whereas Edge AI concentrates on local processing. This allows for a more thorough and centralized perspective on health data.
- **Role in Smart Cities:**
  - **Continuous Monitoring:** IoMT helps to facilitate ongoing health monitoring by enabling the real-time gathering of patient data from both inside and outside of medical facilities.
  - **Data-Driven Insights:** Because of the interconnectedness of IoMT, rich datasets can be created, which helps administrators and healthcare professionals gain insights based on data.
  - **Improved Accessibility:** Through the use of telemedicine and remote patient monitoring, IoMT helps to make healthcare services more accessible.

### 21.1.4.3   Integration of Edge AI and IoMT
- **Complementary Nature:**
  - **Proximity Computing:** Edge AI's confined analyzing powers mesh well with IoMT devices' ongoing data generation and monitoring capabilities.

- **Real-time Decision Support:** Edge AI improves the IoMT framework by offering real-time decision support, which is especially important in situations involving healthcare where prompt interventions are essential.
- **Interconnected Healthcare Ecosystem:**
  - **Unified Data Flow:** Edge AI and IoMT work together to build an integrated healthcare ecosystem in which information moves easily between cloud infrastructure, edge nodes, and devices.
  - **Scalability:** The integrated framework can be adjusted to the changing needs of healthcare in smart cities because it is made to grow along with the growing need for healthcare services.

## 21.2 SYNERGY IN CONNECTED HEALTHCARE

### 21.2.1 PROXIMITY COMPUTING IN HEALTHCARE

Instead of depending on centralized cloud servers, proximity computing in healthcare provides a revolutionary technique where computational operations are carried out in proximity to the data source, devices, or sensors (Amin & Hossain, 2021). When it comes to the healthcare ecosystem's embrace of Edge AI, this idea is very important. Key elements of proximity computing in healthcare are as follows:

- **Real-Time Processing:** Healthcare data can be processed in real time at or close to the place of creation thanks to proximity computing. This is important in situations like observing vital signs or examining diagnostic imaging where quick decisions are required.
- **Decreased Latency:** Proximity computing reduces latency by processing data locally, guaranteeing that crucial healthcare information is examined and responded to promptly. This is particularly crucial in scenarios like emergencies where patient care may be negatively impacted by delays.
- **Bandwidth optimization:** Less data must be transferred to centralized servers when calculations are done closer to the data source. By optimizing bandwidth utilization and reducing the strain on network infrastructure, this improves the effectiveness of healthcare services.
- **Improved Security and Privacy:** By placing sensitive medical data closer to the source, proximity computing can improve security and privacy in the healthcare industry. This creates a more secure environment for data processing and lowers the dangers involved in sending sensitive information over networks.
- **Local Decision-Making:** Using processed data, medical equipment with Edge AI capabilities is able to make local judgments. This is helpful when there is an urgent need to take action, such changing prescription dosages or setting off alarms for life-threatening diseases.
- **Flexibility with Edge Devices:** Medical sensors, wearable technology, and point-of-care diagnostic instruments are just a few examples of the edge devices that proximity computing can be used with. This flexibility guarantees a smooth assimilation of computational powers into the current healthcare framework.
- **Offline Functionality:** When devices are offline or have poor connectivity, proximity computing enables some computations to still take place. This ensures ongoing performance and is advantageous in healthcare contexts where continuous data access may not be assured.
- **Proximity Computing Using Edge AI:** Proximity computing is further enhanced by the incorporation of edge AI technologies, which allow intelligent decision-making at the edge. Without relying on remote servers, machine learning models can be implemented locally to analyze and forecast complicated medical data.

### 21.2.2 ADVANCED DIAGNOSTICS THROUGH EDGE AI

A novel approach in healthcare involves modern diagnostics via edge AI, which uses artificial intelligence at the network's edge to provide more accurate and timely medical evaluations (Alrazgan & Jan, 2022). The following are the main ways that edge AI advances sophisticated diagnostics:

- **Regionalized Information Analysis:** Medical data can be analyzed immediately on the device or at the network edge wherein the data is created thanks to edge AI. Because less data must be transferred to centralized servers as a result of this local processing, diagnostic procedures are able to proceed more quickly and effectively.
- **Real-Time Decision Support:** Healthcare equipment may now offer prompt decision support thanks to Edge AI's real-time processing capabilities. This is especially helpful in urgent cases where prompt judgments have a big influence on the course of treatment for patients.
- **Algorithms for Machine Learning:** Edge AI uses algorithms for machine learning that are able to recognize patterns in medical data and adjust accordingly. These algorithms are very good at finding intricate patterns across a wide range of datasets, which helps with more precise and detailed diagnosis.
- **Enhanced Imaging Analysis:** Edge AI is capable of locally analyzing and interpreting radiological images, including MRIs, CT scans, and X-rays, in the field of medicine. Faster image processing, anomaly detection, and the creation of diagnostic insights are all made possible by this, all without requiring large-scale data transfer.
- **Reduced Diagnostic Latency:** Edge AI dramatically lowers diagnostic latency by cutting down on the amount of time needed to locally process and analyze data. This allows medical professionals to make well-informed decisions quickly, which is especially beneficial in situations where time is of the essence.
- **Predictive Analytics and Continuous Monitoring:** Edge AI facilitates the creation of predictive analytics by allowing for the continuous monitoring of patient data. Prevention strategies and individualized treatment plans are made possible by this proactive approach, which enables the early detection of trends or anomalies.
- **Diagnostic Models That Can Be Customized:** Edge AI makes it easier to implement diagnostic models that can be customized to fit particular medical needs. Because of their flexibility, diagnostic instruments can be adjusted to suit the particular needs of various medical situations.
- **Diagnostics That Preserve Privacy:** Edge AI makes privacy-preserving diagnostics possible by storing sensitive patient data locally on the device or in a restricted network. Data security and privacy issues are addressed here, which is important to take into account in healthcare settings.
- **Integration with Wearables and IoT Devices:** Edge AI enables ongoing health parameter to be used monitoring through integration with wearables and Internet of Things (IoT) devices in an effortless way. This integration offers a comprehensive, real-time picture of a person's health, which improves diagnostic capabilities.
- **Scalability and Resource Efficiency:** Healthcare systems' scalability and resource utilization are enhanced by Edge AI's local data processing capabilities. By reducing the load on centralized servers, it opens up access to and makes advanced diagnostics practical in a range of healthcare environments.

### 21.2.3 PERSONALIZED TREATMENT AND PROACTIVE HEALTHCARE

#### 21.2.3.1 Tailoring Treatments with Edge AI

Personalized and adaptive medical care has advanced significantly with the use of edge AI to tailor treatments (Khaled, 2022). The following are the main ways that edge AI helps with treatment customization:

- **Analyzing patient data in real time:** Edge AI makes it possible to analyze patient data in real time right at the source—from wearable technology to medical sensors to monitoring apparatus. Healthcare professionals can get real-time insights into a patient's health status thanks to this instant analysis.
- **Adaptive Treatment Plans:** Edge AI continuously monitors and analyzes patient data to promote the development of adaptable treatment plans. The treatment plan is able to be rapidly modified as the patient's health changes to make sure it continues to be efficient and in line with the person's evolving medical needs.
- **Machine Learning for Personalization:** Edge AI may benefit from past patient data and patterns by applying machine learning algorithms, which enables the customization of treatment plans. Treatment plans are customized to meet the unique requirements and responses of every patient thanks to adaptive learning.
- **Medication Dosage Optimization:** By using real-time data, edge AI can help optimize medication dosages. Edge AI helps create more accurate and individualized dosing strategies by taking into account variables like a patient's present health status, the effectiveness of their medication, and any possible side effects.
- **Remote Patient Monitoring:** The effectiveness of remote patient monitoring is increased with edge AI. The capacity to perform local data analysis enables ongoing patient monitoring outside of conventional healthcare settings, giving medical staff current data to modify patient care as necessary.
- **Notifications for Critical Circumstances:** Edge AI has the ability to instantly produce notifications for critical circumstances or departures from the anticipated health parameters. By guaranteeing that medical professionals are promptly notified of any problems, this early warning system enables prompt interventions and treatment plan modifications.
- **Integration with Electronic Health Records (EHR):** Edge AI easily links with EHRs, guaranteeing that patient history is easily accessible for examination. By taking long-term trends and responses into account, this thorough understanding of a patient's medical history improves the accuracy of treatment customization.
- **Personalized Therapy Recommendations:** Edge AI is able to provide personalized therapy recommendations by analyzing a variety of data sources, such as genetic information, lifestyle factors, treatment outcomes, and patient demographics. Healthcare that is more patient-centered and efficient is facilitated by this holistic approach.
- **Privacy and Security Considerations:** By limiting the need for large-scale data transfers, edge AI minimizes privacy concerns by keeping sensitive patient data localized. Patient confidentiality is critical in the healthcare industry, where this privacy-preserving strategy is essential.
- **Patient Empowerment and Engagement:** By allowing patients to take an active role in their own care, edge-AI-tailored treatments promote patient engagement. Individualized advice, education, and insights can be given to patients, enabling them to take an active role in their own health management.

In final analysis, edge AI's local data processing and analysis capabilities support customized and adaptive patient care by helping to customize healthcare treatments. This not only increases patient outcomes and overall satisfaction with healthcare services, but it also improves the effectiveness of treatment.

### 21.2.3.2  Developing Proactive Healthcare Systems

Using technologies like edge AI and the IoMT to predict, avoid and deal with health issues prior to the exacerbate is a key component of establishing proactive healthcare systems (Lakshminarayanan et al., 2023). The following are essential elements of proactive healthcare system development:

- **Predictive analytics:** Examine past and present patient data using machine learning algorithms and sophisticated analytics. Healthcare professionals can take preventative action by using predictive models to foresee possible health problems.
- **Continuous Remote Monitoring:** Use IoMT devices to keep an eye on patients continuously from a distance. This covers wearable technology, intelligent medical equipment, and sensors that gather and send health data in real time. The continuous flow of data makes it possible to identify patterns and discrepancies promptly on.
- **Early Intervention Strategies:** Using the information from predictive analytics, formulate preliminary intervention strategies. Establish procedures and automated alerts to cause prompt interventions, like changing prescription dosages or planning preventive screenings.
- **Personalized Preventive Care:** Customize preventive care regimens according to each patient's health history and risk factors. In order to prevent the development of chronic conditions, utilize edge AI to evaluate a variety of patient data and offer specific suggestions for lifestyle modifications, screenings, and vaccinations.
- **Health Risk Assessments:** Make use of digital tools and surveys to conduct proactive health risk assessments. Examine the gathered information to find possible dangers, then create focused treatments to reduce them prior to they become major health problems.
- **Interconnected Healthcare Ecosystem:** Fostering integration and interoperability throughout healthcare systems, equipment, and data sources is the goal of the interconnected healthcare ecosystem. Proactive decision-making by healthcare providers is made possible by seamless data flow facilitated by an interconnected ecosystem.
- **Initiatives for Community Health:** Develop outreach and health education programs to bring preventive healthcare initiatives to the community level. Identify health trends within particular populations, perform screenings, and distribute information using technology.
- **Data Security and Privacy Measures:** Use extra care to protect privacy and data security while managing sensitive health information. Proactive healthcare systems must ensure adherence to all standards in order to protect patient confidentiality.
- **Population Health Management:** Analyze health behaviors and trends within larger groups by utilizing population health management strategies. Healthcare professionals may carry out focused interventions and make effective use of resources thanks to this data-driven approach.
- **Continuous Improvement through Feedback Loops:** In order to continuously assess the efficacy of preventive measures, create feedback loops throughout the healthcare system. Evaluate the results, modify your plan of action in light of them, and put continuous improvement procedures into place.

A comprehensive strategy integrating data-driven insights, patient-centered care, and technological innovation is needed to build proactive healthcare systems. Healthcare systems may transition from a reactive to a proactive model by adopting proactive strategies, which will eventually improve population health and patient care by anticipating and addressing health issues before they arise.

### 21.2.4 Challenges and Considerations

#### 21.2.4.1 Security in Edge AI for Healthcare

Given the sensitivity of medical data and the possible consequences of hacking attempts on patient privacy and healthcare delivery, it is critical to ensure security in edge AI for healthcare (Rahman et al., 2022). The following are important factors to take into account and actions to improve security in edge AI healthcare applications:

- **Encrypt data:** Use strong encryption techniques to safeguard data while it's being transferred and stored. This covers both the encryption of data maintained in order to avoid unwanted access and the encryption of data transferred between servers and edge devices.
- **Secure Communication Protocols:** To protect data transfers between edge devices, cloud services, and other infrastructure elements in the healthcare system, use secure communication protocols. Protocols like HTTPS can improve data transmission security.
- **Authentication and Authorization:** To guarantee that only authorized users and devices are able to utilize edge AI systems, implement robust authentication procedures. Use role-based access controls to limit access according to the function of the user in the healthcare system.
- **Device Security:** By implementing security standards, such as frequent software updates, firmware validation, and the adoption of secure boot mechanisms, edge devices' security can be improved. In which appropriate, think about adding hardware-based safety precautions.
- **Privacy-Preserving Edge Processing:** Use edge AI processing methods that preserve privacy. Encouraging techniques like federated learning can preserve confidentiality for patients while promoting model advancement. Federated learning involves training models across dispersed edge devices with no sharing raw data.
- **Secure Edge Gateways:** Put in place protect edge gateways to serve as a bridge among central servers and edge devices. These gateways have to make sure that solely permitted data is sent to centralized systems, enforce security policies, and validate data. **Secure Model Deployment:** Use virtualization or secure containerization to safeguard the deployment of AI models at the edge. By isolating the AI models, this assists in preventing manipulation and unwanted access.
- **Monitoring and Audits for Security:** Perform routine security audits and surveillance of edge AI systems in order to detect and address possible security risks. Use monitoring tools and intrusion detection systems to find anomalies or questionable activity.
- **Respect for Regulations:** Make sure that healthcare data protection laws, such as the General Data Protection Regulation (GDPR) and the Health Insurance Portability and Accountability Act (HIPAA), are followed. Keep abreast of changing regulatory requirements so that you can modify security measures appropriately.
- **Incident Response Planning:** Create an incident response strategy tailored to edge AI in healthcare and modify it frequently. This plan should specify what should be done in the case of a security incident, including ways to communicate and mitigate the damage.
- **Employee Training:** Give administrators, AI developers, and healthcare workers continuous education on privacy best practices. This involves being conscious of possible dangers, phishing schemes, and the significance of following security procedures.
- **Safe Data Disposal:** When decommissioned or reused, make sure sensitive data is anonymized or destroyed appropriately by establishing secure data removal procedures for edge devices.

Healthcare companies can build a strong and durable security framework for edge AI applications by taking these security factors into account. Proactive safety precautions that leverage edge AI technologies not only safeguard patient data but additionally promote belief in the confidentiality and dependability of healthcare services.

### 21.2.4.2 Interoperability Challenges

The healthcare industry faces significant interoperability challenges that impede the smooth transfer and use of data among various systems and devices. These difficulties intensify as the sector develops to include cutting-edge technologies like edge AI (Kamruzzaman et al., 2023). A fully interconnected healthcare ecosystem is hampered by a number of issues, including inconsistent data formats and standards and disjointed data silos. The variety of data formats and standards used by healthcare systems is one of these main challenges. It is challenging for different platforms, such as those integrating edge AI applications, to interact effectively in a lack of standardized formats. The lack of standard communication protocols makes this lack of cohesiveness even worse and prevents the development of standardized interfaces for reliable data exchange.

Another major issue is data fragmentation, which frequently exists in separate divisions inside healthcare organizations. Applications utilizing edge AI, which seek to utilize extensive patient data, face challenges when data is scattered among various departments or healthcare providers. An additional level of complexity is introduced by combining the integration of edge AI with heterogeneous system architectures that include both contemporary and legacy technologies. The interfaces needed for seamless interoperability may be absent from older systems. Ensuring precise patient identification throughout various systems is an essential consideration. Standardized patient matching algorithms are required because mismatches in patient identification can lead to errors in diagnosis and treatment plans. Furthermore, maintaining privacy and security requires careful balancing.

Even though interoperability is desired, it is still critical to uphold strong security protocols and protect patient privacy. The lack of standardized terminology and semantic models poses a challenge to semantic interoperability, which guarantees consistent understanding of shared information across systems. Vendor lock-in presents financial and operational difficulties for healthcare organizations because it occurs when proprietary solutions from various vendors prevent system switching or upgrading. There are obstacles in the way of edge AI's integration with current healthcare workflows. Successful adoption of interoperable systems requires their seamless integration without hiccups or major alterations. Inconsistencies in regulations among various regions or healthcare organizations pose additional challenges that must be resolved to facilitate successful cross-system collaboration.

## 21.3 IMPACT ON RESOURCE UTILIZATION AND PATIENT OUTCOMES

### 21.3.1 Optimizing Resource Allocation in Healthcare

For successful delivery service, healthcare resource allocation must be optimized. This is especially true when integrating technologies like edge AI (Mishra & Singh, 2023). Key tactics for maximizing the distribution of resources in healthcare are as follows:

- **Making Decisions Based on Data:** Make decisions about the distribution of resources more informed by using data analytics, such as predictive modeling and business intelligence tools. It is possible to spot trends, predict demand, and assign resources more effectively by analyzing both historical and current data.
- **Analytical Forecasting for Patient Movement:** To predict patient admissions, discharges, and bed usage, apply predictive analytics. This makes it possible for healthcare providers to plan ahead and assign resources—like hospital beds, personnel, and equipment—to match projected demand.
- **Edge AI for Real-Time Monitoring:** Use edge AI to keep an eye on healthcare data in real time at the network's edge. This makes it possible to make timely resource adjustments by providing instant insights into patient conditions, equipment status, and other important factors.
  - Use dynamic staff scheduling by planning your schedule according to patient volume, acuity, and expected workload. By ensuring that staffing levels are in line with the changing needs of patient care, adaptive scheduling helps to avoid shortages or overstaffing.

- The integration of telemedicine and remote monitoring solutions can expand the reach of healthcare services beyond conventional settings. By decreasing the need for in-person visits, particularly for routine check-ups and follow-ups, this strategy maximizes resources.
- **Inventory Management Systems:** To streamline the supply chain for pharmaceuticals, consumables, and medical equipment, implement strong inventory management systems. In order to minimize waste, avoid deficits, and guarantee the accessibility of necessary resources, automation and real-time tracking are beneficial.
- **Centralized Command Centers:** Set up command centers that are centralized and have access to communication and real-time data analytics. Inside a healthcare system, these centers facilitate effective resource allocation and coordination amongst different departments and facilities.
- **Capacity Planning and Expansion:** To ascertain whether additional resources or expanded facilities are required, regularly conduct capacity planning assessments. By taking a proactive stance, healthcare infrastructure is guaranteed to keep up with the population's increasing demands.
- **Collaboration and Information Sharing:** Encourage healthcare institutions to work together and share information. It is possible to maximize shared resources—like specialized machinery or knowledge—across several sites, cutting down on redundancy and enhancing overall resource efficiency. Investing in community health initiatives can help decrease the demand on severe healthcare services and encourage the use of preventive care. The community level approach to health issues allows healthcare providers to more effectively allocate resources.
- **Mobile Health Units:** Send out mobile health units that are outfitted with the tools they need to places where there is little access to medical facilities. By delivering basic services, screenings, and preventive care, these units can maximize resources in the most critical areas.

Establish a culture of continuous process improvement within healthcare organizations by routinely evaluating and improving their procedures. This entails getting input, examining performance indicators, and modifying resource allocation plans in light of discovered insights. Healthcare organizations can improve patient care, operational efficiency, and responsiveness to changing healthcare demands by optimizing resource allocation through the integration of data-driven insights, technological innovations like edge AI, and strategic planning.

## 21.3.2 Improving Patient Outcomes with Data-Driven Insights

Using data-driven insights to improve patient outcomes is a core objective of contemporary healthcare (Kelly et al., 2020). Using data to inform decisions, improve treatment plans, and personalize care is possible for healthcare providers, especially when technologies like edge AI are integrated. The following are essential tactics for enhancing patient outcomes via insights derived from data:

- **Predictive Analytics for Early Intervention:** Predictive analytics can be used to find high-risk individuals and possible health problems before they get worse. Improved patient results along with more efficient treatments may result from early intervention determined by data-driven predictions.
- **Patient Risk Stratification:** Classify patients according to their health risks by using data-driven risk stratification models. This enables healthcare providers to concentrate on interventions for high-risk patients and preventive measures for lower-risk patients, thereby allocating resources more effectively.

- **Personalized Treatment Plans:** Utilize data-driven insights to develop individualized treatment programs that are specific to each patient's profile. Healthcare professionals can provide more individualized and efficient care by analyzing patient data, such as genetic information, lifestyle factors, and treatment responses.
- **Edge AI Real-Time Monitoring:** Include edge AI to track patient data in real time at the network's edge. This makes it possible to instantly analyze vital signs, medication adherence, and other important metrics, which enables prompt intervention and treatment plan modifications.
- **Patient Risk Stratification:** Use data-driven risk stratification models to categorize patients based on their health risks. This makes it possible for medical professionals to focus on treating high-risk patients and preventing diseases in patients who are not as likely to need them, which improves resource allocation.
- **Personalized Treatment Plans:** Make use of data-driven insights to create treatment plans that are unique to the needs of every patient. By evaluating patient data, including genetics, lifestyle factors, and treatment outcomes, healthcare providers can deliver more customized and effective care.
- **Real-Time Edge AI Monitoring:** Integrate edge AI to monitor patient data at the edge of the network in real time. This facilitates immediate intervention and treatment plan modifications by enabling the instantaneous analysis of vital signs, medication adherence, and other critical metrics. Utilize outcome analytics and benchmarking to evaluate the efficacy of interventions and treatments. To enhance patient outcomes, care protocols can be refined and areas for enhancement can be identified by benchmarking toward established standards and best practices.
- **Patient Engagement Platforms:** Provide patient engagement tools that enable people to take an active role in their own care. These platforms can support a team-based approach to healthcare by offering self-monitoring tools, educational materials, and personalized health insights. Establish feedback loops with patients, healthcare professionals, and data analysts to promote continuous enhancement. Review patient experiences, results, and comments on a regular basis to hone data-driven tactics and raise the standard of care.
- **Interoperability for Comprehensive Data Access:** To accomplish comprehensive data access, ensure that healthcare systems and devices are interoperable. More comprehensive insights are made possible by having a single view of patient data from all of the touchpoints, which helps with better decision-making.
- **Patient-Reported Results and Questionnaires:** Include surveys and patient-reported outcomes in the process of gathering data. Feedback from patients gives medical professionals important information about how treatments affect their quality of life, allowing them to adjust their interventions.

Healthcare providers may enhance patient satisfaction and overall healthcare quality by adopting data-driven insights and technologies like edge AI. This will also help providers deliver more efficient, timely, and personalized care.

### 21.3.3 Future Directions and Innovations

Technological innovations, changing care models, and a persistent dedication to providing individualized, patient-centered care are expected to come together to shape the coming decades of healthcare. Looking ahead, a number of significant paths and innovations have the potential to completely transform the healthcare experience, improving the standard and accessibility of medical care. Machine learning and artificial intelligence (AI) are at the forefront of transformative technologies (Sundaravadivazhagan et al., 2021). Predictive analytics, treatment planning, and diagnosis are all being revolutionized by developments in these domains. The notable aspect of AI integration at the edge is its ability to facilitate real-time data analysis, which lowers latency and increases the effectiveness of healthcare applications.

The way that edge computing is being adopted is going to change healthcare delivery in a big way. Real-time medical data analysis is made possible by edge devices, which are heavily powered by AI. By doing this, latency is reduced and the ability to provide individualized healthcare interventions is improved. The delivery of healthcare is going to depend even more on telemedicine and remote patient monitoring. While advancements in remote patient monitoring technologies allow for continuous health tracking outside of traditional healthcare settings, telemedicine makes it easier for people to obtain medical consultations remotely and promotes proactive and preventative care (Rathi et al., 2021). The field of genomic medicine is expanding quickly and holds the possibility of tailored treatments. It is expected that treating patients according to their genetic composition will become more common, maximizing therapeutic benefit and reducing side effects. Electronic health records (EHRs), wearables, health apps, and other health technologies are all becoming seamlessly integrated through the development of digital health ecosystems.

This connectivity fosters proactive and cooperative care by offering a thorough, up-to-date picture of each person's health. Blockchain technology is starting to show promise as a security measure for health data. Its decentralized and impenetrable ledger system improves data integrity, safeguards patient confidentiality, and makes it easier for various stakeholders to securely share health information. Applications of virtual reality (VR) and augmented reality (AR) are becoming more prevalent in patient education, surgical planning, and medical training. These innovations offer patients and healthcare providers immersive experiences that improve the interpretation of medical imaging. With the development of 3D printing, personalized implants, prosthetic limbs, and even tissues or organs are now possible, completely changing the healthcare industry. This invention has the power to completely rethink patient-specific treatment approaches. It is anticipated that a greater emphasis on the socioeconomic determinants of health will change healthcare tactics.

Patient-centered care will be more comprehensive if lifestyle, socioeconomic status, and environmental influences are taken into account. Automation and robotics are becoming essential parts of healthcare, helping with routine tasks, medication dispensing, and surgeries. These innovations improve accuracy, lower mistakes, and maximize overall effectiveness in the provision of healthcare. An abundance of real-time health data is promised by continuous biometric monitoring, which includes keeping track of vital signs continuously. With timely interventions and prompt health issue detection made possible by this information, patient outcomes are eventually improved. Simulations and analytics in healthcare could undergo a radical change thanks to quantum computing. Drug discovery could be expedited, treatment algorithms could be optimized, and complex healthcare issues could be resolved with the help of this technology. All of these innovations work together to bring about a more connected, efficient, and personalized healthcare environment that will open up new possibilities for personal growth and better health outcomes.

## 21.4  CONCLUSION

In general, a combination of cutting-edge technologies and a dedication to patient-centered care will propel transformative innovation that will revolutionize the healthcare industry in the near future. Several significant trends and advancements stand out as we navigate this shifting terrain, influencing the direction of healthcare delivery. Predictive analytics, treatment planning, and diagnosis stand to be completely transformed by the combination of artificial intelligence (AI) and machine learning. With its ability to process data in real time, edge AI becomes a vital facilitator of effective and individualized healthcare interventions. With the ability to track health over time and provide medical consultations outside of traditional settings, telemedicine and remote patient monitoring are soon to be essential parts of healthcare delivery.

These technologies promote proactive and preventative care by improving accessibility, especially in underserved or remote areas. Developments in genomics support the move toward personalized medicine, in which treatment regimens are customized based on each patient's unique genetic profile. This holds out the possibility of more focused and efficient therapeutic approaches, reducing side effects and improving patient outcomes. Real-time, comprehensive views of an individual's health are provided by digital health ecosystems, which are distinguished by the seamless integration of wearables, health apps, and electronic health records. Because of this interconnection, patients and healthcare professionals can receive proactive and collaborative care. Blockchain technology is emerging as a key component for protecting patient privacy, data integrity, and secure information sharing in the context of health data security.

Because it is decentralized, it effectively addresses important issues with data security and public confidence in healthcare systems. Applications for virtual reality (VR) and augmented reality (AR) improve patient education, surgical planning, and medical training. Immersion technologies improve patient comprehension and engagement while also advancing the skills of healthcare professionals. The field of 3D printing has the potential to transform patient-specific treatment modalities through the creation of personalized implants, prosthetics, and even tissues. This invention represents a paradigm change in medical device production. The significance of addressing variables outside of conventional clinical care is highlighted by the increased attention being paid to the social determinants of health. A strategy to healthcare that is additionally patient-centered and holistic takes into account lifestyle, environments, and socioeconomic factors. Automation and robotics are becoming more and more essential to the delivery of healthcare because they provide accuracy in procedures, medicine administration, and daily duties. These innovations lower the possibility of errors and improve operational efficiency.

A steady stream of real-time health data is provided by continuous biometric monitoring, allowing for the early identification of health problems and the prompt implementation of interventions. Proactive care contributes to better patient outcomes and healthcare prevention. Drug discovery, treatment optimization, and the resolution of complex healthcare challenges are all made possible by quantum computing's capacity to handle sophisticated analytics and simulations. This new technology has the potential to unleash previously untapped computational power for improvements in healthcare. The future of healthcare is clearly defined by the convergence of technological prowess, data-driven insights, and a dedication to patient well-being, as we embrace these innovations. With the potential to completely reshape healthcare delivery in this revolutionary age, making it more efficient, individualized, and accessible, improved outcomes for patients and a healthier global population.

## REFERENCES

Alrazgan, M., & Jan, N. (2022). Internet of Medical Things and Edge Computing for Improving Healthcare in Smart Cities. *Mathematical Problems in Engineering, Hindawi*, 2022, 1–10.

Amin, S.U., & Hossain, M.S. (2021). Edge Intelligence and Internet of Things in Healthcare: A Survey. *IEEE Access*, 9, 45–59.

Kamruzzaman, M.M., Alrashdi, I., & Alqazzaz, A. (2023). Healthcare Engineering JO. Retracted: New Opportunities, Challenges, and Applications of Edge-AI for Connected Healthcare in Internet of Medical Things for Smart Cities. *Journal of Healthcare Engineering*, 9823658.

Kelly, J., Campbell, K., Gong, E., & Scuffham, P. (2020). The Internet of Things: Impact and Implications for Health Care Delivery. *Journal of Medical Internet Research*, 22(11), e20135.

Khaled, A. (2022). Internet of Medical Things (IoMT): Overview, Taxonomies, and Classifications. *Journal of Computer and Communications*, 10, 64–89.

Lakshminarayanan, V., Ravikumar, A., Sriraman, H., Alla, S., & Chattu, V.K. (2023). Health Care Equity Through Intelligent Edge Computing and Augmented Reality/Virtual Reality: A Systematic Review. *Journal of Multidisciplinary Healthcare*, 16, 2839–2859.

Lim, S.-J. (2023). Remote Monitoring of Health Using Artificial Intelligence and Internet of Things in Smart Cities. *International Journal of Intelligent Systems and Applications in Engineering*, 11(7s), 649–654.

Mantey, E.A., Sundaravadivazhagan, B., et al. (2022). Integrated Blockchain-Deep Learning Approach for Analyzing the Electronic Health Records Recommender System. *Frontiers in Public Health*, 10, 905265.

Mishra, P., & Singh, G. (2023). Internet of Medical Things Healthcare for Sustainable Smart Cities: Current Status and Future Prospects. *Applied Sciences*, 13(15), 8869.

Rahman, A., Hossain, M.S., Muhammad, G., et al. (2022). Federated Learning-Based AI Approaches in Smart Healthcare: Concepts, Taxonomies, Challenges and Open Issues. *Cluster Computing*, 1–41.

Rathi, V.K., Rajput, N.K., Mishra, S., Grover, B.A., Tiwari, P., Jaiswal, A.K., & Hossain, M.S. (2021). An Edge AI-Enabled IoT Healthcare Monitoring System for Smart Cities. *Computers & Electrical Engineering*, 96, Part B, 107524. ISSN 0045-7906.

Rejeb, A., Rejeb, K., Treiblmaier, H., Appolloni, A., Alghamdi, S., Alhasawi, Y., & Iranmanesh, M. (2023). The Internet of Things (IoT) in Healthcare: Taking Stock and Moving Forward. *Internet of Things*, 22, Article 100721.

Rodrigues, V.F., da Rosa Righi, R., da Costa, C.A., et al. (2023). Digital Health in Smart Cities: Rethinking the Remote Health Monitoring Architecture on Combining Edge, Fog, and Cloud. *Health Technology*, 13, 449–472.

Sundaravadivazhagan, B., Subashini, B., & Ashik, M. (2021). A Review on Internet of Things (IoT): Security Challenges, Issues and the Countermeasures Approaches. *Psychology and Education*, 58(2), 6544–6560.

# Index

**0-9**

3D printing, 174, 311

**A**

access control, 217, 218
activity monitoring, 209, 210, 215
adaptive data rates, 186, 189
advection-diffusion equation, 27
agriculture, 153
AI Algorithms, 120–123
AI edge device deployment and real-time inferencing, 38–42
    integration with CT scanners, 37–38, 42
      NVIDIA Jetson TX2, 42
      potential for healthcare optimization, 39, 42
AI-enabled monitoring, 88
AI encapsulated, 104
AI ethics
    privacy considerations, 149
    regulatory compliance, 149
AI in healthcare, 81
AI-powered diagnostic tools advantages for radiologists, 36–37, 39
    embedded AI capabilities, 37–38
    reduction in diagnostic workload, 38
algorithm explainability, 181, 183
algorithmic accountability and transparency, 113
analytical solution, 27
anomaly detection
    customizable models, 148
    integration with edge AI, 148
anonymization, 217
applications
    of blockchain technology, 269
    of Edge AI, 122–124, 209, 211, 215
    edge AI in real-time detection, 145
    harassment prevention, 147
architecture, 221
artificial intelligence (AI), 18–19, 27, 144, 153, 155, 172, 173, 175, 185, 187, 299–301, 303–307, 310, 311
artificial intelligence (AI) applications in medical imaging, 36–37
    integration with quantum neural networks, 37–38
artificial intelligence (AI) and blockchain, 273
artificial-intelligence-assisted, 241
artificial intelligence in edge computing, 119–121
artificial neural networks, 153, 154
asset tokenization, 270
audit trails, 271
augmented reality, 311, 312
authentication and authorization, 307
automated inventory management, 161
automation, 173
automation and robotics, 122
autonomous vehicles, 153, 236

**B**

bandwidth, 221
bandwidth management, 122
bandwidth optimization, 185
Banking, 154
battery life extension, 192
benefits of combining fuzzy clustering and C, 137
bias
    mitigation strategies, 180, 181
bias mitigation, 180
big data analytics, 18
big data processing, 121
biomarkers classification using transfer learning, 37–38
    detection in COVID-19 CT scans, 36–39
    ground-glass opacity lesions, 37, 40–41
    progression to crazy-paving patterns, 38–41
bitcoin transaction, 252
black bird attack (BBA), 258
Black Box AI systems, 101
block, 252
blockchain, 251, 252
    applications, 269
    decentralization, 269
    features, 269
    Future of trust, 278
    integration with edge AI, 273
    integration with machine learning, 273
    Network security, 274
    role in governance, 271
    role in voting, 271
    Scalability issues, 275
    transparency and immutability, 269
blockchain-based businesses, compliance costs, 274
blockchain development tools, 276
blockchain security, 275–276
blockchain technology, 19–20, 311
blockchain technology, scalability issues, 275
block withholding (BWH) attack, 257
blood pressure sensors, 163
breast cancer detection, 94
Business Intelligence, 231

**C**

cancer development process, 129
care coordination, 22, 191
caregivers feedback, 216
challenges
    in Brain Tumour Detection, 129
    data quality and noise, 183
    data security, 149
    in Edge AI, 123–125
    interoperability, 183
    privacy protection, 148
    scalability, 183
    scalability of edge AI systems, 146

chronic disease management, 193
Class Activation Mapping (CAM), 94
Clinical Decision Support, 172
Clinical Decision Support Systems (CDSS), 91
clinical research, 158
cloud computing alternatives, 119–120
cloud infrastructure, 201
cloud integration, 302
cloud services in blockchain, 273–274
CNN, 199, 203
CNN Models, 217, 218
CNN Overview, 127
Cobots, 244
collaboration and information sharing, 309
communication networks, 220
compassionate care, 22
compliance, 217
compliance with regulations, 274
concept of digital twin, digital model, digital shadow, 2
conclusions, 14
confidentiality, 217
connected devices, 302
connection, 220
connectivity, 201
consensus, 238
consensus algorithm, 252
consensus mechanisms, 273
consent
    informed data usage, 180
conventional imaging techniques, 130
convolutional neural networks (CNNs), 120, 134
cost management, 123
cost reduction in blockchain, 269
cost and resource constraints, 277
COVID-19 diagnosis challenges in radiological
        interpretation, 36–37
    framework using hybrid quantum neural networks, 36–39
    integration with AI edge devices, 37–42
cross-referencing
    healthcare sentiments, 178–180
cryptocurrency, 269
CT scans AI-enabled analysis, 36–39
    biomarkers of lung abnormalities, 37–39
    data collection and orchestration, 38–39
customized medicine169
cutting-edge technology, 220
Cyber Security, 153
cyberbullying
    detection using NLP, 147
    online safety strategies, 145–146

**D**

data
    governance practices, 149, 183
    privacy compliance, 149, 180
    protection and consent, 180
    protection and informed consent, 149
    quality and noise, 183
data analytics, 170, 201
data augmentation techniques and applications, 38–40
    importance for transfer learning, 38–39
data carrier, 236

data collection and preprocessing, 201
data collection COVID-19 CT scan datasets, 38–39
    open-source datasets, 38–39
data driven decision making, 172, 173
Data Driven Product Improvement, 162
data encryption, 217
data gathering, 202
data integrity, 269
data minimization, 217
data privacy, 170
data privacy and security, 185, 195
data privacy, 276
data protection measures, 217
data security and privacy, 19, 23, 122–124
data transmission, 220
data transmission reduction, 192
data transparency, 24
data-driven decisions, 242
decentralized applications (DApps), 273
decentralized finance (DeFi), 270
decision-making
    enhanced with sentiment analysis, 182
    in healthcare, 182
deep convolutional neural network, 28
deep learning, 153–156
deep learning Models, 120
demand estimation, 273
detection mechanisms
    reinforcement through AI, 147–148
device, 220
device Monitoring, 211
diagnosing rare diseases, 92
diagnostic applications in healthcare, 122–123
Differential privacy, 273
digital health tools, 21
digital signature, 252
digital twin as an emerging technology, 3
digital twin in healthcare, 6
digital twins in manufacturing industries, 8
digital twin in smart cities, 4
digital twin in supply chain management, 7
disaster relief, 240
dispersion coefficient, 27
distributed computing, 121
driverless cars, 241
drug discovery, 87
drug discovery, 156
dynamic evolution, 114

**E**

early detection, 156
edge AI, 299, 301, 303, 305–308, 310, 311
    anomaly detection, 148
    applications in harassment prevention, 145
    applications in healthcare, 179–180
    enhanced decision-making, 182
    ethical considerations, 180–181
    explainability, 181
    integration with blockchain, 273
    interoperability challenges, 183
    personalization of care delivery, 180
    privacy and security, 273

privacy considerations, 149
   real-time decision making, 273
   real-time processing, 146
edge AI Frameworks, 120–121
edge AI technology, 178–182
edge computing, 200, 204
edge devices, 209, 210, 217
efficiency in AI systems, 119
elderly care, 193, 209, 215
Electronic health records (EHR), 18, 22, 155, 253, 305, 311
electronic health record systems, 100
emergency management, 122
energy efficiency, 185, 186, 189
environmental sustainability, 123
ethical AI, 19, 23
ethical considerations
   responsible data use, 180–181
   transparency in AI-driven decisions, 181
   user privacy and data protection, 149
evaluation metrics, 210, 215
explainability and accountability, 183
explainable AI, 84
explainable AI models in healthcare, 100
explainable artificial intelligence (XAI), 28, 106, 154, 155
explainable boosting machine (EBM), 109

**F**

fall detection, 209, 210, 215
faster RCNN Inception-V3 performance in transfer
      learning, 39–41
   integration with hybrid quantum layers, 40–42
   validation accuracy and training time, 41–42
feature Based Methods, 154
federated Learning, 120–121
feedback Mechanisms, 216
finance sector
   blockchain applications in, 270
   Future of blockchain, 269
   tokenization in real estate, 270
Flowchart of CNN, 128
frameworks for AI Models, 124
fraud detection, 273
Fuzzy, 27
Fuzzy Clustering in Medical Image Analysis, 134
Fuzzy C-Means Clustering Algorithm, 135
Fuzzy form solution, 27
Fuzzy model, 27

**G**

gas and chemical sensors, 165
genetic testing, 155
A Glance of IIoT, 4
glucose sensors, 164
greater faith, 111

**H**

Hansen Robotics, 116
harassment prevention
   anomaly detection strategies, 148
   using edge AI, 145

Hash, 251
healthcare, 154–156, 299–301, 303, 305, 306
   blockchain applications in, 270
   interoperability, 271
   MedRec system, 271
   Patientory, 271
   secure data sharing, 271
healthcare, 5.0, 17–19, 82
healthcare applications, 121–124
healthcare data
   patient-generated insights, 178–179
healthcare datasets, 83
healthcare equity, 19, 24
healthcare monitoring, 209, 215, 218, 240
healthcare organizations
   resource allocation, 182
healthcare system, 27
health monitoring, 156
heart rate sensors, 163
heterogeneous data handling, 123
heterogeneous network, 228
HIPAA Compliance, 217
human-centric smart manufacturing system, 245
hybrid Approaches, 155
hybrid quantum neural networks (QNNs) benefits for
      COVID-19 diagnostics, 37–41
   integration with transfer learning, 37–38
   quantum layer design and retraining, 40–41

**I**

Image Analysis, 199
Image Processing, 121–122
Image segmentation, 28, 200
imaging sensors, 165
Incident Response, 217
Incorporating Fuzzy Clustering into CNN Architecture, 136
Industrial Automation, 235
industry 5.0, 169–171, 173, 175
Industry 5.0 Applications, 120
infectious diseases, 27
inferencing real-time capabilities, 38–42
   implementation on AI edge devices, 37–42
information and communication technology, 226
infrared and thermal sensors, 168
inhomogeneity parameter, 32
Integrating Fuzzy Clustering With CNN, 138
intellectual property protection, 271
interconnected healthcare, 303
interconnected healthcare ecosystem, 304, 306
Internet of Medical Things (IoMT), 299, 300, 301
Internet of Things (IoT), 18–19, 158, 159, 170, 171, 173,
      185, 186, 221
interoperability, 161
   challenges, 183, 275
   in healthcare, 271
InterPlanetary File System (IPFS), 253
interpretable machine learning models, 90
introduction, 1
investment, fractional ownership in real estate, 270
IoT Devices, 201
IoT in blockchain, 273–274
IoT Integration, 209, 210, 217, 218

## L

lack of standardization, 276
Laplace transformation, 29
legal frameworks, 277
licensing processes, 271
LIME and SHAP, 91
local data processing, 302, 303
local edge storage, 241
LoRa technology, 186–188

## M

machine learning (ML), 18–19, 153, 175, 304, 305, 310
machine learning algorithms, 98, 120, 273
    blockchain improvement, 273
    fraud detection, 273
    predictive analytics, 273
machine learning in blockchain, 273
manufacturing, 153
mass customization, 249
medical data analysis, 311
medical engineering, 174
medical equipment manufacturing, 161
medical imaging, 122–123, 155, 156, 172
medical practitioners, 115
micro-transactions, 275
mobile AI models, 120
mobile broadband, 222
mobile network, 220
model agnostics method, 154
model training accelerated using hybrid QNNs, 37–41
    challenges in scalability, 36–37
    transfer learning pipeline, 37–39
model-agnostic, 91
modern sensors, 162
monitoring, 198
Morris sensitivity analysis, 108
motion sensors, 165
multi-signature contracts, 254

## N

Narrow AI, 153
Natural Language Processing (NLP), 153, 231
    applications in cyberbullying detection, 147
    sentiment analysis, 147
    text classification methods, 147
network congestion, 275
Network security, 274
non-fungible token (NFT), 255
NVIDIA Jetson TX2 use in AI edge devices, 42
    hardware and software accelerators, 42

## O

object detection, 200
obstacles and prospects, 198
oxygen sensors, 163

## P

Pathology, 156
patient outcomes, 309, 310

patient satisfaction
    enhanced through sentiment analysis, 182
patient-centered care, 191, 193
patient-centric treatment, 18, 21
patient-generated health data (PGHD), 21
perceptual AI, 105
performance comparison of old and proposed
    algorithms, 140
personalization
    care delivery improvement, 180
personalized healthcare, 191
personalized health services, 301, 306
personalized medicine, 18, 21, 98, 122, 172
personalized treatment, 304
pH sensors, 166
post-quantum cryptography (PQC), 260
predictions, machine learning in blockchain, 273
predictive analytics, 23, 156, 172, 173, 191, 216, 304, 306,
    309, 311
predictive maintenance, 122, 161
pressure sensors, 166
preventive care, 18, 22, 160
privacy
    and anonymity, 276
    blockchain and, 273
    compliance frameworks, 149
    enhancement through edge AI, 148
Privacy compliance
    data protection, 180
privacy concerns, 122–124
Privacy Considerations, 210, 217
privacy preservation in blockchain, 273
proactive healthcare, 304
Proof of Stake (PoS), 276
Proof of Work (PoW), 276
protocol, 271
proximity computing, 302, 303
proximity and contact Sensors, 166
public health surveillance, 88
public trust in blockchain, 269

## Q

quality control, 161
quality of life, 209, 216
quantum blockchain, 260
quantum computer, 259
quantum layers design and training, 40–41
    integration with classical neural networks,
        40–41
qubits, 260

## R

Radiology, 156
reactive Healthcare Systems, 301
real estate, blockchain in, 270
real-time data processing
    edge AI applications, 146
real-time decision-making, 185, 192, 232
Realtime Decision Support, 303
Realtime Diagnostics, 302
Real Time Health Data Connection, 159
recommendation systems, 153

Recurrent learning, 239
regulations, blockchain in finance, 270
regulatory compliance
    adherence to GDPR and CCPA, 149
reinforcing detection mechanism, 148
remote monitoring, 185, 190, 193, 209, 210
remote patient monitoring, 112, 159, 162, 173, 174, 305,
    306, 308
research in blockchain applications, 270
resource allocation
    improved by edge AI, 182
resource constraints, 195
resource management, 122–123
resource utilization, 308
Responsible artificial intelligence
    (RAI), 106
Results of Using FCM and with C, 141
RMSE, 211, 216
robotic process automation, 234
robotics, 156, 171
robotics in Industry, 122
robotic surgery, 155
role of machine learning in medical imaging, 131
rule based methods, 154

**S**

scalability
    edge AI systems, 146, 183
scalability and efficiency, 304
Secure communication protocols, 307
security, blockchain in healthcare, 271
security in edge AI, 123–124
security measures, 217
security and privacy, 174, 175, 299, 304–307
sensitivity, 210, 215
sensor nodes, 202
sentiment analysis
    applications in healthcare, 179–180
    real-time feedback, 180
    role in cyberbullying detection, 147
sentiment analysis applications, 179–180
shared contract, 238
significance of Brain Tumour Detection, 127
slicing network, 223
smart cities, 121, 241, 301, 302
smart contract, 252, 270
Smart devices, 121
smart healthcare, 248
smart hospital, 173
smart thermostats, 231
social media
    patient-generated healthcare data, 179
specificity, 210, 215
Stakeholder feedback, 216
standardization challenges, 276
supply chain management (SCM), 256
supply chain optimization, 273

**T**

telemedicine, 155, 159, 169, 174, 191, 193
telesurgery, 171
temperature sensors, 163
TensorFlow Lite, 123
TLS Protocol, 217
tokenization, 270
training the integrated model, 139
training and model optimization, 120–121
transfer learning, 209, 210, 218
transfer learning application in COVID-19 detection, 37–39
    data preparation and augmentation, 38–40
    hybrid QNN integration, 40–42
transparency, 175
    AI-driven decision-making, 181
    in blockchain, 269
    informed consent practices, 149
transportation, 153
trapezoidal fuzzy number, 28
treatment, 198
treatment recommendations, 92
triangular fuzzy number, 28

**U**

uniform velocity, 27
urban health monitoring, 301
user interface, 201

**V**

versatile production systems, 12
virtual care, 159, 174
virtual network functions, 225
virtual personal assistants, 232
virtual power plant, 221
virtual reality, 311, 312
vital sign tracking, 209, 210, 215
voice assistance, 153
voting and governance, blockchain in, 271
vulnerabilities, 259

**W**

wallet management, 276
weak AI, 153
wearable devices, 155, 156, 169, 185, 193, 300, 304
wearable health monitoring, 122
wearable sensors, 110
wireless communications, 220
wireless networking, 202
workflow automation, 243
workflow optimization, 158

**X**

XAI in healthcare 5.0, 117

For Product Safety Concerns and Information please contact our EU
representative  GPSR@taylorandfrancis.com
Taylor & Francis Verlag GmbH, Kaufingerstraße 24, 80331 München, Germany